Progress in

Obstetrics and Gynaecology

Progress in Obstetrics and Gynaecology
Edited by John Studd

Contents of Volume 12

ISBN 0 443 05307 3

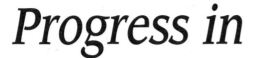

Progress in

Obstetrics and Gynaecology

VOLUME 13

Edited by

John Studd DSc MD FRCOG

Consultant Gynaecologist
Fertility and Endocrinology Centre
Chelsea and Westminster Hospital and
The Lister Hospital, London, UK

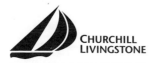

EDINBURGH LONDON NEW YORK PHILADELPHIA SYDNEY TORONTO 1998

CHURCHILL LIVINGSTONE
An imprint of Harcourt Brace & Company Limited

Robert Stevenson House, 1–3 Baxter's Place, Leith Walk, Edinburgh, EH1 3AF

© Harcourt Brace & Company Limited 1998

First published 1998

ISBN 0 443 05868 7
ISSN 0261 0140

British Library Cataloguing in Publication Data
A catalogue record for this book is available from the British Library

Library of Congress Cataloging in Publication Data
A catalog record for this book is available from the Library of Congress

Medical knowledge is constantly changing. As new information becomes available, changes in treatment, procedures, equipment and the use of drugs become necessary. The editors and the publishers have, as far as possible, taken care to ensure that the information given in this text is accurate and up to date. However, readers are strongly advised to confirm that the information, especially with regard to drug usage, complies with current legislation and standards of practice.

The publisher's policy is to use paper manufactured from sustainable forests

Produced by BA & GM Haddock
Printed in China
GCC/01

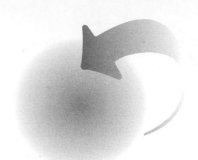

Contents

Contents

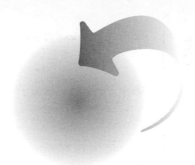

Contributors

J. Aagaard MD
Department of Obstetrics and Gynecology, Skejby Sygehus, Aarhus
University Hospital, Aarhus, Denmark

Phillip R. Bennett BSc MB BS MD PhD MRCOG
Professor in Obstetrics and Gynaecology, Imperial College School of
Medicine, Queen Charlotte's and Chelsea Hospital, London, UK

Jennifer M. Best PhD
Reader in Virology, The Richard Dimbleby Laboratory of Cancer Virology,
Department of Virology, The Rayne Institute, St Thomas' Hospital Campus,
London, UK

Susan Bewley MRCOG MD MA
Director of Obstetrics, Guy's and St Thomas' Hospital Trusts, Department of
Obstetrics and Gynaecology, St Thomas's Hospital, London, UK

Catherine Bobrow MRCOG
Research Fellow, Fetal Medicine Research Unit, University of Bristol, St
Michael's Hospital, Bristol, UK

Deborah C. M. Boyle MB ChB
Research Fellow, Academic Department of Obstetrics and Gynaecology,
Charing Cross and Westminster Medical School, Chelsea and Westminster
Hospital, London, UK

Stephen G. Carroll MB BCh BAO MRCOG MRCP(I)
Subspecialty Trainee in Maternal and Fetal Medicine, St Michael's Hospital,
Bristol, UK

John Cason PhD
Senior Lecturer in Virology, The Richard Dimbleby Laboratory of Cancer
Virology, Department of Virology, The Rayne Institute, St Thomas' Hospital
Campus, London, UK

Brian M. Chin BSc
Visiting Research Fellow, Department of Biology, University of Richmond, Virginia, USA

Michael de Swiet MD FRCP
Academic Sub-Dean/Consultant Physician, Institute of Obstetrics and Gynaecology, Queen Charlotte's and Chelsea Hospital, London, UK

William J. B. Dennes MB BS
Research Fellow/Registrar, Imperial College School of Medicine, Queen Charlotte's and Chelsea Hospital, London, UK

Demetrios L. Economides MRCOG MD
Senior Lecturer and Consultant Obstetrician and Gynaecologist, University Department of Obstetrics and Gynaecology/Haemophilia Centre, The Royal Free Hospital, London, UK

Ignac Fogelman MD FRCP
Consultant in Nuclear Medicine, Guy's Hospital, Guy's and St Thomas' Hospital Trust, London, UK

Malcolm I. Frazer MD FRCOG
Department of Urogynaecology, Women's Health Directorate, Warrington Hospital NHS Trust, Warrington, UK

Alain Gregoire DRCOG MRCPsych
Honorary Senior Lecturer and Director, Mental Health Service, The Old Manor Hospital, Salisbury, Wiltshire, UK

Nigel Holland MD MRCOG
Department of Urogynaecology, Women's Health Directorate, Warrington Hospital NHS Trust, Warrington, UK

Rob Holmes MRCOG
Specialist Registrar, Fetal Medicine Research Unit, University of Bristol, St Michael's Hospital, Bristol, UK

Thomas Ind MBBS MD MRCOG
Senior Registrar, The St George Hospital, Kogarah, Sydney, New South Wales, Australia

Margaret A. Johnson MD FRCP
Consultant in Thoracic Medicine, Director of HIV and AIDS Services, Royal Free Hospital, London, UK

Rezan A. Kadir ABCOG FRCS MRCOG
Clinical Research Fellow, University Department of Obstetrics and Gynaecology/Haemophilia Centre, The Royal Free Hospital, London, UK

Gautam Khastgir MD FRCS MRCOG
Subspecialty Senior Registrar in Reproductive Medicine, Academic Department of Obstetrics and Gynaecology, Chelsea and Westminster Hospital, London, UK

U. B. Knudsen MD PhD
Department of Obstetrics and Gynecology, Skejby Sygehus, Aarhus
University Hospital, Aarhus, Denmark

Ezzat L. Kozman MRCOG
Associate Specialist in Gynaecology, Department of Urogynaecology,
Women's Health Directorate, Warrington Hospital NHS Trust, Warrington,
UK

Ronnie F. Lamont BSc MD FRCOG
Consultant in Obstetrics and Gynaecology, Northwick Park Hospital,
Middlesex, UK and Honorary Senior Lecturer, Institute of Obstetrics and
Gynaecology, Royal Postgraduate Medical School, Hammersmith Hospital,
London, UK

Christine A. Lee MA MD DSc(Med) FRCP FRCPath
Professor of Haemophilia and Director of Haemophilia Centre and
Haemostasis Unit, The Royal Free Hospital, London, UK

Robert D. Macdonald MB ChB
Obstetric Research Fellow, Department of Women's Health, Southmead
Hospital, Bristol, UK

S.D. Maguiness MD MRCOG
Consultant, Department of Gynaecology, The Princess Royal Hospital, Hull,
UK

Michael Maresh MD FRCOG
Consultant Obstetrician and Gynaecologist, Saint Mary's Hospital for Women
and Children, Central Manchester Healthcare NHS Trust, Manchester, UK

Edward P. Morris BSc MRCOG
Research Fellow, HRT Research Unit, Guy's Hospital, Guy's and St Thomas'
Hospital Trust, London, UK

Patrick Neven MD
Consultant Gynaecologist, Department of Obstetrics and Gynaecology,
Algemene Kliniek St Jan, Brussels, Belgium

Kypros H. Nicolaides MD MRCOG
Professor of Fetal Medicine, Harris Birthright Research Centre for Fetal
Medicine, King's College Hospital, London, UK

Adeola Olaitan MRCOG
Specialist Registrar/Consultant Gynaecologist, Gynaecological and
Colposcopy Services, Department of Obstetrics and Gynaecology, Royal Free
Hospital Medical School, London, UK

Nicholas Panay BSc MRCOG MFFP
Research Fellow in Obstetrics and Gynaecology, Academic Department of
Obstetrics and Gynaecology, Chelsea and Westminster Hospital, London, UK

K. Shanti Raju MD
Senior Lecturer in Obstetrics and Gynaecology, Department of Obstetrics and
Gynaecology, St Thomas' Hospital Campus, London, UK

Janice M. Rymer MD MRCOG FRNZCOG
Senior Lecturer/Consultant in Obstetrics and Gynaecology, UMDS, Guy's Hospital, Guy's and St Thomas' Hospital Trust, London, UK

Robert J. Sawdy BSc MB BS MRCOG
Research Fellow/Senior Registrar, Imperial College School of Medicine, Queen Charlotte's and Chelsea Hospital, London, UK

Gurleen Sharland BSc MD FRCP
Senior Lecturer in Fetal and Paediatric Cardiology, Honorary Consultant, Fetal Cardiology, Guy's Hospital, London, UK

J. Richard Smith MD MRCOG
Senior Lecturer/Consultant, Academic Department of Obstetrics and Gynaecology, Charing Cross and Westminster Medical School, Chelsea and Westminster Hospital, London, UK

Sue Smith MRCPsych
Consultant, Sully Hospital, Sully, Vale of Glamorgan, UK

Peter W. Soothill
Professor of Maternal and Fetal Medicine, Fetal Medicine Research Unit, University of Bristol, St Michael's Hospital, Bristol, UK

John Studd DSc MD FRCOG
Consultant Gynaecologist, Academic Department of Obstetrics and Gynaecology, Chelsea and Westminster Hospital, London, UK

David W. Sturdee MD DA FRCOG
Consultant Gynaecologist and Senior Clinical Lecturer, Department of Obstetrics and Gynaecology, Solihull Hospital, Solihull, West Midlands, UK

Jackie Tan MB BS MRCP
Registrar, Institute of Obstetrics and Gynaecology, Queen Charlotte's and Chelsea Hospital, London, UK

J. Guy Thorpe-Beeston MA MD MRCOG
Consultant Obstetrician, Chelsea and Westminster Hospital, London, UK

Austin H. N. Ugwumadu MBBS MRCOG
Research Fellow/Honorary Senior Registrar, Department of Obstetrics and Gynaecology, St George's Hospital Medical School, London, UK

Sanjay K. Vyas MD MRCOG
Consultant Obstetrician and Gynaecologist, Department of Women's Health, Southmead Hospital, Bristol, UK

James J. Walker MD FRCP(G) FRCP(E) FRCOG
Department of Obstetrics and Gynaecology, St James's University Hospital, Leeds, UK

A.J.S. Watson MRCOG
Senior Registrar, Department of Gynaecology, The Princess Royal Hospital, Hull, UK

Susan Bewley

Medical law made easy

Although obstetricians and gynaecologists receive letters from lawyers with some trepidation, this should not be allowed to put them off understanding the basic principles of law! It must be emphasised from the start that although complaints will always occur, practising medicine to a high standard offers the best protection to doctors.

WHAT IS THE PURPOSE OF LAW?

Law is a practical mechanism by which society attempts to settle grievances between people who have come into conflict. It is also used in an attempt to limit the most unacceptable behaviour by human beings. This second function is also achieved by defining activities that are considered actually 'criminal'.

Law in the UK divides into two main branches – civil and criminal law. The first largely deals with grievances between two parties, and issues of compensation. The second deals with individuals whose behaviour is so serious that the State has an interest and may require punishment as well as compensation.

Law is determined in two ways: by Acts of Parliament where new law is written down; and by Common Law (the slow accretion of precedents and interpretations made in judgements by the courts). Another branch, Family Law, deals with intra-familial disputes.

As far as daily medical practice goes, the law is usually 'behind the scenes'. The law, and lawyers, are only invoked to sort out disputes when something has gone wrong. Law tries to deal with the lowest standard of medical behaviour, or the most extreme of conditions when doctors have abused their position. It is right that the profession is regulated not only internally, by

Dr Susan Bewley MRCOG MD MA, Director of Obstetrics, Guy's and St Thomas' Hospital Trusts, Department of Obstetrics and Gynaecology, St Thomas's Hospital, Lambeth Palace Road, London SE1 7EH, UK

Table 1.1 Types of accusations that might be made against an obstetrician/gynaecologist

Criminal	Civil
Murder and manslaughter	Battery
Assault and battery	Negligence
Illegal abortion	Damages

employers and professional codes of behaviour, but also externally with the law determining the lowest acceptable standards of behaviour. In this respect, it is quite different from ethics which is a more theoretical discipline that considers what it is to be a 'good' doctor. Table 1.1 gives examples of the types of accusations that might be made against an obstetrician/gynaecologist.

RELATIONSHIP OF LAW TO THE DOCTOR–PATIENT RELATIONSHIP

If law defines the parameters of acceptable behaviour, it might help to consider the doctor–patient relationship in the form of the **three Cs**: (i) confidentiality; (ii) consent; and (iii) competence. Law on these three aspects corresponds to standard parts of our clinical practice in use every day with every patient (Table 1.2).

Table 1.2 Medical practice and legal constraints

Medical practice	Legal constraint
History	Confidentiality
Examination	Consent
Diagnosis and management	Competence (negligence)
Treatment	To which the patient agrees or gives consent

No special knowledge of ethics or law is required to practice medicine. Good doctors who care about their patients, are knowledgeable and communicate well will rarely encounter extreme ethical or legal problems. There is, indeed, a danger that legal worries may inhibit good medical practice by disrupting the doctor–patient relationship and the flow of communication in both directions.

When, however, a doctor strays into very unfamiliar territory or unusual situations that may have a legal implication, it is always wise to ask for help: either from a colleague, a senior, or a medical defence agency. In the following sections we will look at the three main areas of law in everyday practice.

CONFIDENTIALITY

A promise on the doctor's part to maintain a patient's confidentiality is central to allow patients to speak freely. The diagnostic process will be less efficient if our patients keep information hidden, or if they fear that disclosure of private information may reach the ears of others. It is important for all doctors to realise that information obtained in the context of a doctor–patient relationship is **privileged**. This means that the information would not otherwise have been obtained and, however interesting or shocking, the doctor is necessarily under an obligation to maintain confidentiality, even if other people would be greatly interested in the information, or possibly even harmed by not knowing about it (for example, a doctor knowing that a person has a sexually transmitted disease). The doctor would never have obtained the information in the first place were there not a promise not to tell. In general, it is wrong to break promises we have made to others. In addition, there is the danger that if a few promises were broken, the whole belief and faith of the general public in their doctors would be forfeited. So there is also a public interest in doctors maintaining the highest degree of confidentiality.

The obligation of confidentiality

The legal obligation of confidentiality is recognised both in common law and via specific legal obligations.[1,2] Thus, we can see there is a legal duty created to maintain confidence and, if confidence is broken, there are several ways in which a doctor can be admonished: (i) a civil claim can be made for damages against the discloser; (ii) breaches of confidentiality are also considered professional misconduct, and a doctor may be required by the General Medical Council to explain his or her actions; and (iii) before the event, an injunction can be taken out to stop disclosure (this has been used to stop newspapers breaching medical confidentiality).

Legal exceptions

There are some legal exceptions to the duty of confidentiality. Some diseases and physiological states are statutorily notifiable (for example, certain infectious diseases,[3] births, deaths and terminations of pregnancy.[4] The courts and coroners (and occasionally the police) may issue a summons to reveal what is in medical records. Confidentiality may be breached if it is in the public interest (for example, if a person is at risk of death or serious harm if a doctor did not breach confidentiality). Even in these cases a doctor must break confidentiality to the minimum and only to these people with 'a need to know' and be prepared to defend the action.

Conflicts of interest

At times doctors are involved with patients in relationships that are not strictly for the benefit of the patient. In some cases, conflicts of interest may arise and these are best considered beforehand and explained to the patient so there is no misunderstanding about the confidential nature of the information given or otherwise. For example, if doctor performs a medical examination as part of an occupational health assessment, the employer is entitled to know the results. People may not wish to reveal the same things to their general practitioners as their occupational health doctors, and it is better that they are aware beforehand of the distinction between the two situations.

Researchers may discover diseases or problems that were not apparent when a person or patient volunteered to take part in research. Details may be circulated to other people. In addition, patients who become the subject of case studies or whose photographs appear in journals or books have to be protected from breaches of confidentiality. A recent GMC ruling has led many journals to ask authors to provide written permission from the subjects of case reports.

There is also the thorny issue of children's confidentiality, although in obstetrics and gynaecology this has been reviewed in the context of the Gillick judgement.[5] Once a child has reached the age of 16 years, he or she is considered mature enough to make adult decisions. The question posed by Gillick was whether children under 16 years have the right to confidentiality? If a child is sufficiently mature to make decisions to consent to treatment, then they are certainly mature enough not to have their confidentiality breached. For example, if a 15 year-old came to discuss contraception and went away deciding that she was too young to start having sexual intercourse, she should still have her confidentiality respected.

Another intriguing problem occurs when tests for prenatal diagnosis or other genetic tests reveal unexpected information regarding paternity (or lack of it), or disease in other family members. Whose information is it? The important thing for doctors is to realise **before** they perform tests that there may be problems, so that they may anticipate what they will do afterwards. Although geneticists and general practitioners often see people in families and obstetricians often see couples, it must be remembered that doctors have duties to patients as **individuals**, not couples or groups. Although a doctor may have a duty to several individuals, and they conflict, the patients should be regarded separately and seen one at a time. Therefore, the result of a test that a person may not wish other people to know should really only be given to that person alone, however much other people may wish to know it.

Doctors must take care not to speak too freely or glibly about their patients, particularly in a public setting. It must be remembered that most commonly upsetting breaches of confidentiality happen accidentally, in public places (such as hospital lifts) or socially (such as parties). Or they occur because doctors in good faith reveal secret information, such as details about previous pregnancies, sexual activity or contraception to partners or parents who appear to be more familiar and intimate with the patient than they are really. Be careful – loose talk causes harm.

CONSENT

What is consent?

The fundamental value that consent refers to is the respect we have for bodily integrity and personal autonomy. As human beings we have a general human right not to be interfered with either physically or mentally. This means doctors have to have agreement before they can touch patients and patients can take treatment. Consent is an integral part of every single consultation, although it is usually in the background and taken for granted.

The components of consent

There are three components of consent:

Competence

Competence is assumed once children are over 16 years old. A patient has to have the mental ability to understand the 'nature and purpose' of procedures, whether that be taking their clothes off to be examined, taking tablets, or being given an anaesthetic for an operation. Mental ability can be affected by illness or disease. Autonomy can be diminished through fear, delirium, anxiety, etc. It may be that a person is competent for some things, but not others. For example, a mentally handicapped person may understand the need to take off her socks for her feet to be examined, but she may not be able to participate in a research trial with a complex information sheet. The doctor has to assess competence and understanding.

Information

Information is required for people to make decisions. This has been tested most notably in the Sidaway case.[6] People are unable to make real decisions about their lives or treatments if they are unaware of the consequences of the action (for example, the side effects and risks of success and failure). Therefore, doctors must explain the risks and side effects if they are important. Both the likelihood and seriousness of the risks are relevant to the patient. An important side effect might be one that is common (e.g. dry mouth with anticholinergics) or very serious even when rare (e.g. hysterectomy to control bleeding after myomectomy). Extremely remote risks may not have to be explained, but if a patient asks questions they must be answered fully and truthfully. Although the British courts in their judgements have traditionally been very favourable to doctors, the standard of information required is going up gradually, and quite rightly, as the population becomes more informed and sophisticated.

Duress

If consent is obtained under duress, it may be completely invalid. One, therefore, has to be very careful if patients are being offered something 'in return', for example, when they donate eggs, receive payments or volunteer for research projects at the same time as having treatments. It is all too easy for people to agree to things through fear or desperation without being fully aware of the implications to themselves. Doctors are powerful and authoritative figures and have to be particularly wary of wittingly or unwittingly manipulating agreement.

Situations in which consent is not possible

1. Some patients are *not competent*. This group would include some (but not all) children and mentally handicapped adults. In these cases, someone else has to make the decisions on behalf of the patient, and they must use what is called the 'best interests test'. A parent can be a proxy decision-maker for a child but cannot make a decision that is against the child's interest (for example, parents refusing life-saving treatment for their

child). No one can legally act as a proxy for the mentally handicapped adult, and very important decisions, such as sterilisation, have then to be referred to the courts.

2. When patients are *unconscious* and there is an emergency decision needed, doctors may act without consent using the doctrine of 'necessity' and again, try to act according to 'best interests'. Consent cannot be obtained, but doctors are unlikely to be prosecuted for assault and lack of consent as this would prevent them from looking after some of the very sickest patients. However, if circumstances change or there are unexpected findings at an operation, it would be an unwise doctor who did more than the minimum to save the patient's life. There are many cases in gynaecology in particular, where something is found at operation when the patient is unconscious but it is not an emergency. If a patient's life is not in danger, and the situation has not been discussed beforehand, it is important not to make assumptions as to what the patient would decide. Doctors who think that they can 'put themselves into someone else's shoes' will eventually get into trouble! Relatives cannot consent on behalf of the unconscious patient though it is wise to inform them what is going on.

3. Sometimes patients make irrational, or ill-understood *refusals*. Sometimes doctors have great difficulty accepting the beliefs of other people, for example, Jehovah's Witnesses' refusal to receive blood, even in life-threatening situations. There can easily be a temptation on the doctor's part to act without consent as they feel it must be in the patient's best interest to live, or that the reason given is stupid or wayward. Unfortunately, to act against consent may violate someone's most deeply and sincerely held beliefs and thus violate who they are and their deepest sense of self. This violation of autonomy may be considered an assault[7] and it is a mark of the respect in which we hold autonomy that we do not override another person, even when we do not agree with them. What is small to the doctor (the transfusion) may be massive to the patient (a loss of integrity or hope of eternal life). On the other hand, doctors have got to be careful about too easily accepting a refusal when it may be that a patient has misunderstood the seriousness of the situation or if fear, anxiety or ignorance are clouding their judgement or indeed they are mentally unfit to decide. The important thing is to keep the trusting doctor–patient relationship open. Keep talking to the patient in simple language to clarify what are areas of misunderstanding about medical matters and what are areas of disagreement about the fundamental meaning of existence. Be careful not to accept refusals at face value as they too must be 'informed refusals'.

4. At present, the woman who refuses treatment that is *lifesaving for her unborn child* (e.g. intra-uterine transfusion or caesarean section for fetal distress) cannot be forced to take the treatment, although we can appeal to her better nature and apply heavy moral pressure to try and persuade her. The fetus does not exist legally as a person who can be a party at law. Although there was one case of caesarean without consent (Re S),[8] which was lifesaving for the mother and performed after the babies' death, legal

commentators generally agree that it was anomalous. RCOG guidelines recommend that obstetricians do not perform caesarean sections without consent.[9] Recent cases have confirmed that competent mothers have a right to refuse caesarean even if that leads to the death of the baby.[10] If there is a question about competence, it is best to seek psychiatric and legal evidence well in advance.

NEGLIGENCE

We have to accept that many patients are harmed during the course of medical treatment. Some are harmed by the progression of their disease, some by unavoidable side-effects of treatment and some are avoidable harms secondary to medical incompetence. If a patient is harmed, she has a right to question what occurred and a right to redress if it was caused negligently. It is not possible to redress everyone who has disease or damage, as illness and death come to every member of society.

Other methods of redress have been considered but 'no-fault' compensation can still only be given to those people whose harm is caused by accidents, rather than nature, whereas negligence limits compensation only to those cases where there is fault. In our specialty, we may see three equally brain-damaged babies, one through prenatal cerebral palsy (illness), one through cord prolapse in labour (accident) and one through the ignoring of an abnormal cardiotocograph for many hours during an obstructed labour (negligence). At present, the children and their burdened families are not all equally entitled to compensation.

Legal claim for negligence

When a person makes a claim (or possibly a guardian makes a claim on a child's behalf) what is being said in law is 'but for your negligence, I would not have been harmed'. Table 1.3 shows the steps that need to be made in a negligence claim.

Duty of care
It is usually clear in obstetrics and gynaecology that a duty of care is owed. As soon as doctors take on the care of patients (even if it is by a telephone consultation or in a social context) they are accepting the duty and the responsibilities that flow from it.

Breach of duty
The test by which a breach of duty is judged is that of your peers, the 'Bolam test'.[11] If a respectable body of medical opinion would have acted in the same

Table 1.3 Steps in a negligence claim

A duty of care has to be owed
The duty has to have been breached
Harm flowed from the breach of the duty (causation)
Amount of damages

way, a doctor may not be found negligent. The standard expected is that of someone in the same situation. This means that a registrar is not expected to perform manoeuvres to the same standard as a consultant, but a 'reasonable registrar' would assess their own limitations, and refer for advice if they were out of their depth.

Causation

Many cases fall at the point of causation as, to prove negligence, the plaintiff (the patient making the claim) has to show that the damage would not have occurred if the care had been better. Even though care may have been extremely sparse and negligent during a consultation or hospital admission, it may be that the damage sustained was inevitable, a result of underlying disease and unrelated to the poor quality care.

Although obstetricians and gynaecologists are worried about negligence claims, the process of finding a doctor negligent is long, drawn out and expensive (even when the plaintiff has the help of Legal Aid) and this deters most claims. We should be humble enough to realise that many actions are negligent and luckily are picked up by other colleagues before harm occurs. In addition, many patients who are harmed by negligent mistakes never sue. Only a small number of mistakes make it as far as a claim. There is evidence from the US that complaints about doctors are less related to objective measures of competence than to communication skills and patients feeling seriously cared for as opposed to tolerated or processed.[12,13]

LAW SPECIAL TO OBSTETRICS AND GYNAECOLOGY

In view of advances in medical technology and the precious nature of genetic inheritance, fertility, embryos and fetuses, special law has been required to limit medical endeavour. By having special laws, society makes a symbolic statement about the importance of the care with which its newest and most vulnerable members will be treated.

Human Fertilisation and Embryology Act 1990 (HFEA)

This Act was the result of the Warnock Committee and sets up a framework by which an embryo in vitro is neither a simple piece of property, nor a legal person, but a precious object that has to be dealt with in a limited number of ways. It cannot be grown in a laboratory nor experimented upon after 14 days (the time considered important when the neural streak develops and implantation has usually occurred). Centres performing assisted conception have to be licensed and visited for approval by the HFE Authority thus allowing public reassurance about medial practices.

Abortion

The intentional termination of a pregnancy (or procurement of a miscarriage) was made a crime with a mandatory life sentence for both the doctor and mother under the 1861 Offences against the Person Act. Although some abortions were performed (and most notably the law was extended by the Bourne judgement in 1939[14]) abortion became much more available after the 1967 Abortion Act (since amended by the HFEA 1990), although the Act does not apply in Northern Ireland. The framework remains that abortion is a crime except when it is legal. What makes a particular abortion legal is that two medical practitioners are of the opinion, made in good faith, that: (i) one of the clauses of the Abortion Act has been fulfilled; (ii) that the abortion is performed in an NHS hospital or otherwise licensed premises; and lastly (iii) that it is notified. Although some consider that effectively abortion is available 'on demand' in the UK, this is not the case legally. At the moment, the law is unclear as to the exact meaning of the words of one of the clauses without gestation limit; 'substantial risk that if the child were born it would suffer from such physical or mental abnormalities as to be seriously handicapped', and it would be unsurprising if a case were not brought to court in the future. For difficult late terminations for fetal abnormality, refer to recent RCOG guidelines.[15,16]

WHY DO SO MANY LEGAL CASES ARISE IN OBSTETRICS AND GYNAECOLOGY?

Our specialty is not so much numerically worse compared to other disciplines, but we have a peculiarity that many of the sums payable in obstetrics are so large that cases are fought to the bitter end. However, legal cases occur with increasing frequency and are often of great interest in the media. Are obstetricians and gynaecologists particularly arrogant or poor communicators? Is the context of our work, which includes maternal and fetal deaths, abortion, sexuality and fertility, exceptionally emotional? We deal with the most intimate stuff of people's lives, and it is not to be treated lightly. There is also a new tension between women being considered as 'patients' or 'clients'. There is a widespread belief that in this century many physiological variations have been 'medicalised'. We have obstetricians and gynaecologists who are experts in pregnancy, birth, menstrual variations and the menopause. It is true that many women who attend for care are normal, young and healthy and, therefore, are both demanding of the medical system and particularly disappointed if they are worse off after their encounters. It may be that at a fundamental philosophical level our specialty is right on the interface of the conflict between old notions of 'medical paternalism' and new notions of 'informed consumerism'. Practitioners should be alert to all these concerns but not overwhelmed by them. Good communication and high standards are the keystones to keeping out of trouble.[17] The law is absolutely vital to protect the general public and sets limits to unacceptable behaviour within medicine.

KEY POINTS FOR CLINICAL PRACTICE

- Practise obstetrics and gynaecology to a high standard at whatever level you are and always aspire to do better
- Have a good knowledge base, work on problem solving and improving your attitudes and communication skills with patients

KEY POINTS FOR CLINICAL PRACTICE (continued)

- Listen to patients, midwifery and nursing staff and medical colleagues

- Keep legible, meticulous and contemporaneous notes

- Spot trouble early and ask for help

- Check that patients understand your explanations and proposed courses of action

- Respect what patients tell you and assume that everything is confidential

- Do not worry about lawyers!

REFERENCES

1 The National Health Service (Venereal Diseases) Regulations (SI 1974 No 29). London: HMSO, 1974
2 The Human Fertilisation and Embryology Act 1991. London: HMSO, 1991
3 Public Health (Infectious Diseases) Act 1984. London: HMSO, 1984
4 The Abortion Regulations 1968 (SI 1968 No 390 as amended). London: HMSO, 1968
5 Gillick v West Norfolk and Wisbech Area Health Authority [1985] 3 All ER 402 HL
6 Sidaway v Board of Governors of the Bethlem Royal and the Maudsley Hospital [1984] 2 WLR 778, [1985] 2 WLR 480
7 Malette v Schulman (1988) 63 OR (2d) 243 (Ontario High Court)
8 Re S (Adult: refusal of medical treatment)[1992] 4 All ER 671
9 Royal College of Obstetricians and Gynaecologists. A consideration of the law and ethics in relation to court-authorised obstetric intervention. RCOG Guidelines Ethics April 1994; 1
10 Re MB [1997] 8 Med LR 217
11 Bolam v Friern Hospital Management Committee [1957] 2 All ER 118, [1957] 1 WLR 582
12 Hickson G B, Clayton E Q, Entman S S et al. Obstetricians' prior malpractice experience and patients' satisfaction with care. JAMA 1994; 272: 1583–1587
13 Entman S S, Glass C A, Hickson G B, Githens P B, Whetten-Goldstein K, Sloan F A. The relationship between malpractice claims history and subsequent obstetric care. JAMA 1994; 272: 1588–1591
14 R v Bourne [1939] 1 KB 687, CCC
15 Royal College of Obstetricians and Gynaecologists. Termination of pregnancy for fetal abnormality. RCOG 1996 in England, Wales and Scotland
16 Royal College of Obstetricians and Gynaecologists. A consideration of the Law and Ethics in relation to late termination for fetal abnormality. RCOG 1998
17 General Medical Council. Duties of a doctor. London: GMC, 1995

FURTHER READING

Much more detailed information about medical law can be obtained from the following books:

Dyer C (Ed) Doctors, patients and the law. Oxford: Blackwell, 1992. *Several specialists analysing medical law and practice*
Kennedy I, Grubb A (Eds) Medical Law – Text and Materials. London: Butterworth, 1994. *A huge textbook with relevant cases and judgements. Really for students or experts.*
Brazier M. Medicine, patients and the law. London: Penguin, 1987. *An easy-to-read wide ranging book*

William Dennes   Robert Sawdy   Phillip Bennett

Molecular biology in obstetrics

The central dogma of molecular genetics is that a gene, consisting of double stranded DNA, is transcribed into single stranded messenger RNA (mRNA), and this is translated into a protein. Each DNA molecule is made up of two strands in a double helix. The bases on each strand pair by hydrogen bonding, adenine (A) with thymine (T) and cytosine (C) with guanine (G). Each three bases, known as a codon, codes for a single amino acid. A gene consists of a 5′ untranslated region, which contains controlling elements, to which modulating proteins may bind, followed by the transcribed sequence. The coding portion of the gene is usually interrupted by non-coding intervening sequences The expressed coding parts of the gene are known as the exons, whilst the intervening sequences are known as introns. The introns in mRNA are spliced out so that cytoplasmic mRNA consists only of coding regions and an untranslated region at the extreme 3′ end. A polyadenine tail, which may act to control mRNA degradation is added to most mRNA molecules at their 3′ end (Fig. 2.1). Once in the cytoplasm the mRNA message is translated into protein by a ribosome. In lower organisms, the majority of DNA which constitutes the genome is coding. In higher species, the vast majority of the genome is non-coding. The amount of human DNA which actually functions as genes may be less than 10%, and much of the remainder consists of regions of DNA with repeating motifs.

OBTAINING HUMAN DNA FOR STUDY

DNA can be obtained from nucleate cells. The commonest source is white blood cells. Blood is collected for DNA analysis in EDTA tubes, to inhibit the

Dr William J. B. Dennes, Research Fellow/Registrar, Imperial College School of Medicine, Queen Charlotte's and Chelsea Hospital, Goldhawk Road, London W6 0XG, UK

Dr Robert J. Sawdy, Research Fellow/Senior Registrar, Imperial College School of Medicine, Queen Charlotte's and Chelsea Hospital, Goldhawk Road, London W6 0XG, UK

Prof. Phillip R. Bennett, Professor in Obstetrics and Gynaecology, Imperial College School of Medicine, Queen Charlotte's and Chelsea Hospital, Goldhawk Road, London W6 0XG, UK

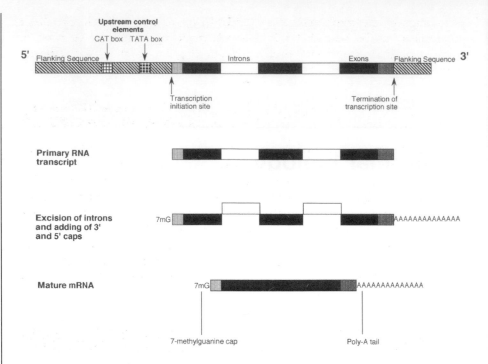

Fig. 2.1 Generalized structure of a human gene, showing the results of transcription and processing to form mature RNA.

action of DNAses. Leucocytes are separated from the anucleate erythrocytes and lysed. DNA is extracted by mixing the cellular lysate with phenol. Proteins and lipids dissolve in phenol whilst DNA and RNA remain in the aqueous phase. The DNA is then isolated by precipitation with alcohol. A similar procedure will extract DNA from most tissues, including amniocytes and chorion villus biopsies.

RESTRICTION ENDONUCLEASES

An enzyme which cuts within a DNA molecule is referred to as an endonuclease. The restriction endonucleases, or restriction enzymes, only cut at sites within specific sequences of DNA, and are part of the primitive immune system of bacteria. Their names are derived from their bacterial source, for example *EcoR1* from *Escherichia coli*, and *Tac1* from *Thermus aquaticus*. Restriction enzymes cut DNA molecules into consistent, and predictable pieces. For example, digestion of bacteriophage lambda by a particular restriction enzyme will consistently yield a series of fragments of specific sizes depending upon the sites of the recognition sequence within the lambda genome. Since the entire nucleotide sequence of bacteriophage lambda is known, the size of the fragments can be predicted and may be used as standards to compare with DNA of unknown size. Similarly digestion of total human DNA with a single restriction enzyme also results in a series of fragments of varying size. The number of fragments is so large that, after separation by electrophoresis, the total DNA appears as a streak. On closer analysis it can be seen that this streak is made up of a large number of individual DNA fragments, each corresponding in length to the distance between two restriction sites.

ELECTROPHORESIS

DNA fragments, generated by polymerase chain reaction (PCR) or by restriction enzyme digest, can be separated using electrophoresis. The commonest electrophoretic media are agarose, a gelling polysaccharide purified from agar, and polyacrylamide. Agarose is used to separate DNA fragments varying in size from about 50 000 to 200 base pairs. Polyacrylamide gels allow separation of smaller DNA fragments to as little as a few base pairs. The rate of migration of DNA through gel is a function of both its molecular size, and the concentration of agarose or polyacrylamide. Once the DNA has been separated, the gel is stained with ethidium bromide and DNA can be visualized under UV light.

SOUTHERN BLOTTING

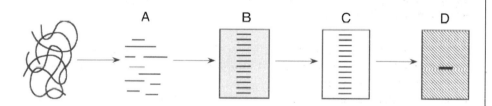

Fig. 2.2 Southern analysis. (**A**) High molecular weight DNA is digested by a restriction enzyme, producing a series of smaller molecules, each representing the distance between recognition sites. (**B**) DNA molecules are separated by electrophoresis. Small molecules travel further down the gel than larger molecules. (**C**) DNA is transferred to a nylon membrane by Southern blotting. (**D**) The Southern blot is hybridised to a radiolabelled DNA probe which detects only a specific restriction fragment.

Southern blotting, developed by Professor E.M. Southern[1], is a technique which allows DNA in an electrophoretic gel to be transferred onto a charged nylon membrane where it can be hybridized to a complimentary DNA probe (Fig. 2.2). The gel is placed onto a filter paper wick on a raised support with the nylon membrane on top of it. On top of this is placed a stack of paper towels compressed by a weight. A high salt solution rises up through the paper wick by capillary action, taking the denatured DNA through to the membrane to which it binds (Fig. 2.3). Thus the filter becomes a replica of the original gel. The Southern blot can then be hybridized to a radiolabelled DNA probe, specific for the gene or region of DNA under study. The location of bound probe on the filter can then be identified by autoradiography. To determine the size of restriction fragment bearing the sequence of interest, comparison can be

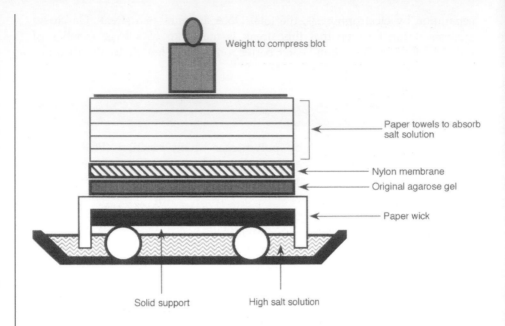

Fig. 2.3 Southern blot. High-salt solution is drawn up the paper wick by capillary action and through the gel to the membrane. DNA in the agarose gel is drawn with the solution to the nylon membrane. The DNA initially binds to the membrane electrostatically, and can be later fixed permanently by baking or cross-linking under UV light.

made with known molecular weight DNA standards. Similar techniques for analysis of RNA and proteins are known as Northern and Western blotting, but as yet there is no Eastern blotting!

POLYMERASE CHAIN REACTION

Polymerase chain reaction (PCR) is a technique for the amplification of specific DNA sequences, essentially by making multiple copies of the initial 'template' molecule. PCR relies on the ability of a DNA polymerase to make a complimentary copy of a single stranded DNA molecule in the 5′ to 3′ direction, but only when primed from a stretch of double stranded DNA at the 5′ end. To perform amplification of DNA using PCR requires the nucleic acid sequence of the region at either end of the fragment to be known. Usually the sequence in between will also be known, but in diagnostic applications it is often the polymorphism which is found between the two primer sites which is to be examined. The PCR requires primers which are specific for the region of DNA to be amplified. Two primers are needed, one on each complementary strand, at each 5′ end of the region to be amplified. The reaction mix also contains all four single nucleotides and the DNA polymerase. The DNA is first heated to 92°C which breaks the bonds between the two complementary strands, forming single stranded DNA. The reaction is then cooled to a temperature at which the specific primers will anneal to the DNA at each 5′

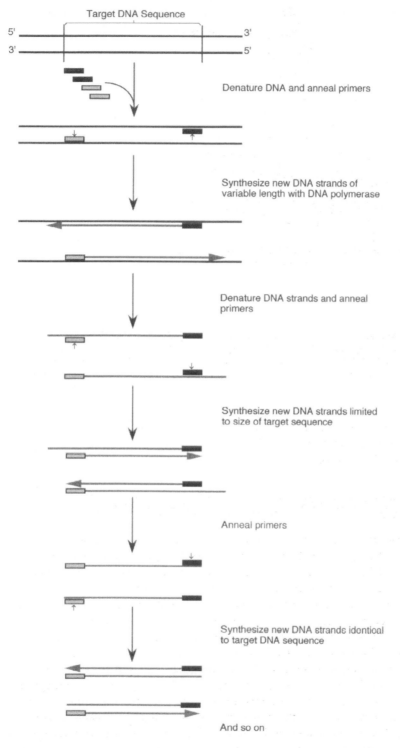

Fig. 2.4 Schematic representation of the polymerase chain reaction (PCR). Further cycles of denaturing, annealing and synthesis yield an exponential increase in the amount of PCR product.

end. This temperature varies between primers, but ideally primer pairs are designed to have similar annealing temperatures. The primer's concentration in the reaction mixture is in great excess over the template DNA, so template/primer hybridization is favoured over re-annealing of the two template strands. The temperature is then changed to 72°C, the optimal temperature for DNA polymerase. The DNA polymerase synthesizes a new strand of DNA complementary to the template, beginning at the primer site (Fig. 2.4). The number of molecules of the specific region of DNA has now doubled. Repeating the temperature cycle denatures the newly formed double stranded DNA, allows the primers to anneal to the single strand templates and again doubles the amount of specific DNA present. If the temperature cycle is repeated 20 or 30 times, the specific region of DNA, originally present in nanogram quantities, can be amplified to microgram quantities, sufficient to be seen on an ethidium bromide stained agarose gel. PCR is automated using commercially available cycling heat blocks. PCR is extremely sensitive, allowing amplification of minute amounts of DNA such as those found in single cells. The extreme sensitivity of PCR makes it essential to avoid contamination of reactions with template DNA from other sources.

IN SITU FLUORESCENCE HYBRIDIZATION FOR DIAGNOSIS OF ANEUPLOIDY

A major disadvantage of amniocentesis for the diagnosis of fetal aneuploidy is the 2–3 week delay whilst amniocytes grow in culture, prior to the preparation of metaphase spreads. Direct visualization of the chromosomes at any stage of the cell cycle using fluorescence in situ hybridization (FISH) may allow diagnosis to be made more quickly. In the classical technique, large DNA probes of several thousand base pairs are labelled with fluorochromes and hybridized to the cell nucleus. The fluorescence can then be viewed, using a fluorescence microscope, which can be linked to a cooled charge coupled (CCD) camera for digital imaging. It would be expected that when a probe specific for chromosome 21 is used, a euploid cell would have two spots of fluorescence, whereas a trisomy 21 cell would have three spots of fluorescence. Unfortunately hybridization artifacts mean that a proportion of the cells from a normal culture may show more than two signals. The first major prospective study to report on the comparative deficiency of FISH with classical cytogenetic diagnosis for aneuploidies correctly identified all 21 abnormalities in a total study size of 526.[2] Later Ward et al,[3] in a study of 4,500 patients, showed that FISH was informative in 90% of cases, with overall diagnostic accuracy of 99.8% in autosomal, and 99.9% in sex chromosome abnormalities. A major limitation to the sole use of FISH for the diagnosis of aneuploidy is that it is limited to abnormalities of chromosomes 13, 18, 21, X and Y, whereas traditional cytogenetics can show the full range of karyotypic abnormalities in one examination. FISH provides a rapid diagnosis of aneuploidy which should, at present, be confirmed by traditional karyotyping, and would also exclude other rarer chromosomal abnormalities.

FISH can also be used to identify small chromosomal deletions which are not visible on a standard metaphase spread. Probes specific for the potentially deleted region can be hybridized to a chromosome preparation, which will only be successful if that region is present. Chromosome painting is performed using fluorochrome labelled collections of DNA sequences, which either span part of, or the entire, human chromosome. This approach is particularly useful for identification of translocations, since a chromosome paint should normally only light up two chromosomes. However, if a small part of one chromosome has been translated onto another, that region will also light up with the chromosome paint. At present FISH has not superseded PCR for diagnosing small chromosome region or single copy sequence abnormalities. However, it is likely that in the future amplification techniques, such as primed in situ labelling (PRINS) or in situ PCR, may enable FISH to be used for the diagnosis of single gene disorders.

PRENATAL DIAGNOSIS: SINGLE GENE DEFECTS

The use of molecular biological techniques, and PCR in particular, has had a profound effect on the ability to detect single gene defects prenatally. There are broadly two approaches to the prenatal diagnosis of single gene defects, either detection of the genetic mutation (direct analysis), or analysis of a DNA sequence that is closely linked with that mutation (linkage analysis). Direct analysis is appropriate if the disease process is a result of the same mutation, or one of a limited number of mutations, but relies on knowledge of the gene sequence. Linkage analysis, or more accurately gene tracking, was initially used where the gene sequence of an inherited disorder was not known, but where its mutation was known to be inherited with a closely linked DNA polymorphism. Thus, whilst the mutation itself was not identified, a risk of inheriting that mutation could be calculated. In some conditions, such as β-thalassaemia, which arise as a result of a number of different mutations, linkage analysis may be preferable to direct analysis.

Direct analysis

As knowledge of the human genome expands, the number of mutations that can be identified by direct analysis rapidly increases. There are a number of different methods available to detect a specific DNA sequence change. The simplest relies on the presence or absence of a restriction site created by the mutation. After PCR amplification, digestion with the appropriate restriction endonuclease will generate products of different sizes. For example, in sickle cell anaemia, the mutation is a single base pair substitution from valine to glutamine in the β globulin gene, abolishing a site for the restriction enzyme Mst II. PCR amplification with primers designed to amplify a 110 bp product which spans the mutation site and subsequent digestion with Mst II, will generate two bands in an unaffected case and a single band in an affected case (Fig. 2.5).[4]

In cystic fibrosis, some 500 different mutations have been described, but different populations vary in the proportions of each mutation. In Northern Europe, the ΔF508 mutation (a 3 bp deletion which causes loss of a phenylalanine at position 508 of the cystic fibrosis protein) accounts for some

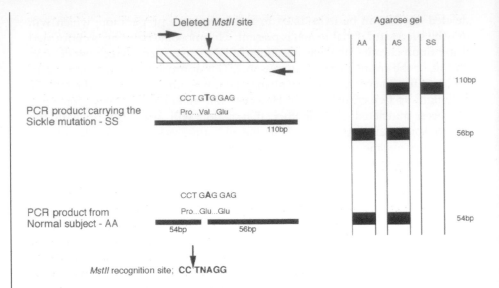

Fig. 2.5 Diagnosis of sickle cell disease using PCR, followed by restriction digest with *Mst* II. The point mutation deletes an *Mst* II site within the PCR product. PCR product from a chromosome carrying the sickle mutation will not therefore cut, and will be seen as a single band, whereas normal DNA will cut and will be seen as two smaller bands.

70% of cases.[5] For diagnosis of this mutation, PCR primers have been designed that span the mutation site and generate a 98 bp product in unaffected cases and a 95 bp in affected cases.[6]

Several diseases have now been identified as resulting from expansion of a trinucleotide repeat. Expanded trinucleotide repeat diseases are ideal for direct testing because the mutation is almost always the same, the only question being how many repeat units are present. Huntington's disease (HD) is a result of a CAG repeat in the HD gene on the short arm of chromosome 4. There is a range of 30–70 repeats in affected individuals and 9–34 in normals.[7] Amplification of the trinucleotide repeat sequence will generate products of different sizes, depending on the number of repeats, which can then be resolved by gel electrophoresis.

Alternative techniques have been developed for gene mutations which do not involve alterations in restriction sites or changes in the size of PCR products. Amplification refractory mutation system (ARMS) uses allele-specific oligonucleotides to detect point mutations.[8] One primer (the common primer) is the same in both reactions, the other is either specific for the normal sequence, or includes the point mutation change. Generation of product in either reaction implies successful annealing and presence or absence of the mutation. Control primers are usually required. Allele-specific oligonucleotide (ASO) hybridization is an alternative technique for identifying single base pair changes. ASO probes are normally 15–20 nucleotides long, and are designed to hybridize to specific regions containing the putative mutation site. The DNA duplex generated by hybridization is only stable at high hybridization stringency, if both target and probe have identical sequences. If there is a single mismatch, then the duplex will be unstable and hybridization will not occur.[9]

For many diseases, no single mutation is particularly frequent. In Duchenne muscular dystrophy (DMD), for example, the mutation represents a number of different deletions involving one or more exons in the dystrophin gene. The size of the exons as a whole would be too large to amplify by conventional PCR, therefore, multiplex PCR is employed. This involves designing primers to amplify each of the exons concerned individually, and including them all in one reaction. Each exon is, therefore, amplified individually and deletions can be identified.

Linkage analysis

Providing the chromosomal location of a gene is known, gene tracking using linked markers can be performed, even if the specific DNA mutation has not been identified. Most commonly for diagnosis by linkage analysis, a restriction fragment polymorphism (RFLP) or microsatellite repeat polymorphism is used. For any specific restriction enzyme there will be thousands of recognition sites within the human genome. It has been estimated that within non-coding DNA, between individuals, or individual chromosomes, there is a single base pair difference every 300 base pairs. These differences may either introduce or remove restriction sites and, in so doing, generate fragments of DNA of different length – an RFLP. During prophase of meiosis, homologous chromosomes line up and 'crossing over' can occur between chromosomes, with resultant exchange of genetic material (recombination). Therefore, for a particular allele of an RFLP to be consistently co-inherited with the mutation, the RFLP must be located close to the gene of interest, such that recombination takes place in 1% or less of meioses.[10] It is then said to be linked (hence linkage analysis). In the absence of recombination between the RFLP and the disease, it can be assumed that an individual who inherits a linked RFLP allele will also inherit the mutation. Analysis of family members for RFLPs and clinical presence of disease, enables a determination of which of the RFLP alleles is on the chromosome carrying the mutation. This is termed 'establishing phase'. For diagnosis by linkage analysis family members must be informative for the RFLP involved. For autosomal recessive disorders this means both parents must be heterozygous; for autosomal dominant conditions the individual at risk of transmitting the disease must be heterozygous; and for X-linked disorders the mother must be heterozygous.

Linkage analysis was originally carried out on DNA obtained from amniocentesis or chorionic villous sampling, using Southern analysis. Recently, analysis of microsatellite repeat polymorphisms by PCR has begun to replace RFLP analysis for gene tracking. Microsatellite DNA regions are small sequences of simple tandem repeats distributed throughout the genome. Mononucleotide and dinucleotide repeats are common. CA tandem repeats, for example, account for about 5% of the total genome, and are highly polymorphic in their number of repeat units. Trinucleoide and tetranucleotide repeat sequences are comparatively rare, but often display higher degrees of polymorphism. The significance of these microsatellite regions is unknown, although as previously discussed in Huntingdon's disease, these sequences are subject to pathogenic expansion. Primers can be designed to amplify the locus, and will generate different size products depending on the number of repeat

2

Molecular biology in obstetrics

sequences at that locus. PCR can, therefore, be used to amplify small amounts of DNA obtained from amniotic fluid or trophoblast samples.

PRENATAL DETERMINATION OF FETAL RED BLOOD CELL AND PLATELET ANTIGEN TYPE

Rhesus D (RhD) alloimmune disease occurs when a RhD negative mother, carrying a RhD positive fetus, produces anti-RhD antibodies which cross the placenta and destroy fetal red cells. Where the father is heterozygous RhD positive, and the mother is RhD negative, there is a 50% chance that the fetus will be RhD negative, and thus will be unaffected by maternal antibodies. The fetal RhD type may be determined by fetal blood sampling, but this carries a 1–2% risk of fetal loss, risk of fetomaternal haemorrhage and increased sensitization. Serial amniocentesis, for spectrophotometric quantitation of bilirubin is less accurate, is unable to distinguish a RhD negative from a mildly affected positive fetus, and exposes the RhD negative fetus to the risks of multiple invasive procedures

The Rh blood group antigens are carried by a series of three homologous, but distinct membrane-associated proteins. Two of these have immuno-logically distinguishable isoforms, designated C, c, and E, e, whereas the principal protein, D, has no isoform d. The rhesus locus, on chromosome 1p34-p36 consists, on RhD positive chromosomes, of two homologous structural genes designated *CcEe* and *D*. The first gene, *CcEe*, encodes both the C/c and E/e proteins, by alternative splicing of a primary transcript. The second gene, *D*, encodes the major antigen RhD, and is absent on both chromosomes of RhD negative individuals. These two genes show a high degree of similarity but there are regions in which there are differences. Several strategies have been designed to determine RhD type using PCR based on the region of difference between the two genes. The originally described technique used PCR to amplify a unique region in the 3′ untranslated part of the RhD gene.[11] Re-arrangements and deletions have recently been discovered in the RhD and C/E genes of certain individuals which would make a PCR based test at a particular position in the gene incorrect. It is, therefore, usual now in clinical practice to use at least two different tests simultaneously.

Kell alloimmune disease is similar to RhD, and is based upon a single base pair change, leading to one amino acid substitution in the Kell protein. Perinatal alloimmune thrombocytopenia (PAIT) is an analogous diseases of fetal platelet destruction. Of the five platelet antibodies identified to date, HPA1 is the principal cause of PAIT. The HPA1 positive individuals express the HPA1a protein. HPA1 negative individuals are homozygous for the HPA1b isoform. 98% of the population are HPA1 positive, of whom 30% are heterozygotes. In the 30% of alloimmunised HPA1 negative woman with a heterozygous partner, there is a 50% chance that the fetus will be unaffected. Since amniocentesis cannot be used to determine the platelet count, fetal blood sampling is currently required for fetal HPA1 type determination. The HPA1b gene differs from the HPA1a gene by having a C to G base pair change at position 196. This creates a restriction site for *Nci* I which has been used as the basis for HPA1 typing. Since restriction analysis may be made inaccurate by partial digestion, this technique has been superseded by the use of site specific oligonucleotide probes. Similar techniques have been developed for prenatal determination of Kell type, as well as for other platelet polymorphisms, and RhCc and RhEe types.

MINIMALLY AND NON-INVASIVE PRENATAL DIAGNOSIS

Currently, a definitive prenatal diagnosis of aneuploidy or a single gene disorder cannot be performed without obtaining fetal cells or DNA by an invasive procedure, which places the pregnancy at risk. Chorion villus biopsy carries a miscarriage rate of 2% over background. Amniocentesis and fetal blood sampling are associated with 0.5–2% pregnancy loss rates. Many groups are now applying molecular biological techniques to identify and analyse fetal DNA non-invasively.

Transcervical harvesting of cells for prenatal diagnosis from the lower pole of the uterus, involves the introduction of a cannula into or beyond the cervical canal, and aspiration of cells with or without saline flushing.[12] These techniques can retrieve adequate numbers of fetal or placental cells for DNA analysis.[13] However, these procedures are 'minimally-invasive' rather than 'non-invasive' and have the potential to cause pregnancy loss, through infection or rupture of the amniotic sac. There are currently no published series in ongoing pregnancies. In a large study, Overton et al[14] were unable to detect fetal cells in over 60% of transcervical aspirates or flushings. With further development, this technique may prove to have a role in prenatal diagnosis although its usefulness may be limited by both poor cell and DNA yields, and the risk of pregnancy loss.

A technique for the reliable isolation of fetal cells or DNA from the maternal circulation would eliminate the risk to the fetus and represents an important goal in prenatal diagnosis. It has been known for over a century that fetally derived cells might be found in the maternal circulation.[15] Studies using detection of specific fetal cell DNA suggest that a degree of fetomaternal cell transfer occurs in all pregnancies,[16] although estimates of the number of fetal cells in the maternal circulation vary, the most recent estimate suggests 19 fetal cells in 16 ml of maternal blood.[17]

Most techniques currently proposed for the separation of fetal cells rely on different physical characteristics of the target fetal cells, or on specific antibodies, or usually on a combination of both. An important primary consideration is the target fetal cell type. Trophoblast cells have a unique, and easily identifiable, morphology. Although they can be found in the circulation of women with severe pre-eclampsia, the effective clearance of trophoblast cells by the maternal lungs makes them difficult to isolate in normal pregnancies. Specific anti-trophoblast monoclonal antibodies have been difficult to develop, although Mab340 appears promising.[18] Trophoblasts may shed cell surface proteins which are re-presented by maternal leukocytes, causing maternal, rather than fetal, cells to be enriched.[19] The use of fetal leukocytes as a target is complicated by the lack of specific antibodies, not shared with maternal cells. Paternal HLA polymorphisms might be used, but this requires knowledge of the father and his HLA type. Fetal lymphocytes persist in the maternal circulation for many years[20] so isolated fetal leukocytes may not represent the current pregnancy.

Fetal nucleated erythrocytes (NRBCs) are currently the most popular candidates for identification in the maternal circulation, as they are common in fetal blood, are well differentiated and have a limited lifespan. Most strategies for enrichment of maternal blood for fetal NRBCs involve two steps. Firstly, the entire nucleated cell population is enriched, either by selective lysing of maternal anucleate erythrocytes, or by single, double or triple density gradient centrifugation through Histopaque layers of different densities. NRBCs are then selected by binding to a monoclonal antibody to the transferrin receptor (CD71),[21] glycophorin-A,[22] or thrombospondin receptor.[23] Separation of antibody-labelled cells can then be performed using fluorescence activated cell sorting (FACS) or magnetic cell sorting techniques (MACS). At present, the majority of the NRBCs which are enriched using these techniques prove to be maternal in origin.[24]

Once a population of cells has been enriched, a method for identification of specific cells, or of at least proving that there are fetal cells present in the sample, is needed. PCR, to amplify fetal specific genomic sequences, can demonstrate the presence of fetal DNA, without visualization of fetal cells. Nested PCR for Y specific sequences has been used,[25] but this can only apply to male pregnancies. Paternally inherited HLA-DQ alpha sequences have been used to demonstrate fetal DNA in sorted fetal cells.[26] Where the father carries a polymorphism not present in the mother, detection of fetal single gene disorders may be possible. For example, fetal inheritance of haemoglobin Lepore-Boston has been demonstrated using PCR, targeting fetal DNA from the maternal circulation.[27] Targeting of fetal RNA is an alternative strategy[28] and may not require prior separation of fetal cells from the maternal background. Diagnosis of anueploidy (usually by chromosome specific fluorescence in situ hybridization or FISH) requires specific visualization of fetal cells. Whilst fetal cells might be identified using 'specific' antibodies, such as anti-HbF, the pretreatment needed for FISH damages most antigenic epitopes. Synchronous viewing of immunocytochemical and FISH markers is, therefore, not possible. This problem has been partly overcome by using a computer matrix which can 'remember' the location of a cell identified using immunocytochemistry, and find it again following hybridization of FISH probes. Alternatively, fetal cell 'specific' antibodies may be used to identify fetal cells allowing them to be collected by micromanipulation. Cheung et al,[29] identified fetal cells using anti-HbF, and then microselected single cells PCR diagnosis of β-thallasaemia.

PRE-IMPLANTATION GENETIC DIAGNOSIS

Pre-implantation genetic diagnosis has enabled the birth of more than 100 unaffected children, born to couples at high risk of single gene or chromosome abnormalities, by selective transfer of embryos which have undergone single cell diagnosis, usually using PCR, following micro-manipulation and embryo biopsy. Pre-implantation diagnosis avoids the risks and ethical dilemmas of amniocentesis or chorion villus biopsy and pregnancy termination. Following in vitro fertilisation, the fertilised zygotes are grown to day 3, typically the 6–10 cell blastomy stage, when one or two cells are removed. This is carried out by drilling a hole through the zona pellucida, using an acidified medium in a micropipette, and aspiration through a second pipette filled with culture medium.[30] Embryo biopsy does not appear to affect subsequent viability and, after diagnosis by polymerase chain reaction, unaffected embryos can be transferred later the same day.

The first cases of pre-implantation diagnosis used PCR to amplify a multi-copy Y chromosome-specific repeat.[31] This allowed sex selection and the transfer of only female embryos in mothers at high risk of an X-linked disease. The first single gene defect to be diagnosed pre-implantation was cystic fibrosis.[32] Because of the very small concentration of template DNA, just one copy of each allele in a single cell, a nested technique is used. In nested PCR, two pairs of primers are designed to flank the mutation. The first, outer pair of primers is used in PCR with an annealing temperature lower than the optimal. This allows considerable non-specific priming and the generation of non-specific PCR products. It does, however, ensure that there is priming of the target sequences. Specificity is introduced by using the inner primer pair in a more stringent reaction, so that only the specific target sequence products of the first reaction are amplified in the second reaction. A further problem with the use of PCR for pre-implantation diagnosis is that of allele drop out. If PCR primers fail to hybridize properly with both alleles at the start of a polymerase chain reaction, then the products of one allele will gain a head start over the products of the other. Because PCR is an exponential amplification process, this essentially means that products will only be visible at the end of the reaction from one allele. To reduce the risk of allele drop out, a technique known as primer extension pre-amplification has been developed. This is a method for pre-amplifying the entire genome with random primers, and increases the number of target sequences at the start of the diagnostic PCR. Primer extension pre-amplification also allows more than one diagnostic PCR to be performed on a single cell. So, for example, the products of primer extension pre-amplification can be divided into two aliquots. One can be used for direct diagnosis of the suspected mutation, whilst the second can be used to examine linked informative polymorphisms simultaneously.

Over 50% of miscarriages are known to be due to aneuploidy and aneuploidy is probably a significant cause of unsuccessful IVF. Aneuploidy may be determined in pre-implantation embryos using FISH chromosome painting techniques. Application of these techniques in couples who have undergone multiple unsuccessful IVF attempts has been shown to improve the pregnancy rate. Although not currently a routine part of in vitro fertilisation, it is possible that in the future FISH may be used to exclude chromosome abnormalities.

FETAL INFECTION

The ability to detect fetal infection prenatally has important clinical implications. Whilst maternal infection is usually readily detectable, transplacental transmission is by no means inevitable. For example, in maternal *Toxoplasma* infection, only approximately 20% of fetuses will be infected transplacentally. If termination of pregnancy is to be considered an option as a result of suspected fetal infection, prior diagnosis must be reliably established. In addition, maternal antibiotic therapy is effective treatment for a *Toxoplasma* infected fetus, but is not without risks to the fetus, and should be reserved for cases where fetal infection has been established.

PCR based tests are available for prenatal detection of most of the TORCH-type infections. Primers have been designed that amplify the *Toxoplasma* B1 gene in cells pelleted from amniocentesis.[33] The role of this gene is unknown, but it is repeated 35 times in the *Toxoplasma* genome and, therefore, makes a better target than a single-copy gene. A similar test is available for detecting cytomegalovirus (CMV) in amniotic fluid.

Estimates of transplacental transmission of HIV vary between 20–70%, dependent on the use of Zidovudine therapy and elective caesarean section.[34] Although the incidence of transmission correlates with maternal disease status,[35] the predictive value of maternal CD4 lymphocyte counts, p24 antigen status or viral load are limited. Direct diagnosis of fetal HIV infection has been performed by PCR following fetal blood sampling.[36–38] Fetal blood sampling, however, increases the risk of viral transmission and placental transmission may occur late in pregnancy limiting the use of mid-trimester prenatal diagnosis.[39] There is also a role, therefore, for neonatal testing by PCR.

PCR has also been used to demonstrate the presence of hepatitis B DNA in sero-negative at-risk individuals. Single point mutations in the genome may significantly alter its antigenicity and, therefore, complicate serological testing. PCR will still amplify sequences containing point mutations.

THE FUTURE

The rate of development of molecular biological techniques, and their application to clinical practice, has exploded over the last two decades. It is less than 20 years since Southern blotting was invented and only 10 years since the first prenatal diagnosis of single gene disorder by direct detection of the mutation. At the beginning of this decade, the molecular basis of only a handful of diseases was known, whereas now the genetic defect causing most well-known single gene disorders has been determined. Development in molecular biology is likely to continue to be exponential, and many of the goals of prenatal diagnosis, such as the rapid determination of aneuploidy, or the reliable separation of fetal cells from the maternal circulation, are likely to be realized in the next decade. The genes for a large number of known proteins have been cloned and as we begin to understand the molecular basis for more esoteric human differences, such as memory, appearance and intelligence, a whole new series of ethical questions surrounding prenatal diagnosis are likely to be raised.

REFERENCES

1 Southern E M. Detection of specific sequences among DNA fragments separated by gel electrophoresis. J Mol Biol 1975; 98: 503–517

2 Klinger K, Landes G, Shook D et al. Rapid detection of chromosome aneuploidies in uncultured amniocytes by using fluorescence in situ hybridization (FISH). Am J Hum Genet 1992; 51: 55–65

3 Ward B E, Gersen S L, Carelli M P et al. Rapid prenatal diagnosis of chromosomal aneuploidies by fluorescence in situ hybridization: clinical experience with 4,500 specimens. Am J Hum Genet 1993; 52: 854–865

4 Huang S Z, Sheng M, Zhao J Q et al. Detection of sickle cell gene by analysis of amplified DNA sequences. I Chuan Hsueh Pao 1989; 16: 475–482

5 Kerem B, Rommens J M, Buchanan J A et al. Identification of the cystic fibrosis gene: genetic analysis. Science 1989; 245: 1073–1080

6 Taylor G, Noble J, Hall J, Quirke P, Stewart A, Mueller R. Rapid screening for ΔF508 deletion in cystic fibrosis. Lancet 1989; ii: 1345

7 Snell R G, MacMillan J C, Cheadle J P et al. Relationship between trinucleotide repeat expansion and phenotypic variation in Huntington's disease. Nat Genet 1993; 4: 393–397

8 Newton C R, Heptinstall L E, Summers C et al. Amplification refractory mutation system for prenatal diagnosis and carrier assessment in cystic fibrosis. Lancet 1989; ii: 1481–1483

9 Saiki R K, Chang C A, Levenson C H et al. Diagnosis of sickle cell anemia and beta-thalassemia with enzymatically amplified DNA and nonradioactive allele-specific oligonucleotide probes. N Engl J Med 1988; 319: 537–541

10 Lathrop G M, Lalouel J M, Julier C, Ott J. Strategies for multilocus linkage analysis in humans. Proc Natl Acad Sci USA 1984; 81: 3443–3446

11 Bennett P R, Le V K C, Colin Y et al. Prenatal determination of fetal RhD type by DNA amplification. N Engl J Med 1993; 329: 607–610

12 Griffith-Jones-M D, Miller D, Lilford R J, Scott J, Bulmer J. Detection of fetal DNA in trans-cervical swabs from first trimester pregnancies by gene amplification: a new route to prenatal diagnosis? Br J Obstet Gynaecol 1992; 99: 508–511

13 Rodeck C, Tutschek B, Sherlock J, Kingdom J. Methods for the transcervical collection of fetal cells during the first trimester of pregnancy. Prenat Diagn 1995; 15: 933–942

14 Overton T G, Lighten A D, Fisk N M, Bennett P R. Prenatal diagnosis by minimally invasive first-trimester transcervical sampling is unreliable. Am J Obstet Gynecol 1996; 175: 382–387

15 Schmorl G. Pathologisch–anatomische untersuchungen uber puerperal eklampsie. Leipzig, Germany: Vogel, 1893

16 Bianchi D W. Prenatal diagnosis by analysis of fetal cells in maternal blood. J Pediatr 1995; 127: 847–856

17 Bianchi D W, Williams J M, Sullivan L M, Hanson F W, Klinger K W, Shuber A P. PCR quantitation of fetal cells in maternal blood in normal and aneuploid pregnancies. Am J Hum Genet 1997; 61: 822–829

18 Martin W, Bruce J, Smith N, Liu D, Durrant L. A magnetic colloid system for isolation of rare cells from blood for FISH analysis. Prenat Diagn 1997; 17: 1059–1066

19 Bertero M T, Camaschella C, Serra A, Bergui L, Caligaris C F. Circulating 'trophoblast' cells in pregnancy have maternal genetic markers. Prenat Diagn 1988; 8: 585–590

20 Bianchi D W, Zickwolf G K, Weil G J, Sylvester S, DeMaria M A. Male fetal progenitor cells persist in maternal blood for as long as 27 years postpartum. Proc Natl Acad Sci USA 1996; 93: 705–708

21 Ganshirt A D, Borjesson S R, Burschyk M et al. Detection of fetal trisomies 21 and 18 from maternal blood using triple gradient and magnetic cell sorting. Am J Reprod Immunol 1993; 30: 194–201

22 Simpson J L, Elias S. Isolating fetal cells from maternal blood. Advances in prenatal diagnosis through molecular technology. JAMA 1993; 270: 2357–2361

23 Simpson J L, Elias S. Isolating fetal cells in maternal circulation for prenatal diagnosis. Prenat Diagn 1994; 14: 1229–1242

24 Slunga T A, El R W, Keinanen M et al. Maternal origin of nucleated erythrocytes in peripheral venous blood of pregnant women. Hum Genet 1995; 96: 53–57

25 Lo Y M, Bowell P J, Selinger M et al. Prenatal determination of fetal RhD status by analysis of peripheral blood of rhesus negative mothers. Lancet 1993; 341: 1147–1148

26 Geifman H O, Holtzman E J, Vadnais T J, Phillips V E, Capeless E L, Bianchi D W. Detection of fetal HLA-DQa sequences in maternal blood: a gender-independent technique of fetal cell identification. Prenat Diagn 1995; 15: 261–268

27 Camaschella C, Alfarano A, Gottardi E et al. Prenatal diagnosis of fetal hemoglobin Lepore-Boston disease on maternal peripheral blood. Blood 1990; 75: 2102–2106

28 Hamlington J, Cunningham J, Mason G, Mueller R, Miller D. Prenatal detection of rhesus D genotype. Lancet 1997; 349: 540

29 Cheung M C, Goldberg J D, Kan Y W. Prenatal diagnosis of sickle cell anaemia and thalassaemia by analysis of fetal cells in maternal blood. Nat Genet 1996; 14: 264–268

30 Bolton V N, Wren M E, Parsons J H. Pregnancies after in vitro fertilization and transfer of human blastocysts. Fertil Steril 1991; 55: 830–832

31 Handyside A H, Kontogianni E H, Hardy K, Winston R M. Pregnancies from biopsied human preimplantation embryos sexed by Y-specific DNA amplification. Nature 1990; 344: 768–770

32 Handyside A H, Lesko J G, Tarin J J, Winston R M, Hughes M R. Birth of a normal girl after in vitro fertilization and preimplantation diagnostic testing for cystic fibrosis. N Engl J Med 1992; 327: 905–909

33 Grover C M, Thulliez P, Remington J S, Boothroyd J C. Rapid prenatal diagnosis of congenital *Toxoplasma* infection by using polymerase chain reaction and amniotic fluid. J Clin Microbiol 1990; 28: 2297–2301

34 Connor E M, Sperling R S, Gelber R et al. Reduction of maternal-infant transmission of human immunodeficiency virus type 1 with zidovudine treatment. Pediatric AIDS Clinical Trials Group Protocol 076 Study Group. N Engl J Med 1994; 331: 1173–1180

35 Mayaux M J, Blanche S, Rouzioux C et al. Maternal factors associated with perinatal HIV-1 transmission: the French Cohort Study: 7 years of follow-up observation. The French Pediatric HIV Infection Study Group. J Acquir Immune Defic Syndr Hum Retrovirol 1995; 8: 188–194

36 Krivine A, Firtion G, Cao L, Francoual C, Henrion R, Lebon P. HIV replication during the first weeks of life. Lancet 1992; 339: 1187–1189

37 Burgard M, Mayaux M J, Blanche S et al. The use of viral culture and p24 antigen testing to diagnose human immunodeficiency virus infection in neonates. The HIV Infection in Newborns French Collaborative Study Group. N Engl J Med 1992; 327: 1192–1197

38 Daffos F, Forestier F, Mandelbrot L, Pialoux G, Rey MA, Brun VF. Prenatal diagnosis of HIV infection: two attempts using fetal blood sampling. J Acquir Immune Defic Syndr 1989; 2: 205–207

39 Mandelbrot L, Brossard Y, Aubin J T et al. Testing for in utero human immunodeficiency virus infection with fetal blood sampling. Am J Obstet Gynecol 1996; 175: 489–493

Adeola Olaitan   Margaret A. Johnsont

Human immunodeficiency virus in obstetrics

The World Health Organization (WHO) estimates that at least 50% of the 17 million people infected with the human immunodeficiency virus worldwide are female and that, by the year 2000, 13 million women will be infected with HIV.[1] In the UK, 3645 women had been reported as HIV positive by the end of September 1995,[2] and the number is increasing.[3] The majority of these women are in their reproductive years and many still elect to have children after their HIV diagnosis.[4] Data from the unlinked anonymous testing programme indicate that, although the rate outside London remains lower, each London obstetric unit has managed at least one woman found to be HIV positive on anonymous testing. However, HIV infection was clinically recognised in only 17% of women identified by anonymous testing, with 6% identified by voluntary named antenatal testing.[5] It is evident, therefore, that obstetricians need to be familiar with the clinical manifestations of HIV disease so that at-risk and infected women can be recognised. It has also become increasingly important for obstetricians to be conversant with the management of pregnancy in women with HIV infection, in order to minimise the risk of vertical transmission, and ensure that the woman receives optimal medical care for her condition.

BACKGROUND AND EPIDEMIOLOGY

The causative virus of AIDS, the human immunodeficiency virus, is an RNA virus characterised by the enzyme, reverse transcriptase, which allows its RNA content to be transcribed backwards to viral DNA which is randomly

Miss Adeola Olaitan, Specialist Registrar/Consultant Gynaecologist, Gynaecological and Colposcopy Services, Department of Obstetrics and Gynaecology, Royal Free Hospital Medical School, Pond Street, London NW3 2QG, UK

Dr Margaret A. Johnson, Consultant in Thoracic Medicine, Director of HIV and AIDS Services, Royal Free Hospital, Pond Street, London NW3 2QG, UK

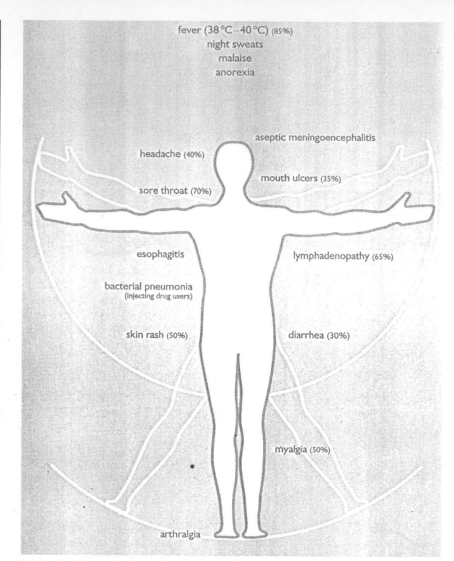

fever (38 °C–40 °C) (85%)
night sweats
malaise
anorexia

aseptic meningoencephalitis

headache (40%)

mouth ulcers (35%)

sore throat (70%)

esophagitis

lymphadenopathy (65%)

bacterial pneumonia
(injecting drug users)

skin rash (50%)

diarrhea (30%)

myalgia (50%)

arthralgia

Fig. 3.1 Diagrammatic representation of the manifestations of HIV seroconversion (reproduced with the permission of Parthenon Publishing Ltd from an Atlas of Differential Diagnosis in HIV Disease).

incorporated into the host nucleic DNA. The envelope glycoproteins confer the ability for the virus to attach to cells bearing the CD4+ antigen, particularly T-helper (CD4) lymphocytes which have a co-ordinating effect on other elements of the immune system (for review, see Webster and Johnson[6]).

Most cases of AIDS in the Western world are associated with HIV-1. HIV-2 affects sub-Saharan Africa, and some West European countries, especially Portugal, but remains uncommon in the UK. Infection is from blood, semen, saliva, female genital tract secretions and breast milk. In Britain and Ireland, 59% of infection in women is acquired from heterosexual intercourse. Other risk factors are intravenous drug use (37%), and the use of infected blood and blood products (3%).[7] The proportion of heterosexually-acquired HIV

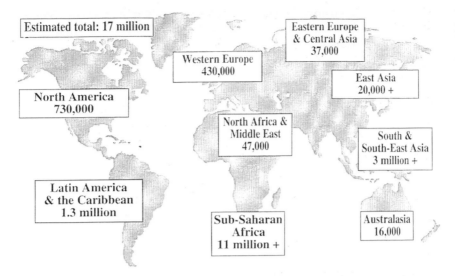

Fig. 3.2 Estimation of prevalent HIV infections in adults calculated by WHO from multiple sources and methods (reproduced with the permission of Mediscript Limited from HIV & AIDS Current Trends).

infections would be higher if Britain alone is considered, as the majority of infected women from Ireland acquired HIV through intravenous drug use.

Initial HIV infection may be asymptomatic, or produce an acute glandular fever-type illness, often associated with a characteristic rash (Fig. 3.1). Antibodies are usually detected in the serum within 3 months of infection. The mean time from infection to the development of AIDS in men is 8–10 years from seroconversion,[8] and current evidence indicates that the same applies to women.[9–11] As an estimated 10–20% of infected individuals have AIDS, there is a large pool of asymptomatic, unknown infection in the community.

Although, in the Western world, HIV infection is presently confined to defined at-risk groups with a male predominance, in sub-Saharan Africa and other under-developed countries, it is more widespread with an equal number of men and women being affected, and heterosexual spread being the main mode of transmission (Fig. 3.2). However, even in developed countries, including the UK, heterosexual transmission is becoming increasingly important in the spread of HIV infection. Data from the anonymous, unlinked antenatal screening programme have shown an increase in the prevalence of HIV infection amongst pregnant women, with the rise more marked in inner London.[3] Although this may be, in part, accounted for by the influx of refugees from sub-Saharan Africa into London,[12] there is evidence of a rise in prevalence amongst the indigenous population also. These women may, therefore, not consider themselves to be at risk, and HIV infection may not be suspected until the woman becomes symptomatic. A retrospective review of gynaecological case-notes showed that, in a majority of HIV-infected women undergoing invasive gynaecological procedures, neither the doctor nor the woman were aware of the possibility of HIV infection.[13] Studies have shown that women are less likely than homosexual men to be aware of their HIV status before AIDS is diagnosed[14] and anonymous testing programmes have revealed that the majority of HIV positive women are unaware of their status. The recognition of this fact, and the knowledge that early diagnosis of HIV infection improves outcome, both in terms of disease-free survival and in pregnancy, the reduction of the risk of vertical transmission, has led to the introduction of voluntary, named antenatal screening for HIV infection.

SCREENING

The WHO recommends that when screening for any condition, the benefits of a positive test should outweigh the risks. Early recognition of HIV disease is particularly important in pregnancy, as, in addition to ensuring that the woman receives optimal medical care for her condition, various strategies can be employed to minimise the risk of HIV transmission to the fetus. It also enables the woman to be counselled about the implications of pregnancy with HIV infection and to discuss the option of pregnancy termination where appropriate. The paediatrician can be involved early in the management, should the woman elect to continue with her pregnancy.

The obvious argument against antenatal screening is that early pregnancy is a traumatic time for a woman to discover HIV infection and to have to face both the dilemmas of pregnancy and HIV infection at the same time. However, while pre-pregnancy diagnosis is ideal, not all women have access to pre-pregnancy health care and, indeed, not all pregnancies are planned. The overall benefits of early detection of HIV infection in pregnancy far outweigh the emotional trauma, which, with proper counselling, the woman will ultimately overcome.

A concern often voiced by several women, and some health care professionals is that the mere fact of undergoing HIV antibody testing, even when the result is negative, can adversely affect assessment for life insurance. However women can now be reassured as changes in the wording of insurance forms now mean that an individual only need declare an HIV test if the result is positive.[15]

Universal screening, where HIV antibody testing is offered to all pregnant women regardless of their history, is not always feasible, mainly because of the cost. Yet, a policy of selectively targeting high risk cases on the basis of their history, will lead to some cases of HIV infection being missed, particularly in areas of high HIV prevalence. Goldberg and Johnstone have suggested that voluntary named testing of pregnant women should be performed on a selective basis in settings where unlinked anonymous testing have shown a low prevalence of HIV.[16] Where the seroprevalence is greater, universal named testing should be considered.

The potential implications of a positive HIV antibody test make it inappropriate to offer screening without some form of prior discussion, the main object being to provide the woman with the relevant knowledge for her to make an informed decision about whether she wishes to undergo the test, and to obtain explicit consent. The General Medical Council[17] has stated that the need to obtain consent 'is particularly important in the case of testing for HIV infection, not because the condition is different in kind from other infections but because of the possible serious social and financial consequences which may ensue from the mere fact of having been tested for the condition'. The pre-test discussion is within the remit of most obstetricians, who, as part of their role, counsel women for complicated pre-natal diagnostic tests.

IMPLICATIONS OF HIV IN PREGNANCY

Earlier reports suggested that pregnancy, which has a suppressive effect on cell-mediated immunity, may accelerate the course of HIV disease. Indeed, the first six reported cases were all fatal.[18] This has not been supported by more recent studies which have shown that the markers of disease progression are not adversely affected in women who have had a pregnancy compared to those who have not.[20,21]

Similarly, it was thought that babies born to HIV infected women experienced more obstetric and neonatal complications, with an excess of prematurity and intra-uterine growth retardation. A specific HIV-related syndrome was even described.[21] However, when confounding factors are excluded or controlled for, it becomes apparent that there are no more adverse fetal effects than in an HIV negative pregnancy.[22,23]

Transmission to the offspring is the issue that dominates current thinking about HIV infection. Estimates of vertical transmission have been revised downwards as more information has become available. The largest follow-up study of pregnancy with HIV infection has reported a vertical transmission rate of 14.4% in the Western world.[24] Higher transmission rates have been reported in Africa.[25] Of the children infected by maternal transmission, 26% had developed AIDS, and 17% had died of an HIV-related illness by 12 months of age.[26] The management of the pregnancy is made more difficult by the fact that, at present, there is no practical method of pre-natal diagnosis to predict which infants are affected. The reasons for this are 2-fold. Methods of definitive pre-natal diagnosis such as cordocentesis are invasive, and carry a theoretical risk of paradoxically infecting the fetus with HIV by inoculating maternal blood into the fetal compartment, and should, therefore, be avoided. Second, there is growing evidence that most neonatal infection occurs during the delivery process[24,27] and, therefore, even if there was an available diagnostic method, it may be impossible in early intra-uterine life, to determine which neonates will be ultimately infected. Early diagnosis of HIV infection in the neonate may also be difficult: maternal HIV IgG antibodies cross the placenta and may persist in fetal circulation for up to 18 months (median 10 months[24]), and HIV infection may not be conclusively excluded for this time period. Unfortunately, IgM estimations are not helpful in this situation as the presence or absence of this antibody has not been shown to correlate with other evidence of infection.[28]

However, there are certain predictors of probable neonatal infection. The risk of vertical transmission is increased by advancing maternal disease (P24 antigenaemia, CD4 count $< 700/\mu m$), and this may reflect a high viral load. HIV seroconversion during pregnancy is associated with a higher risk of vertical transmission, again probably because of a high viral load. Breast feeding and prematurity (birth before 34 weeks' gestation) are also associated with increased vertical transmission rates.[24] Recent studies[29] in which maternal serum viral load was directly measured have demonstrated a positive correlation between viral load and maternally-acquired HIV infection in the off-spring. Reducing viral load by the administration of anti-retroviral medication diminished the risk of vertical transmission.[30,31]

It is still not clear how and when maternal–fetal transmission of HIV infection occurs. While circumstantial evidence indicates that infection occurs during parturition, there have been reports of isolation of HIV by polymerase chain reaction (PCR) from aborted fetuses in the second trimester of pregnancy.[32] A recent study[33] of 100 aborted fetuses from HIV positive pregnancies detected HIV infection by PCR in only 2 fetuses, and concluded that the low frequency of early *in utero* HIV transmission observed suggests that transmission occurs mostly later in pregnancy and/or at delivery, and that specific risk factors may have implications in the occurrence of early as opposed to late transmission. The presence of high levels of HIV neutralising antibodies in the maternal plasma has also been shown to reduce the risk of vertical transmission, independent of viral load.[34,35] The mode of transmission, whether by intact cells or by cell-free virus, has also not been elucidated, but cervico-vaginal secretions from non-menstruating HIV infected women have been found to contain both cell-free and cell-associated HIV,[36,37] supporting the potential for intrapartum transmission of HIV. Several reports indicate that the frequency and quantity of HIV in genital secretions may be higher in infected women who are pregnant than in non-pregnant HIV positive women.[38] It is clearly important that these issues are resolved if effective strategies to reduce intra-uterine infection are to be devised.

ANTENATAL CARE

The care of pregnant women known to be infected with HIV should be multidisciplinary, involving the obstetrician, the HIV physician, the general practitioner, the paediatrician, mid-wives, health visitors and social workers. The woman should be referred for booking as early as possible and counselled about the implications of pregnancy with HIV disease, including the risks of vertical transmission (Table 3.1). She should be made aware as early as possible that breast feeding, which may increase vertical transmission rates by a further 14%,[39] is contra-indicated. Illicit drug use should discussed where relevant as there is evidence that this may increase perinatal transmission.[40] The option of pregnancy

Table 3.1 Counselling pregnant HIV positive women

Personal prognosis based on lymphocyte sub-sets (and (?) HIV viral load)
Illicit drug use (where relevant)
Vertical transmission rates
No method of pre-natal diagnosis
Option of pregnancy termination
Breastfeeding contra-indicated
Neonatal prognosis
Death of HIV-infected parent(s) in child's infancy

Table 3.2 Screening and follow-up tests in pregnancy

Test	Frequency	Changes with HIV disease
FBC	3-monthly	Anaemia, lymphopaenia, thrombocytopaenia
LFTs	3-monthly	Concurrent hepatitis or drug treatment may affect
Hepatitis B and C markers	Baseline	May be acquired via same route as HIV
Toxoplasma serology	Baseline	Seropositives at risk of reactivation if immunosuppressed
Syphilis serology	Baseline	High endemicity may correspond with high HIV prevalence
Cervical cytology	Baseline/yearly	Higher rate of abnormality and faster progression in HIV positive women
T Cells	3-monthly	CD4 fall with increasing immunosupression
p24 Ag	3-monthly	Rises with disease progression
HIV viral load	3-monthly	Predictor of vertical transmission and need for anti-retroviral therapy. Still experimental

termination should be available, where appropriate. Data from Edinburgh indicates that HIV infection alone is not usually the deciding factor for a termination,[41] and HIV positivity *per se* should not be assumed to justify an abortion on request.[42] Appropriate specialist counselling should be available and care must be taken to avoid a hasty and regretted decision to terminate a previously wanted pregnancy, especially when HIV status is discovered during pregnancy.

In addition to routine antenatal tests, screening for hepatitis B and C, which are also blood-borne viruses with similar epidemiology, should also be carried out. As HIV is often a sexually transmitted infection, women presenting with HIV in pregnancy should also be offered screening for other STDs, which may independently affect pregnancy outcome. In addition, any associated mucosal inflammation may increase the potential for vertical transmission. However, the experience in our centre is that a relatively low frequency of other sexually transmitted diseases are detected in HIV positive women.[43] Cervical intra-epithelial neoplasia is more common in HIV positive women and is related the degree of immunosuppression.[44] A cervical smear should, therefore, be taken at the booking clinic if the woman has not had one in the preceding 6 months.

Invasive pre-natal diagnostic procedures should be avoided for the reasons stated above. After appropriate counselling, women in whom there is an age-related or other concern of fetal chromosomal abnormality may be referred to a specialist centre for ultrasound scanning to detect physical markers of chromosomal abnormality.

At each routine obstetric visit, enquiries should be made for symptoms suggestive of HIV-related infection and a full physical examination, including fundoscopy and chest auscultation should be performed at a minimum of 3 monthly intervals by the HIV physician. Any adverse symptoms or signs should prompt a full clinical and laboratory search for HIV associated disease.

Laboratory tests of immune function (Table 3.2) should be undertaken at 3 monthly intervals, or more frequently if there is evidence of deteriorating immune function.

Prophylaxis against pneumocystis pneumonia (PCP) is indicated if the CD4 lymphocyte count falls below 200/mm³ or in women with symptomatic disease. Co-trimoxazole, 960 mg/day, which also offers some protection against toxoplasmosis, or monthly nebulised pentamidine are the most commonly used drugs, with dapsone used less frequently. Although there have been concerns about co-trimoxazole toxicity in the newborn, there is no clear evidence that it is harmful in pregnancy, particularly if the dose is lowered near term to reduce the small risk of neonatal haemolysis and methaemoglobinaemia. Nebulised pentamidine has little systemic absorption but the risk of extra-pulmonary pneumocystis infection and pneumothorax, and the fact that it is less efficacious,[45] make co-trimoxazole the drug of choice.

ANTI-RETROVIRAL MEDICATION

Zidovudine (AZT), a nucleoside analogue which inhibits viral replication, thereby slowing progression of HIV, is the most commonly used anti-retroviral drug. The Concorde trial, a large, double-blinded, multicentre placebo-controlled trial, run in three countries,[46] failed to demonstrate an advantage in the initiation of zidovudine therapy in asymptomatic HIV disease over early symptomatic infection. The early initiation of zidovudine therapy is, therefore, not indicated, particularly in pregnancy where there may be concerns about fetal toxicity. However, zidovudine therapy should be continued after the first trimester in pregnant HIV-infected women with medical indications for antiretroviral therapy.

Attention has recently turned, however, to the use of zidovudine in pregnancy to prevent vertical transmission. The ACTG 076 trial,[47] a double-blind, placebo-controlled, randomised clinical trial was designed to evaluate the efficacy, safety and tolerance of zidovudine for the prevention of maternal–fetal transmission. HIV positive pregnant women meeting the enrolment criteria (Table 3.3), were randomised to receive zidovudine 100 mg 5 times a day, or placebo. Therapy was commenced between 14 and 34 weeks' gestation, with a median time of 26 weeks, and continued through out the remainder of pregnancy, followed by intrapartum zidovudine given by

Table 3.3 ACTG 076 trial: criteria for enrolment

Pregnant
HIV positive
No previous zidovudine use
No medical indication for zidovudine use
CD4 lymphocyte count > 200/mm³
14–34 weeks' gestation

continuous intravenous infusion (loading dose 2 mg/kg and then 1 mg/kg/h) until delivery. Oral zidovudine syrup, 2 mg/kg, 6 hourly, was then given to the neonate, starting 8–12 h after birth and continued for 6 weeks. The primary study end point, HIV infection of the infant, was defined by one positive viral culture obtained from peripheral blood. Specimens for viral culture were obtained at birth, 12 and 78 weeks post-partum. The interim analysis showed such a marked reduction in transmission in the study arm that the trial was terminated and all the women in the placebo arm were offered zidovudine: the transmission rate in the placebo arm was 25.5%, compared with 8.3% in the study arm. The only recorded fetal effect was a transient anaemia, with mean decrease in haemoglobin of less that 1 g/dl, which recovered spontaneously.

However, the transmission rate in the placebo arm was high, and HIV transmission still occurred in patients receiving zidovudine. Moreover, the study does not address the question of the optimal dose and timing for zidovudine in pregnancy, and long-term follow-up of children exposed to zidovudine *in utero* is also required. Despite these drawbacks, the study is sufficiently conclusive for its findings and limitations to be discussed with all suitable pregnant women, and for zidovudine to be commenced in those who opt for this form of therapy. However, there has been little experience with the use of zidovudine in the first trimester, and the advice is that its use at this time should be avoided if the sole indication is to avoid vertical transmission.

A second trial (ACTG 185) is evaluating the use of hyper-immune HIV immunoglobulin (HIVIG) in HIV-infected women with late-stage disease (CD4 count $< 500/mm^3$, in whom antiretroviral therapy is medically indicated). All women receive the ACTG 076 regimen, and HIVIG, or immunoglobulin without HIV, was given monthly during pregnancy and at birth to the neonate. There has been little or no experience with the use of other anti-retrovirals in pregnancy although trials of these, and of active immunisation with candidate HIV vaccines (ACTG 233, 234, 235) are underway or planned.[48] Evaluating the use of other anti-retrovirals in pregnancy has become even more important in the light of the results of the DELTA trial which showed that combination therapy with AZT and ddI or ddC is superior to AZT alone in prolonging disease-free survival in HIV-infected women.[49]

THE CONDUCT OF LABOUR AND DELIVERY

When supervising the labour of an HIV-infected woman, precautions should be taken to minimise the risk of nosocomial infection to healthcare workers, and the risk of vertical transmission to the fetus.

The risk of HIV transmission through occupational exposure is small. Needlestick injury with an HIV positive patient carries a sero-conversion rate of 0.2%[50] compared with 25% with a patient who is hepatitis B e antigen positive. Double-gloving, the use of water-proof gowns and the wearing of spectacles all reduce the risk of acquiring infection, particularly if these precautions are universally implemented.[51]

There is growing evidence that maternal–fetal transmission of HIV occurs during parturition, and intervention at this stage may reduce vertical transmission rates. Goedert et al,[27] in their review of vaginal delivery of twins in HIV infected women, demonstrated that the first twin which is usually in contact with maternal fluids for a longer period, had a 2.8-fold greater risk of infection than the second twin. The European Collaborative Study[24] also demonstrated a trend to lowered vertical transmission rates in women undergoing caesarean section, though this was by no means conclusive. A retrospective study has indicated that HIV positive women may be at higher risk of postoperative complications after caesarean section than non-HIV infected women.[52] The difference was more marked in immunosuppressed HIV-infected women, and this factor should be taken into account when deciding the mode of delivery. A prospective, case-controlled, multi-centre randomised trial of elective caesarean section versus spontaneous vaginal delivery is now underway and should resolve the question of the best mode of delivery. At present, the policy is to offer caesarean section for standard obstetric implications.

Another potential obstetric intervention for the prevention of peripartum transmission is vaginal lavage with a microbicidal agent during labour. The use of microbiocidals during labour to prevent neonatal *Streptococcus* group B infection has been reported. Burman et al[53] found that vaginal washing with chlorhexidine significantly lowered the rate of neonatal group B streptococcal infection, with no maternal or fetal toxic effects. Chlorhexidine has been shown to neutralise HIV in vitro,[54,55] but its in vivo application for this purpose is yet to be evaluated.

The risk of maternal–fetal transmission in labour may be reduced by avoiding artificial rupture of membranes, or leaving this till as late as possible, thereby minimising fetal contact with maternal secretions. Chorio-amnionitis has also been shown to increase the vertical transmission rate,[56] so care should be taken to avoid ascending infection. Fetal blood sampling, and the use of fetal scalp electrodes are contra-indicated. The European Collaborative Study[24] found higher vertical transmission rates with vaginal deliveries in which forceps, vacuum extractors and episiotorny were used, but only in centres where the use was not routine.

Caesarean section, if indicated, should be performed by the most experienced person available, to reduce the risk of injury to staff. Smith and Grant[57] have shown that glove puncture in obstetricians occurs in 54% of caesarean sections and, where such perforations are recognised by the surgeon, 60% of them occurred during closure of the lower uterine segment. Double gloving reduces the risk of puncture of the inner glove by a factor of 6,[58] and

Table 3.4 Serological and virological tests in newborns at risk of HIV infection

FBC and differential
T lymphocyte subsets
Urine for CMV
Hepatitis B serology
HIV serology – ELISA
Virus isolation by lymphocyte culture
p24 antigen
Polymerase chain reaction

the use of blunt needles and tissue-handling forceps, further decreases the risk of needlestick injury.[51]

The third stage should be conducted actively to reduce blood loss which, aside from the risk of infection to staff, may lead to maternal anaemia and delay post-partum recovery and discharge. The infant should be washed as soon as possible, to cleanse it of all maternal fluids. Cord blood should be obtained for serological and virological tests for HIV infection (Table 3.4).

THE NEONATAL PERIOD

After birth, the baby should be examined by a paediatrician. Haematological, virological and immunological investigations should be undertaken at birth, 6 weeks and 3 monthly, thereafter. The mother will require advise on immunisations (Table 3.5), and lines of referral if the baby becomes unwell. Many HIV infected women remain reluctant to inform their GP of their HIV diagnosis, but they should be encouraged to do this to ensure continuity of care, particularly for the child, in the community.

Table 3.5 Immunisation for children born to HIV infected mothers

Vaccination	Indication/special caution
Polio	Use killed vaccine, theoretical risk of infecting immunocompromised family members with pathogenic mutation if live vaccine given
MMR	No reported risk
BCG	Withhold from children definitely known to be infected but give all others
Haemophilus influenzae	All HIV-infected children
Pneumococcus	All HIV-infected children
Hepatitis B IG	Within 7 days
Hepatitis B vaccine	1 and 6 months
ZIG, HIG	Promptly after exposure to chickenpox or measles

PCP occurs most frequently in infants under 6 months of age and has a high mortality. Although data are lacking, prophylaxis with co-trimoxazole from 3 weeks of age is recommended.[59] The follow-up schedule should be discussed with the parents. Although maternal antibodies may not disappear until 18 months of age, investigations and clinical examinations enable the majority if infected children to be identified much earlier. If PCP prophylaxis is not given early, close follow-up for the first 6 months of life is essential.

AREAS FOR FURTHER RESEARCH

At the time of the previous review of HIV in pregnancy in *Progress in Obstetrics and Gynaecology*,[6] the use of zidovudine for the prevention of vertical transmission was still experimental, and the prognosis for pregnant HIV-infected women uncertain. The prognosis for HIV infected women who decide to have children has now improved with increasing experience in the medical and obstetric management of the condition. However, there remain several areas in which the care of these women can be enhanced. It has now been established that earlier diagnosis of HIV infection improves outcome,[60] but women are still far less likely to present early for HIV testing, with the consequence that the disease is often diagnosed in a more advanced stage. Better training of medical staff to recognise the manifestations of HIV disease, and more effort at public health education, particularly targeting ethnic minority groups may lead to an earlier diagnosis of HIV. Consequently, more women will be aware of their HIV status, and have access to pre-pregnancy counselling, before a decision for pregnancy is made. Horizontal transmission rates may also be reduced, thereby limiting the spread of HIV within the community.

The decrease in vertical transmission of HIV demonstrated by the ACTG 076 trial of zidovudine in pregnancy is encouraging, but none of the current strategies in use completely eliminate the risk of vertically acquired HIV. In addition, the cost of zidovudine will almost certainly exclude third world countries, which have the highest prevalence rates of HIV, from implementing this regimen. Detailed studies of the immune system of the female genital tract mucosa are urgently required to increase our understanding of the mode and timing of vertical and horizontal transmission, so that more effective, and ideally, inexpensive methods can be devised to prevent maternal–fetal, and male-to-female transmission of HIV. Studies in this department have demonstrated alterations in the distribution and proportions of immunocompetent cells within the cervix before there is evidence of systemic immune suppression in HIV positive women.[61] In addition, the safety of antiretrovirals in pregnancy must be evaluated further by the long-term follow-up of children exposed to zidovudine.

CONCLUSIONS

The rise in heterosexually acquired HIV disease in women, and the introduction of voluntary named antenatal screening will mean that most obstetricians will, at some stage, be involved in the care of an HIV positive woman. It is important, therefore, for every obstetrician to be familiar with the management of pregnancy in women with HIV infection and to be aware of research developments in this field. A good liaison with the woman's GP and HIV physician is essential so that the woman receives optimal care both for her HIV disease and her pregnancy.

REFERENCES

1 World Health Organization AIDS global data. Wkly Epidemiol Rec 1995; 70: 353
2 PHLS HIV Bulletin. December 1995; 7: 14–15
3 Nicoll A, Hutchinson E, Soldan K et al. Survey of human immunodeficiency virus infection among pregnant women in England and Wales: 1990–93. Commun Dis Rep 1994; 4: R115–R119

4 Olaitan A, Reid W, Mocroft, McCarthy K, Madge S, Johnson M A. Infertility among human immunodeficiency virus-positive women: incidence and treatment dilemmas. Hum Reprod 1996; 11(12): 2793–2796

5 PHLS, Communicable Diseases Surveillance Centre. Unlinked Anonymous HIV Seroprevalence Monitoring Programme in England & Wales, 1995

6 Webster A, Johnson M. Human immunodeficiency virus infection. Prog Obstet Gynaecol 1990; 8: 175–190

7 The study group for the MRC collaborative study of HIV infection in women. Ethnic differences in women with HIV infection in Britain and Ireland. AIDS 1996; 10: 89–94

8 Rutherford G W, Lifson A R, Hesson N A et al. Course of HIV infection in a cohort of homosexual and bisexual men: an 11 year follow-up study. BMJ 1990; 301: 1183–1188

9 Melnick S L, Sherer R, Louis T A et al. Survival and disease progression according to gender of patients with HIV infection. JAMA 1994; 272: 1915–1921

10 von Overbeck J, Egger M, Davey Smith G et al. Survival in HIV infection: do sex and category of transmission matter? AIDS 1994; 8: 1307–1313

11 Phillips A N, Antunes F, Stergious G et al. A sex comparison of new AIDS-defining disease and death in 2554 AIDS cases. AIDS 1994 8: 831–835

12 Shah P N, Iatrakis G M, Smith J R et al. Women with HIV presenting at three London clinics between 1985–1992. Genitourin Med 1993; 69: 439–440

13 Olaitan A, Madge S, McCarthy K H, Phillips A N, Johnson M A. Unrecognised HIV infection among gynaecology patients. Br J Obstet Gynaecol 1996; 107: 470–473

14 Porter K, Wall P, Evans B. Factors associated with lack of awareness of HIV infection before diagnosis of AIDS. BMJ 1993; 307: 20–33

15 Byrne L. Insurers relax questions on HIV. BMJ 1994; 309: 360

16 Goldberg D J, Johnstone F D. HIV testing programmes in pregnancy. Ballière's Clin Obstet Gynaecol 1992; 6: 33–51

17 General Medical Council. HIV infection and AIDS: the ethical considerations. Letter to all doctors. 1988

18 Johnstone F D, Willcox L, Brettle R P. Survival time after AIDS in pregnancy. Br J Obstet Gynaecol 1992; 99: 633–636

19 Brettle R P, Leen C L S. The natural history of HIV and AIDS in women. AIDS 1991; 5: 1283–1292

20 Brettle R P. Pregnancy and its effects on HIV/AIDS. Ballière's Clin Obstet Gynaecol 1992; 6: 125–136

21 Marion R W, Wiznia A A, Hutcheon G et al. Human T-cell lymphotrophic virus III (HTLV III) embryopathy: a new dysmorphic syndrome associated with HTLV III infection. Am J Dis Child 1986; 140: 638–640

22 Johnstone F D, MacCallum L, Brettle M, Inglis J M, Peutherer J F. Does infection with the human immunodeficiency virus affect the outcome of pregnancy? BMJ 1988; 296: 467

23 Berrebi A, Kobuch W E, Puel J, Tricoire J, Herne P, Fournie A. Effects of HIV infection on pregnancy [abstract]. 5th International Conference on AIDS, Montreal, 1989; MBP26

24 European Collaborative Study. Risk factors for mother-to-child transmission of HIV-1. Lancet 1992; 339: 1007–1012

25 Datta P, Embree J E, Kreiss J K et al. Mother-to-child transmission of human immuno-deficiency virus type 1: report from the Nairobi study. J Infect Diseases 1994: 170: 1134–1140

26 European Collaborative Study. Children born to women with HIV-1 infection: natural history and risk of transmission. Lancet 1991; 337: 253–263

27 Goedert J J, Duliege A M, Amos C I, Felton S, Biggar R J. High risk for HIV-1 infection for first born twins. Lancet 1991; 338: 1471–1475

28 Ryder R, Nsa W, Hassig S E et al. HIV IgG antibody at the age of 12 and 18 months but not HIV IgM antibody at birth or age 3 months correlates with clinical evidence of perinatally acquired HIV infection [abstract]. 5th International Conference on AIDS Montreal, 1989; B625

29 Dickover R E, Garratty E M, Herman S A et al. Identification of levels of maternal HIV-1 RNA associated with risk of perinatal transmission. JAMA 1996; 275: 599–605

30 Melvin A J, Burchett D H, Watts J. Natural history of viral load in HIV infected women with or without zidovudine treatment [abstract]. 35th ICAAC Meeting, September 1995. San Francisco, 1995; 15

31 Weiser B, Nachman S, Tropper P et al. Quantitation of human immunodeficiency virus type 1 during pregnancy: relationship of viral titer to mother-to-child transmission and stability of viral load. Proc Natl Acad Sci USA 1994; 91: 8037–8041

32 Courgnand V, Laure F, Brossard A et al. Frequent and early in utero HIV-1 infection. AIDS Res Hum Retroviruses 1991; 7: 337–341

33 Brossard Y, Aubin J, Mandelbrot L et al. Frequency of early in utero HIV-1 infection: a blind DNA polymerase chain reaction study on 100 fetal thymuses. AIDS 1995; 9: 359–366

34 Goedert J J, Mendez H, Drummond J E et al. Mother to infant transmission of human immunodeficiency virus type 1: association with prematurity or low anti-gp120. Lancet 1989; i: 1351-1354

35 Devash Y, Calvelli T A, Wood D G, Reagan K J, Rubinstein A. Vertical transmission of human immunodeficiency virus is correlated with the absence of high affinity/avidity maternal antibodies to the gp120 principal neutralising domain. Proc Natl Acad Sci USA 1990; 87: 3445–3449

36 Voght M W, Witt D J, Craven D E et al. Isolation of HTLVIII/LAV from cervical secretions of women at risk for AIDS. Lancet 1986; i: 525–527

37 Clemetson B D, Moss G B, Willerford D M et al. Detection of HIV DNA in cervical and vaginal secretions. Prevalence and correlates among women in Nairobi, Kenya. JAMA 1993; 269: 2860–2864

38 Henine Y, Mandelbrot L, Henroin R, Pradinaud R, Courland J P, Montagnier L. Virus excretion in cervicovaginal secretions of pregnant and non-pregnant HIV-infected women. J Acquir Immune Defic Syndr 1993; 6: 72–75

39 Dunn D T, Newell M L, Ades A E, Peckham C S. Risk of human immunodeficiency virus type I transmission through breastfeeding. Lancet 1992; 340: 585–587

40 Rodriguez E M, Mofenson L M, Chang B et al. Association of maternal drug use with HIV culture positivity and perinatal HIV transmission. AIDS 1996; 10: 273–282

41 Johnstone F D, Brettle R P, MacCallum L R, Mok J, Peutherer F, Burns S. Women's knowledge of their HIV antibody status: its effect on their decision to continue the pregnancy. BMJ 1990; 300: 23–24

42 Bewley S, Mercey D. Obstetric and neonatal implications of HIV infection. Mini-symposium: HIV in obstetrics and gynaecology. Curr Obstet Gynaecol 1994; 4: 193–198

43 Olaitan A, Mocroft A, McCarthy K et al. Cervical abnormality ans sexually transmitted diseases screening in human immunodeficiency virus-positive disease screening in human immunodeficiency virus-poitive women. Obstet Gynecol 1997; 89: 71–75

44 Smith J R, Kitchen V S, Botcherby M et al. Is HIV infection associated with an increase in the prevalence of cervical neoplasia? Br J Obstet Gynaecol 1993; 100: 149–153

45 Hardy W D, Feinberg J, Finkelstein D et al. A controlled trial of trimethoprin-sulfamethoxazole or aerolised pentamidine for secondary prophylaxis of Pneumocystis carinii in patients with acquired immunodeficiency syndrome. N Engl J Med 1992; 327: 1842–1848

46 Concorde Coordinating Committee. Concorde: MRS/ANRS randomised double-blind controlled trial of immediate and deferred zidovudine in symptom-free HIV infection. Lancet 1994; 343: 871–879

47 Connor E M, Sperling R S, Gelbert R et al. Reduction of maternal–infant transmission of HIV type 1 with zidovudine treatment. Paediatric AIDS Clinical Trials Group. Protocol 076 Study Group. N Engl J Med 1994; 331: 1173–1180

48 Minkoff H, Mofenson L M. The role of obstetric interventions in the prevention of paediatric human immunodeficiency virus infection. Am J Obstet Gynecol 1994; 171: 1167–1175

49 Delta Coordinating Committee. Delta: a randomised double-blind controlled trial comparing combinations of zidovudine plus didanosine or zalcitabine with zidovudine alone in HIV-infected individuals. Lancet 1996; 348: 283–291

50 Ippolito G, Puro V, the Italian Collaborative Study Group on occupational risk of HIV infection. Rate of seroconversion after occupational exposure to HIV in health care settings: the Italian multicentric study [abstract]. Sixth International Conference on AIDS, San Francisco, 1990; FC34

51 Smith J R, Kitchen V S. Reducing the risk of infection for obstetricians. Br J Obstet Gynaecol 1991; 98: 124–126

52 Semprini A E, Castagna C, Ravizza M et al. The incidence of complications after caesarean section in 156 HIV-positive women, AIDS 1995; 9: 913–917

53 Burman L G, Christensen P, Christensen K et al. Prevention of excess neonatal morbidity associated with group B streptococci by vaginal chorhexidine disinfection during labor. Lancet 1992; 340: 65–69

54 Harbisson M A, Hammer S M. Inactivation of human immunodeficiency virus by Betadine products and chorhexidine. J Acquir Immune Defic Syndr 1989; 2: 16–20

55 Montefiori D C, Robinson W E, Modliszewski A, Mitchell W M. Effective inactivation of human immunodeficiency virus with chorhexidine antiseptics containing detergents and alcohol. J Hosp Infect 1990; 15: 279–282

56 St Loius M E, Kamenga M, Brown C et al. Risk for perinatal HIV-1 transmission according to maternal immunologic, virologic and placental factors. JAMA 1993; 269: 2853–2859

57 Smith J R, Grant J M. The incidence of glove puncture during caesarean section. J Obstet Gynecol 1990; 10: 317–318

58 Matta H, Thompson A M, Rainy J B. Does wearing two pairs of gloves protect operating theatre staff from skin contamination? BMJ 1989; 297: 597–598

59 Gibb D, Walters S. Guidelines for the management of children with HIV infection. West Sussex: AVERT, 1992

60 Norman S, Studd J, Johnson M. HIV infection in women: needs early identification to limit complications. BMJ 1990; 301: 1231–1232

61 Olaitan A, Johnson M A, Maclean A B, Poulter L W. The distribution of immuno-competent cells in the genital tract of HIV-positive women. AIDS 1996; 10: 759-764

Stephen G. Carroll Kypros H. Nicolaides

Maternal and fetal thrombocytopenia

Thrombocytopenia in pregnancy is associated with risks to both the mother and the fetus. There are essentially four types of thrombocytopenia, which differ in their aetiology, implications and clinical management: gestational, maternal disease or pregnancy complication, autoimmune and alloimmune.

GESTATIONAL THROMBOCYTOPENIA

In normal pregnancy, the maternal platelet count decreases with gestation by about 12% between 20 and 40 weeks.[1] Thrombocytopenia, defined by a platelet count of less than $150 \times 10^9/l$, occurs in 6–15% of pregnancies,[1,2] and in more than 70% of cases the thrombocytopenia is mild, with platelet counts between 70 and $150 \times 10^9/l$.[3] In these cases, in the absence of a history of autoimmune thrombocytopenia, the term gestational thrombocytopenia is used. The cause of this condition is uncertain but may be due to platelet destruction by the placenta or hormonal depression of megakaryocytopoesis. Gestational thrombocytopenia is not associated with maternal haemorrhagic complications or fetal thrombocytopenia, and does not require any treatment.[4,5] The platelet count returns to normal within a few weeks of delivery.

THROMBOCYTOPENIA DUE TO MATERNAL DISEASE

Thrombocytopenia during pregnancy may be secondary to maternal illness, such as systemic lupus erythematosus, antiphospholipid syndrome, human

Dr Stephen G. Carroll, Subspecialty Trainee in Maternal and Fetal Medicine, Fetal Medicine Unit, St Michael's Hospital, Southwell Street, Bristol BS2 8EG, UK

Dr Kypros H. Nicolaides, Harris Birthright Research Centre for Fetal Medicine, King's College Hospital, London, UK

immunodeficiency virus infection, drug ingestion such as heparin or aspirin and pregnancy complications such as pre-eclampsia, abruptio placentae or other causes of disseminated intravascular coagulation. The diagnosis and management will inevitably depend on the underlying cause, but if this is uncertain and the platelet count is less than $70 \times 10^9/l$, examination of the bone marrow may be necessary to exclude diseases such as acute leukaemia.

AUTOIMMUNE THROMBOCYTOPENIA

Autoimmune thrombocytopenia is found in 1–2 per 1000 pregnancies.[4] It is characterised by inappropriate synthesis and binding of immunoglobulin to the platelet surface. In the majority of patients, the antibody is IgG, which crosses the placenta and can, therefore, cause fetal thrombocytopenia.[6] Platelets coated with antibodies are bound by the Fc receptors of macrophages in the reticuloendothelial system, mainly in the spleen, and are phagocytosed. The course of pre-existing thrombocytopenia is not affected by pregnancy, but the disease may influence pregnancy outcome. The main risk to the mother is haemorrhage at the time of delivery, but this is only the case if the platelet count is less than $50 \times 10^9/l$.[2,7] Severe fetal thrombocytopenia (less than $50 \times 10^9/l$) occurs in about 12% of pregnancies and in about 1% of cases there is fetal intracranial haemorrhage.[3]

Diagnosis

The main differential diagnosis is gestational thrombocytopenia. Measurement of platelet associated immunoglobulin (PAIgG) does not reliably differentiate autoimmune from gestational thrombocytopenia, and elevated levels of PAIgG are found in 40–90% of patients with gestational thrombocytopenia and other cases of thrombocytopenia due to non-immunological causes.[7-11] In a study of 90

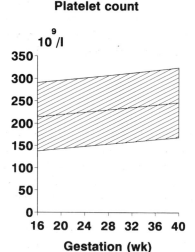

Platelet count

$10^9/l$

Fig. 4.1 Reference range (mean and individual 95% confidence intervals) of fetal platelet count ($10^9/l$) with gestation in normal pregnancies (adapted from Van den Hof et al[18]).

patients with autoimmune and 160 with gestational thrombocytopenia, PAIgG was comparably elevated in the majority of patients in both groups.[11] Similarly, there were no significant differences in the values for platelet-associated complement C3 or indirect IgM between the two groups. The likelihood that a patient suffers from autoimmune rather than gestational thrombocytopenia increases as the platelet count decreases; however, no specific platelet count below which gestational thrombocytopenia may be excluded has been identified.[4] Thus, the most useful means of differentiating autoimmune and gestational thrombocytopenia is, by definition, the presence or absence of thrombocytopenia before the pregnancy, sometimes in association with symptoms including petechiae, bruises and epistaxis. Additionally, in auto-immune, but not in gestational, thrombocytopenia, there is a rapid increase in maternal platelet count following the administration of corticosteroids or immunoglobulin. However, immune thrombocytopenia secondary to HIV infection or the antiphospholipid syndrome are also associated with an increase in platelet count with steroids and immunoglobulins.[2]

Maternal treatment

When the platelet count is above $50 \times 10^9/l$, the risk of bleeding is minimal and there is no need for treatment.[7] When the platelet count is less than this value, corticosteroids (prednisolone, 0.25–1.0 mg/kg/day), which inhibit antibody production and stimulate platelet production in the marrow, are recommended as initial treatment and are given until delivery. A gradual response is seen in 70–90% of patients, usually within 3 weeks.[12,13] Complete normalisation of the maternal platelet count is not required and the aim is to maintain the platelet count above $50 \times 10^9/l$.

In patients that do not respond to steroids, intravenous gamma globulin (IgG; 0.4–1.0 g/kg/day for 5 days) can be used. This treatment acts by interfering with Fc-receptor-mediated clearance of IgG-coated platelets and produces a rise in platelet count in 80% of patients, usually within 5–10 days and the remission lasts for about 3 weeks.[13,14] Splenectomy in pregnancy is used rarely when there is failure to respond to appropriate medical management. Platelet transfusions are only indicated with severe bleeding, because they may stimulate more antibodies and may worsen maternal thrombocytopenia.

Fetal treatment

There is no correlation between fetal platelet counts and maternal platelet antibody titres or maternal platelet counts.[15] Furthermore, administration of corticosteroids or IgG to the mother does not affect the fetal platelet count.[16,17] Therefore, antenatal therapy should be directed toward treating maternal thrombocytopenia because there is no clear evidence that it is of any benefit to the fetus.

In normal pregnancy, the fetal platelet count increases linearly with gestation from a mean of $190 \times 10^9/l$ at 15 weeks' to $280 \times 10^9/l$ at 40 weeks' gestation (Fig. 4.1).[18] When the platelet count drops to below $50 \times 10^9/l$, there is a risk of haemorrhagic complications,[19] the most serious being intracranial haemorrhage. This risk is thought to be greatest at the time of delivery and, therefore, if the fetal platelet count is less than $50 \times 10^9/l$, elective caesarean delivery has been advocated.[12,20] Estimation of fetal platelet count after transcervical fetal scalp blood sampling has been used,[21] but this is possible only after labour has progressed to adequate cervical dilatation. Furthermore, the results may be unreliable because of clotting or contamination with maternal blood or amniotic fluid.[12,22] Therefore, investigators have advised the more accurate measurement of fetal platelet count by performing cordocentesis at 36–38 weeks' gestation.[12,20,23]

However, the use of cordocentesis is controversial,[3] because: (i) the risk of fetal intracranial haemorrhage is low (1%); and (ii) there are risks to the fetus associated with cordocentesis, especially if fetus is severely thrombocytopenic. Although it has been reported that there is no correlation between fetal platelet number and the duration of bleeding from the umbilical cord puncture site following cordocentesis,[24] a previous study demonstrated that the bleeding time from the umbilical cord following cordocentesis is significantly longer in fetuses with thrombocytopenia compared to fetuses with a normal platelet count.[25] Two studies involving 63 cases of autoimmune thrombocytopenia, where cordocentesis was performed, showed procedure-related complications in 5 cases (8%), three of which were attributed to haemorrhagic complications including umbilical cord and subchorionic haematomas; the fetal platelet count was less than $50 \times 10^9/l$ in two of these three cases, and within normal range in the other two.[20,26] However, another study reported no fetal complications among 33 cases undergoing cordocentesis, where four fetuses had severe thrombocytopenia.[27] Thirdly, to support the contention that cordocentesis is not indicated in autoimmune thrombocytopenia, there are no conclusive data that delivery by caesarean section poses less risk of haemorrhage in a thrombocytopenic fetus than a vaginal delivery. In a large review of 15 studies involving 474 patients with autoimmune thrombocytopenia, the authors showed that the prevalence of intracranial haemorrhage in infants with birth platelet counts less than $50 \times 10^9/l$ was 5% after vaginal delivery and 4% after caesarean section.[28] Similarly, in a recent study of 31 patients, of four infants with postpartum cord-blood platelet counts less than $50 \times 10^9/l$, where three were delivered vaginally and one by caesarean section for an obstetrical indication, there were no cases of intracranial haemorrhage.[5] Thus, these data suggest that it is appropriate to follow the recommendations for vaginal delivery without estimation of the fetal platelet count, with caesarean section reserved only for obstetric indications.

ALLOIMMUNE THROMBOCYTOPENIA

This is a serious fetal disorder with no maternal significance and occurs in about 1 per 2000 pregnancies.[29] It is caused by maternal IgG antibodies directed against alloantigens on the fetal platelets, and its mechanism is analogous to red cell alloimmunisation. However, about 50% of cases of alloimmune thrombocytopenia are in primiparous women and the diagnosis is made when a patient with a normal platelet count delivers an infant with severe thrombocytopenia.[30,31] The clinical manifestations of thrombocytopenia are purpura, haematuria or gastrointestinal haemorrhage, but the most serious is intracranial haemorrhage, which occurs in about 20% of cases.[32] The latter results in death and severe neurological impairment in 7% and 19% of cases, respectively.[30,33] The other causes of thrombocytopenia in fetal blood samples include chromosomal abnormalities and infection with toxoplasmosis, rubella and cytomegalovirus.[34]

Platelet immunology

A number of platelet antigen polymorphisms have been reported in association with alloimmune thrombocytopenia, the most common being the PL[A1]/PL[A2] antigen system, which is responsible for 80% of the cases. PL[A1] and PL[A2] are autosomal dominant alleles with differences in the glycoprotein complex represented by a single amino acid change. PL[A1]-negative individuals are PL[A2] homozygous, while PL[A1]-positive individuals are either PL[A1] heterozygous or homozygous. Alloimmunisation occurs when a woman has PL[A2]/PL[A2] platelets and anti-PL[A1] antibodies. The PL[A1]-positive platelets of the fetus trigger the production of PL[A1] antibodies by the mother, which cross the placenta and lead to destruction of fetal platelets. Other antigen systems involved in alloimmune thrombocytopenia include Br[a], Pen[a] and Pen[b].

The distribution of the three possible antigen genotypes in the general population is PL[A1]/PL[A1] in 69% of cases, PL[A1]/PL[A2] in 28% and PL[A2]/PL[A2] in 3%.[35] Therefore, potentially 3% of pregnancies are at risk of sensitisation but the prevalence of alloimmunization is only 1 in 2000. The reason for the vast majority of PL[A1]-negative women not becoming sensitised is because the production of alloantibodies is related to immune-response genes located in the major histocompatibility complex (DR3, DRw52 and DRw6), which are not common.[23]

The rate of recurrence of alloimmune thrombocytopenia depends on the alloantigen involved and the zygosity of the father. In the case of PL[A1]-positive fathers, for example, the distribution of the alleles is such that approximately 75% are homozygous (PL[A1]/PL[A1]) and 25% are heterozygous (PL[A1]/PL[A2]).

Identification of fetuses at risk

The first affected child with alloimmune thrombocytopenia is unexpected as PL[A] typing of mothers is not part of routine antenatal screening. Furthermore, unlike rhesus isoimmunisation, where Rh-antibodies in maternal serum are followed to monitor disease severity, monitoring of maternal anti-PL[A1] antibodies has not proved useful in predicting the severity of fetal thrombocytopenia; high titres have been found in cases of mild thrombocytopenia and conversely low titres with severe haemorrhages.[36] In one series, maternal antibodies were not even detectable in 20% of cases.[37]

Fetal blood sampling is the best way of establishing the diagnosis and also provides a means for intra-uterine transfusion of PL[A1]-negative platelets. Women at high risk include those with a previous history or those with a sister whose child died due to alloimmunisation. If screening of first pregnancies was routine, high risk patients would include those who are PL[A1]-negative and HLA DR3 with PL[A1]-positivity in fathers.

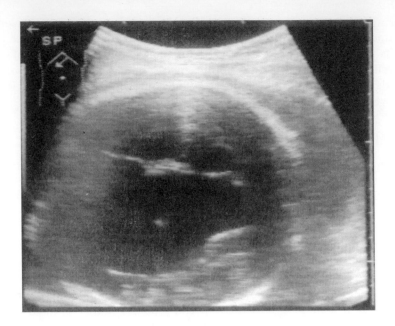

Fig. 4.2 Ultrasound showing hydrocephalus due to a large intraventricular haemorrhage in a fetus at 36 weeks' gestation.

In high risk cases, cordocentesis may be performed at 20 weeks for measurement of fetal platelet count, determination of the platelet group and the detection of platelet-bound antibodies. If the platelet count is very low, serological typing for platelet alloantigens may be impossible, and in such cases typing may be made with DNA amplification techniques.[38] As fetal thrombocytopenia is likely to be present, it is necessary to prepare a platelet concentrate and infuse the fetus with it just after sampling. The platelet concentrate can be prepared from the mother's platelets, which must be washed and irradiated to prevent graft-versus-host disease. Because fetuses with platelet counts below $50 \times 10^9/l$ are at increased risk due to bleeding from the umbilical cord immediately after cordocentesis, it is recommended that the platelets be available at the time of cordocentesis and be transfused before the needle is removed.[39] This requires that the fetal platelet count be completed within 2 min of aspirating the fetal blood.

An alternative approach to cordocentesis in all cases at 20 weeks is to determine the PL^A genotype of the father and, if heterozygous, to perform amniocentesis or chorion villus sampling to examine the fetal PL^A genotype.[40–42] If the father is heterozygous there is only a 50% risk of an affected fetus. If the fetus is found to be PL^{A2} homozygous cordocentesis and maternal treatment are unnecessary.

Antenatal management

Antenatal treatment of at-risk fetuses is indicated because: (i) platelet specific antibodies are able to cross the placenta from 14 weeks' gestation[43] and cordocentesis has demonstrated severe fetal thrombocytopenia as early as

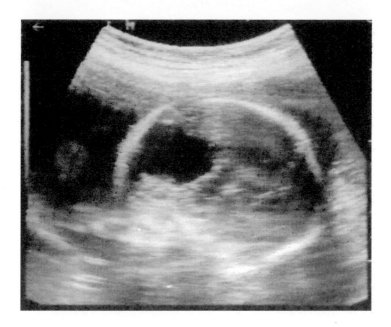

Fig. 4.3 Ultrasound showing a porencephalic cyst due to intracranial haemorrhage in a fetus at 30 weeks' gestation.

16–20 weeks;[44–48] (ii) intracranial haemorrhage occurs *in utero* in up to 50% of cases leading to fetal death, hydrocephalus (Fig. 4.2) or porencephalic cyst (Fig. 4.3);[23] and (iii) the recurrence rate in subsequent pregnancies is 100% if the fetus is antigen (PL^{A1}) positive.

The antenatal therapeutic options for alloimmune thrombocytopenia are a combination of maternal IgG and steroids and fetal platelet transfusions. It is proposed that IgG decreases the destruction of fetal platelets in the placenta or fetal reticuloendothelial system.[23] In a study involving 18 women, who had previously delivered infants with severe thrombocytopenia, where weekly i.v. IgG was given to all cases and corticosteroids to 9, no intracranial haemorrhages occurred in the treated fetuses, compared with 10 cases among the 21 untreated siblings.[49] Only 3 of the 18 fetuses compared with 16 of 20 untreated siblings had platelet counts less than 30×10^9/l. The no steroids group's mean increase from the pretreatment platelet count to the next one at cordocentesis or birth was 33×10^9/l; the steroid group's was 41×10^9/l. The data were suggestive of a benefit with steroids, but the results were not statistically significant because of the sample size. In another study of 54 patients treated with weekly i.v. IgG, where 26 received additional corticosteroids, repeat cordocentesis 4–6 weeks later in 47 of the cases showed that the median platelet increase was 29×10^9/l; corticosteroids had no additive effect beyond that seen with IgG alone. None of the fetuses in this study had intracranial haemorrhages compared to 10 who had haemorrhages in the previous pregnancies.[39]

Some studies have reported that maternal IgG administration is not associated with an increase in the fetal platelet count.[50–52] This may be because the placenta blocks or alters the functional capacity of exogenous immuno-

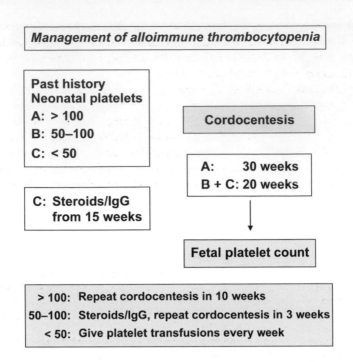

Fig. 4.4 Management of alloimmune thrombocytopenia

globulins because, in two studies, IgG infused via cordocentesis resulted in an increase in fetal platelet counts.[53,54]

When the fetal platelet count is less than $50 \times 10^9/l$, despite the administration of steroids and immunoglobulins to the mother, then it is necessary to give platelet transfusions to the fetus. Since the lifespan of platelets is short, it is necessary to repeat the transfusions at weekly intervals until 32–35 weeks, followed by elective caesarean section.[55,56] Murphy et al[57] described 10 cases managed successfully with combinations of serial platelet transfusions and i.v. IgG and steroids; in 4 of the cases considered to be severely affected (initial fetal platelet count less than $20 \times 10^9/l$) weekly platelet transfusions were given between 18–29 weeks and continued until delivery at 33–35 weeks. The authors concluded that IgG and steroids may be effective in some mildly affected cases, but serial platelet transfusions are the preferred therapy for those who are severely affected.

Recommeded management (Fig. 4.4)

The likely severity of alloimmune thrombocytopenia is based on the history of previous affected pregnancies and the results of cordocentesis. Like rhesus disease, the degree of fetal thrombocytopenia in the current pregnancy is invariably as or more severe than that seen in the previous infant.[58] The disease is considered to be mild, moderate or severe if the neonatal platelet count in the previous pregnancy was greater than $100 \times 10^9/l$, between $50–100 \times 10^9/l$ or less than $50 \times 10^9/l$, respectively. For mild disease, no IgG or steroids are given and cordocentesis is performed at 30 weeks' gestation. Similarly, for moderate disease, no IgG or steroids are given but cordocentesis is carried out at 20 weeks. For severe disease, IgG and steroids are given from 12–16 weeks and cordocentesis is performed at 20 weeks.

At cordocentesis, the fetal platelet count is determined and the same criteria as in the neonate are used to classify the severity of the disease. If the platelet count is greater than $100 \times 10^9/l$, no further treatment is necessary and cordocentesis should be repeated in 10 weeks. If the platelet count is between $50–100 \times 10^9/l$, the patient should receive IgG and steroids weekly, and cordocentesis is repeated 3 weeks later. If the platelet count is less than $50 \times 10^9/l$, then weekly platelet transfusions are given until delivery at 34 weeks.

REFERENCES

1 Kaplan C, Forestier F, Dreyfus M, Morel-Kopp M C, Tchernia G. Maternal thrombocytopenia during pregnancy: diagnosis and etiology. Semin Thromb Hemost 1995; 21: 85–94

2 Cohen D L, Baglin T P. Assessment and management of immune thrombocytopenia in pregnancy and in neonates. Arch Dis Child 1995; 72: F71–F76

3 Silver R M, Branch W, Scott J R. Maternal thrombocytopenia: time for a reassessment. Am J Obstet Gynecol 1995; 173: 479–482

4 Burrows R F, Kelton J G. Thrombocytopenia at delivery. A prospective survey of 6715 deliveries. Am J Obstet Gynecol 1990; 162: 731–734

5 Burrows R F, Kelton J G. Fetal thrombocytopenia and its relation to maternal thrombocytopenia. N Engl J Med 1993; 329: 1463–1466

6 Paidas M J, Haut M J, Lockwood C J. Platelet disorders in pregnancy: implications for mother and fetus. Mt Sinai J Med 1994; 61: 389–403

7 Bussel J B. Management of infants of mothers with immune thrombocytopenic purpura. J Pediatr 1988; 113: 497–499

8 Kelton J G, Powers P J, Carter C J. A prospective study of the usefulness of the measurement of platelet-associated IgG for the diagnosis of idiopathic thrombocytopenic purpura. Blood 1982; 60: 1050–1053

9 Panzer S, Szamait S, Bodeker R H et al. Platelet-associated immunoglobulins IgG, IgM, IgA and complement C3 in immune and nonimmune thrombocytopenic disorders. Am J Hematol 1986; 23: 89–99

10 Samuels P, Bussel J B, Braitman L E et al. Estimation of the risk of thrombocytopenia in the offspring of pregnant women with presumed immune thrombocytopenic purpura. New Engl J Med 1990; 323: 229–235

11 Lescale K, Eddleman K A, Cines D B et al. Antiplatelet antibody testing in thrombocytopenic women. Am J Obstet Gynecol 1996; 174: 1014–1018

12 McCrae K R, Samuels P, Schreiber A D. Pregnancy-associated thrombocytopenia: pathogenesis and management. Blood 1992; 80: 2697–2714

13 Biswas A, Arulkumaran S, Ratnam S S. Disorders of platelets in pregnancy. Obstet Gynecol Survey 1994; 49: 585–594

14 Berchtold P, McMillan R. Therapy of chronic idiopathic thrombocytopenic purpura in adults. Blood 1989; 74: 2309–2317

15 Scott J, Rote N, Cruikshank D. Antiplatelet antibodies and platelet counts in pregnancies complicated by autoimmune thrombocytopenia. Am J Obstet Gynecol 1983; 145: 932–939

16 Christiaens G, Niewenhuis H, Von den Borne A et al. Idiopathic thrombocytopenic purpura in pregnancy: a randomised trial of the effect of antenatal low dose corticosteroids on neonatal platelet count. Br J Obstet Gynaecol 1990; 97: 893–898

17 Burrows R, Kelton J. Thrombocytopenia in pregnancy. In: Greer I, Turpie A, Forbes C. (eds) Haemostasis and thrombosis in obstetrics and gynaecology. London: Chapman & Hall, 1992; 407–429

18 Van den Hof M, Nicolaides K H. Platelet count in normal, small, and anemic fetuses. Am J Obstet Gynecol 1990; 162: 735–739

19 Scott J R, Cruikshank D P, Kochenoor N K, Pitkin R M, Warenski J C. Fetal platelet counts in the obstetric management of immunologic thrombocytopenic purpura. Am J Obstet Gynecol 1980; 136: 494–499

20 Garmel S H, Craigo S D, Morin L M, Crowley J M, D'Alton M E. The role of percutaneous umbilical blood sampling in the management of immune thrombocytopenic purpura. Prenatal Diagn 1995; 15: 439–445

21 Ayromlooi J. A new approach to the management of immunologic thrombocytopenic purpura in pregnancy. Am J Obstet Gynecol 1978; 130: 235–236

22 Moise Jr K J, Patton D E, Cano L E. Misdiagnosis of a normal fetal platelet count after coagulation of intrapartum scalp samples in autoimmune thrombocytopenic purpura. Am J Perinatol 1991; 8: 295–296

23 Menell J S, Bussel J B. Antenatal management of the thrombocytopenias. Clin Perinatol 1994; 21: 591–615

24 Weiner C P. Fetal blood sampling and fetal thrombocytopenia. Fetal Diagn Ther 1995; 10: 173–177

25 Segal M, Manning F A, Harman C R, Menticoglou S. Bleeding after intravascular transfusion: experimental and clinical observations. Am J Obstet Gynecol 1991; 165: 1414–1418

26 Moise Jr K J, Carpenter R J, Cotton D B, Wasserstrum N, Kirshon B, Cano L. Percutaneous umbilical cord blood sampling in the evaluation of fetal platelet counts in pregnant patients with autoimmune thrombocytopenic purpura. Obstet Gynecol 1988; 72: 346–350

27 Kaplan C, Daffos F, Forestier F et al. Fetal platelet counts in thrombocytopenic pregnancy. Lancet 1990; 336: 979–982

28 Cook R L. Miller R C, Katz V L, Cefalo R C. Immune thrombocytopenic purpura in pregnancy: a reappraisal of management. Obstet Gynecol 1991; 78: 578–583

29 Murphy M F, Pullon H W H, Metcalfe P et al. Management of fetal alloimmune thrombocytopenia by weekly in utero platelet transfusions. Vox Sang 1990; 58: 45–49

30 Mueller-Eckhardt C, Grubert A, Weisheit M et al. 348 cases of suspected neonatal alloimmune thrombocytopenia. Lancet 1989; 1: 363–366

31 Shulman NR. Platelet immunology. In: Colman R W, Hirsh J, Marder V J, Saizman E W. (eds) Hemostasis and thrombosis: basic principles and clinical practice. Philadelphia: Lippincott, 1993; 414–468

32 Bussel J B, Berkowitz R L, McFariand J G, Lynch L, Chitkara U. Antenatal treatment of neonatal alloimmune thrombocytopemia. N Engl J Med 1988; 319: 1374–1378

33 Kaplan C, Daffos F, Forestier F, Morel M C, Chesnel N, Tchernia G. Current trends in neonatal alloimmune thrombocytopenia: diagnosis and therapy. In: Kaplan-Gouet C, Schlegel N, Salmon C, MacGregor J (eds) Platelet immunology. Fundamentals and clinical aspects. Paris: John Libbey, 1991; 267–278

34 Hohlfeld P, Forestier F, Kaplan C, Tissot J D, Daffos F. Fetal thrombocytopenia: a retrospective survey of 5,194 fetal blood samplings. Blood 1994; 84: 1851–1856

35 Flug F, Karpatkin M, Karpatkin S. Should all pregnant women be tested for their platelet PLA (Zw, HPA-1) phenotype? Br J Haematol 1994; 86: 1–5

36 Reznikoff-Etievant M F. Management of alloimmune neonatal and antenatal thrombocytopenia. Vox Sang 1988; 55: 193–201

37 Kaplan C, Daffos F, Forestier F et al. Management of alloimmune thrombocytopenia: antenatal diagnosis and in utero transfusion of maternal platelets. Blood 1988; 72: 340–343

38 Kuijpers R W, Faber N M, Kanhai H H, von dem Borne A E. Typing of fetal platelet alloantigens when platelets are not available. Lancet 1991; 336: 1319

39 Bussel J B, Berkowitz R L, Lynch L et al. Antenatal management of alloimmune thrombocytopenia with intravenous gamma-globulin: a randomised trial of the addition of low-dose steroid to intravenous gamma-globulin. Am J Obstet Gynecol 1996; 174: 1414–1423

40 Goldman M, Decary F, David M. Should all pregnant women be tested for their platelet PLA (Zw, HPA-1) phenotype [letter]?. Br J Haematol 1994; 87: 670

41 Sagot P, Bonneville F, Bignon J D, Cesbron A, Boog G, Muller J Y. Management of platelet and RhD maternal immunizations by PCR phenotypes after early amniocentesis. Fetal Diagn Ther 1995; 10: 373–380

42 Madsen H, Taaning E, Georgsen J, Ryder L P, Svejgaard A, Bock J. PCR for fetal platelet HPA-1 alloantigen typing. Lancet 1991; 337: 493

43 Morales J W, Stroup M. Intracranial hemorrhage in utero due to isoimmune neonatal thrombocytopenia. Obstet Gynecol 1985; 65: 20s–21s

44 Daffos F, Forestier F, Kaplan C, Cox W L. Prenatal diagnosis and management of bleeding disorders with fetal blood sampling. Am J Obstet Gynecol 1988; 158: 939–946

45 Taaning E, Killman S-E, Morling N, Ovesen H, Svejgaard A. Post-transfusion purpura (PTP) due to anti-Zw^b (-PL^{A2}): the significance of IgG3 antibodies in PTP. Br J Haematol 1986; 64: 217

46 Waters A, Murphy M, Hambley H, Nicolaides K. Management of alioimmune thrombocytopenia in the fetus and neonate. In: Nance S J. (ed) Clinical and basic aspects of immunohaematology. Arlington, VA: American Association of Blood Banks, 1991; 155

47 Murphy M F, Metcalfe P, Waters A H, Ord J, Hambley H, Nicolaides K. Antenatal management of severe feto-maternal alloimmune thrombocytopenia: HLA incompatibility may affect responses to fetal platelet transfusions. Blood 1993; 81: 2174–2179

48 Johnson J M, McFarland J, Blanchette V S, Freedman J, Siegel-Bartlet J. Prenatal diagnosis of neonatal alloimmune thrombocytopenia using an allele-specific oligonucleotide probe. Prenatal Diagn 1993; 13: 1037–1042

49 Lynch L, Bussel J P, McFarland J G, Chitkara O, Berkowitz R L. Antenatal treatment of alloimmune thrombocytopenia. Obstet Gynecol 1992; 80: 67–71

50 Mir N, Samson D, House M J, Kovar I Z. Failure of high-dose immunoglobulin to improve fetal platelet count in neonatal alloimmune thrombocytopenia. Vox Sang 1988; 55: 188–189

51 Nicolini U, Tannirandorn Y, Gonzalez P et al. Continuing controversy in alloimmune thrombocytopenia: fetal hyperimmunoglobulinemia fails to prevent thrombocytopenia. Am J Obstet Gynecol 1990; 163: 1144–1146

52 Kroll H, Giers G, Bald R et al. Intravenous IgG during pregnancy for fetal (Zw^a) thrombocytopenic purpura? Thromb Hemost 1993; 69: 1625A

53 Zimmermann R, Huch A. In-utero fetal therapy with immunoglobulin for alloimmune thrombocytopenia. Lancet 1992; 340: 606

54 Marzusch K, Wiest E, Pfeiffer K H, Grubbe G, Schnaidt M. Antenatal fetal therapy for neonatal allo-immune thrombocytopenia with high dose immunoglobulin. Br J Obstet Gynaecol 1994; 101: 1011–1013

55 Mueller-Eckhardt C, Kiefel V, Jovanovic V et al. Prenatal treatment of fetal alloimmune thrombocytopenia [letter]. Lancet 1988; 2: 910

56 Nicolini U, Rodeck C H, Kochenour N K, Greco P, Fisk N M, Letsky E. In utero platelet transfusion for alloimmune thrombocytopenia. Lancet; 1988; 2: 506

57 Murphy M F, Waters A H, Doughty H A et al. Antenatal management of fetomaternal alloimmune thrombocytopenia-report of 15 affected pregnancies. Transfus Med 1994; 4: 281–292

58 Bussel J B. Neonatal alloimmune thrombocytopenia (NAIT): a prospective case accumulation study. Pediatr Res 1988; 23: 337a

5

Rezan A. Kadir   Christine A. Lee
Demetrios L. Economides

Inherited bleeding disorders in obstetrics and gynaecology

Hereditary deficiency of each of the 12 coagulation factors have been reported. The most important disorders in terms of frequency and severity are von Willebrand's disease (vWD), haemophilia A [factor VIII (FVIII) deficiency], haemophilia B [factor IX (FIX) deficiency] and factor XI (FXI) deficiency. These four disorders account for 90% of all patients on the UK Haemophilia Centre Directors' Organisation registry.

vWD is far more common than was previously suspected and is the commonest inherited bleeding abnormality affecting women with a prevalence of 0.8%[1] to 1.3%.[2] vWD is the result of quantitative and/or qualitative defects of von Willebrand's factor (vWF). vWF serves as a carrier for FVIII in the circulating blood preventing it from inactivation. It also mediates platelet adhesion and thrombus formation at the site of vascular injury. vWD exhibits significant phenotypic heterogeneity, depending on the particular subtype considered. Two main categories of patients can be identified, distinguished on the basis of whether the main pathogenetic factor is quantitative (type I and III) or qualitative (type II) defect of vWF.[3] Type I is the most common form of the disease, accounting approximately for 70% of all cases. This type is characterised by equally low plasma levels of FVIII, usually between 5–40 IU/dl (normal = 50–150 IU/dl), von Willebrand factor antigen (vWF:Ag) (normal = 50–175 IU/dl) and von Willebrand factor activity (vWF:Ac) (normal = 50–175 IU/dl) as assessed by ristocetin-induced cofactor assay. This is caused by reduced

Mr Rezan A. Kadir, Clinical Research Fellow, Clinical Research Fellow, University Department of Obstetrics and Gynaecology/Haemophilia Centre, The Royal Free Hospital, Hampstead, London NW3 2QG, UK

Prof. Christine A. Lee, Professor of Haemophilia and Director of Haemophilia Centre and Haemostasis Unit, University Department of Obstetrics and Gynaecology/Haemophilia Centre, The Royal Free Hospital, Hampstead, London NW3 2QG, UK

Mr Demetrios L. Economides, MRCOG MD, Senior Lecturer and Consultant Obstetrician and Gynaecologist, University Department of Obstetrics and Gynaecology/Haemophilia Centre, The Royal Free Hospital, Hampstead, London NW3 2QG, UK

production of normally functioning vWF resulting in a secondary defect of FVIII.[4] The pathophysiological basis of type 2 is qualitative abnormalities of vWF. Type 2 comprises many different subtypes and is phenotypically very heterogeneous: subtype 2A is characterised by the absence of large and intermediate size multimers and ristocetin-induced platelet agglutination in platelet rich plasma; subtype 2B, only large multimers are absent and interaction between platelets and vWF is increased;[5] subtype 2M has decreased platelet dependent function but normal multimers and subtype 2N has a defect of FVIII binding. Type 3 is the least common of all forms of vWD and is characterised by very low levels of plasma vWF and FVIII with severe bleeding manifestations.

The prevalence of haemophilia A and B is 1–2/10 000 in the UK.[6] However, the prevalence of carrier women is unknown. As these disorders are X-linked recessive and female carriers have only one affected chromosome, the clotting factor level is expected to be around 50% of normal. However, a wide range of values (22–116 IU/dl) has been reported[7] as a result of random inactivation of one of the two X chromosomes, i.e. lyonization.[8] A significant number of haemophilia carriers may have very low factor levels[9] due to extreme lyonization or homozygosity for haemophilia gene.[10]

FXI deficiency has been described in all racial groups, but is particularly common in Ashkenazi Jews where the carrier rate has been reported to be as high as 9%.[11] FXI levels are severely reduced (< 15 IU/dl) (normal 70-u-150 IU/dl) in homozygotes and partially deficient or low normal in heterozygotes.[12] There is a poor correlation between FXI level and bleeding tendency in patients with FXI deficiency.[12–16] Some patients with severe deficiency may not bleed at all following trauma, while some heterozygotes have excessive bleeding after challenge. The bleeding tendency may also vary in the same individual following haemostatic challenge.[17] This is dependent on patient's genotype, site of surgery and the presence of additional coagulation factor defects, most commonly vWD.

Inherited bleeding disorders are underestimated by obstetricians and gynaecologists in the aetiology of obstetric haemorrhage and menorrhagia. In addition, because these disorders in women are usually mild and only revealed in the majority of cases after a haemostatic challenge, they are probably under-diagnosed. The aim of this review is to highlight obstetric and gynaecological problems and their management in women with inherited bleeding disorders as well as the role of these disorders in obstetric and gynaecological haemorrhage.

GENETICS OF INHERITED BLEEDING DISORDERS

vWF is encoded by a gene located on the short arm of chromosome 12 at 12p12-pter.[18,19] The advances in molecular biology of vWF and the use of polymerase chain reaction have helped to identify the precise molecular defect in a number of patients, however, the molecular basis of the most common type of vWD (Type 1) is still unknown in most cases. Type 1 and 2 vWD are transmitted as autosomal dominant trait, however, type 3 is autosomal recessive in inheritance. The theoretical risk of women with type 1 or type 2A vWD of transmitting the disease to their child is 50%, however, only 33% of children of these women are affected, probably because of variable penetrance and expression of the abnormal gene.[20] The situation is more complicated for the other subtypes of type 2 vWD and extensive family studies are required to assess this risk. Type 3 vWD is an autosomal recessive disorder and affected individuals are either homozygotes or compound heterozygotes. If a child with type 3 has already been born in the family, the risk of a subsequent child being affected is 25%.

Haemophilia A and B are X-linked recessive bleeding disorders. Therefore, in each pregnancy of a carrier, there is 1 in 2 chance that a male fetus have haemophilia and a female fetus will be a carrier of haemophilia. The genes for FVIII and FIX are located near the tip of the long arm of the X chromosome (Xq2.8). Many genetic defects have been identified in haemophilic families including deletions, point mutations, or mutations resulting in stop codons.[21]

The inheritance of FXI deficiency has now been confirmed to be autosomal with severe deficiency in homozygotes and partial deficiency in heterozygotes.[12] The FXI gene is located on chromosome 4 q34-35.[22] Several genetic mutations causing FXI deficiency have been reported.[23-26] In Ashkenazi Jews, FXI deficiency is caused by type II (a stop codon in exon 5) and type III (a single base change in exon 9) mutations in most kindreds.[17,27,28] However, in non-Jews, most mutations remain to be defined.

PRECONCEPTIONAL CARE AND COUNSELLING

Female members of families with inherited bleeding disorders should be reviewed prior to their first pregnancy for identification and counselling of affected or carrier women. The aim of preconceptional counselling is to help these women to understand the genetic implication of their disorder, options of prenatal diagnosis and other aspects of the management of future pregnancy. Genetic counselling should be provided by a team including experts in haemophilia care, molecular genetics and prenatal diagnosis. Psychological support should be available to the women and their families during all aspects of counselling. Women who are likely to require blood product therapy should be immunised against hepatitis A and B.

PRENATAL DIAGNOSIS

The issue of prenatal diagnosis is particularly relevant in carriers of haemophilia because of the severity of the condition in their male offsprings. In addition, the use of polymerase chain reaction (PCR)-based genetic testing for both polymorphism linkage analysis and direct mutation detection has significantly simplified prenatal diagnosis for haemophilia. After appropriate counselling, prenatal diagnosis can be performed in one of three methods, depending on the information available about the family and the couple's plan for the pregnancy.[29] The first involves fetal sex determination. Nowadays, with better resolution of the newer ultrasound machines and the advent of the transvaginal probe this can be determined in the first trimester.[30] Ultrasonic

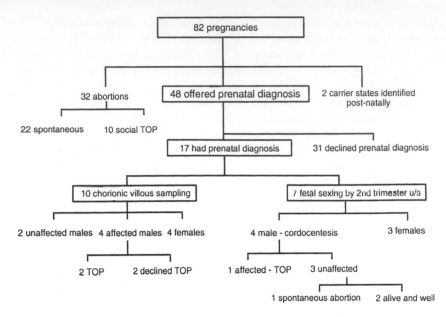

TOP, Termination of pregnancy

Fig. 5.1 Uptake and results of prenatal diagnosis in carriers of haemophilia. TOP, termination of pregnancy; u/s, ultrasound. Reproduced from Kadir et al[33] with permission of Blackwell Science Ltd.

fetal sex determination is helpful in several situations: (i) if a fetus is identified as female then the mother can be reassured and the risks of invasive procedures are avoided; (ii) when specific prenatal diagnosis for haemophilia is not possible for a carrier mother because she is not informative on DNA analysis or because adequate information about the family can not be obtained; and lastly (iii) knowledge of fetal sex is very helpful to the attending obstetrician for labour management of carrier mothers who had not had specific prenatal diagnostic tests (see section on labour). Specific prenatal diagnosis for haemophilia A or B can be performed by chorionic villus sampling (CVS) or amniocentesis for carrier mothers who are informative on DNA analysis. However, with amniocentesis, it is often not possible to obtain adequate DNA for analysis. In addition, with CVS, the patient has the advantage of first trimester termination of pregnancy, if opted for, which is less traumatic and more acceptable to the patient. The other method of specific prenatal diagnosis is clotting factor assay of fetal blood sample obtained by cordocentesis. This procedure is suitable for carriers who are non-informative on DNA analysis, but can only be performed after 18 weeks' gestation.

The uptake of specific prenatal diagnosis is low (between 20–30%) in most centres. Carriers of haemophilia do not consider the disorder to be a sufficiently serious to justify an abortion,[31] and only slightly more acceptable reason for abortion than poor social circumstances.[32] In our centre, the uptake of prenatal diagnosis for haemophilia is 35% and termination of pregnancy is opted for in only 50% of affected male fetuses[33] (Fig 5.1) compared to 71% uptake rate in women at risk for Down's syndrome on biochemical screening and 85% termination rate in affected pregnancies.

Table 5.2 Obstetric management of women with inherited bleeding disorders: general principles*

Prepregnancy diagnosis, counselling, hepatitis B immunisation	
Regular clinical and haemostatic monitoring during pregnancy	
Ultrasound determination of fetal gender**	
Avoid unnecessary invasive procedures	
On admission for delivery	Full blood and platelet count
	Coagulation investigations
	Blood group and retain serum
Minimise maternal and fetal trauma at delivery	
Access to blood product replacement is necessary	
Avoid intramuscular injections	
Collect cord blood for investigation	
Give neonate vitamin K_1 orally	
Immunisation to infant by intradermal route	
Consider hepatitis B immunisation for infant	

*Reproduced from Walker[34] with permission of the *Journal of Clinical Pathology*, BMJ Publishing Group.
**For carriers of haemophilia.

In vWD, the option of prenatal diagnosis is only offered to families affected with severe forms of the disease, mainly type 3. In FXI deficiency, prenatal diagnosis is only possible in Ashkenazi Jews because of the limited number of mutations in this population, and is offered when there is a risk of severe FXI deficiency in the child. To avoid risk of haemorrhage, in any woman with a bleeding disorder, it is essential that maternal clotting factor is checked prior to any invasive prenatal procedure and prophylactic treatment arranged when FVIII, FIX levels are less than 50 IU/dl or FXI is less than 70 IU/dl.

MANAGEMENT OF PREGNANCY

Antenatal care

Pregnancy and labour should be managed in close collaboration with the local haemophilia centre. Advice from the haemophilia team is invaluable for arrangement and interpretation of blood tests, and arrangement of prophylactic or replacement treatment especially when there is a bleeding complication. Management guidelines (Table 5.1) should be enclosed in patients' notes and strictly followed.

Haemostatic response to pregnancy is variable in different types and subtypes of bleeding disorders. There is usually a progressive increase in coagulation factor activity in most patients with vWD and carriers of haemophilia A.[33,35,36] Although the majority of patients develop factor levels within the normal range, the rise is variable, unpredictable and a small proportion still have levels below 50 IU/dl at term.[33,35,36] In contrast, patients with type 3 vWD, FXI deficiency and carriers of haemophilia B do not show significant rise in the factor levels (Figs 5.2–5.4).[33,35–37] Therefore, it is recommended that the mother's coagulation factor activity should be checked

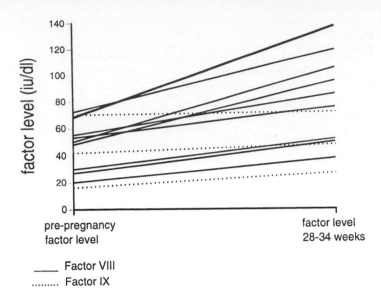

Fig. 5.2 Changes in factor VIII (solid line) and Factor IX (dashes) levels during pregnancy. Reproduced from Kadir et al[33] with permission of Blackwell Science Ltd.

at booking, 28 and 34 weeks. Monitoring during the third trimester is particularly important as prophylactic treatment can be arranged during labour and post-partum to decrease the risk of post-partum haemorrhage, especially in patients at risk of rapid labour, e.g. 'grand multipara' patients and patients with previous history of rapid labours. Some patients with type 2B vWD may develop thrombocytopenia during pregnancy[38] due to increased synthesis of abnormal multimers. This is usually mild and active intervention is not necessary. However, monitoring platelet count in these patients is necessary, as occasionally the platelet count may fall to a dangerous level. In these cases, thrombocytopenia can be treated by vWF concentrate.[39]

Labour and delivery

Labour and delivery are critical periods for women with bleeding disorders and their affected fetuses. At the beginning of labour the maternal blood sample should be sent for full blood count, coagulation screen and appropriate factor assay, as well as saving serum for cross matching when needed. If the factor level is less than 50 IU/dl, an intravenous line should be established and prophylactic treatment for labour and the post-partum period given.

Affected fetuses could be at risk of serious scalp haemorrhage, including scalp abrasions, cephalhaematoma, subgaleal haematoma and intracranial haemorrhage from the process of birth, invasive monitoring techniques or instrumental deliveries. To our knowledge, no serious bleeding complication in affected fetuses and neonates has been reported so far from invasive monitoring techniques, probably they have not been used frequently in these situations. However, it is advisable to avoid their use in fetuses at risk. In 1994, Ljung et al[40] reviewed the mode of delivery and perinatal bleeding in 117 children with moderate or severe haemophilia. They concluded that the risk of

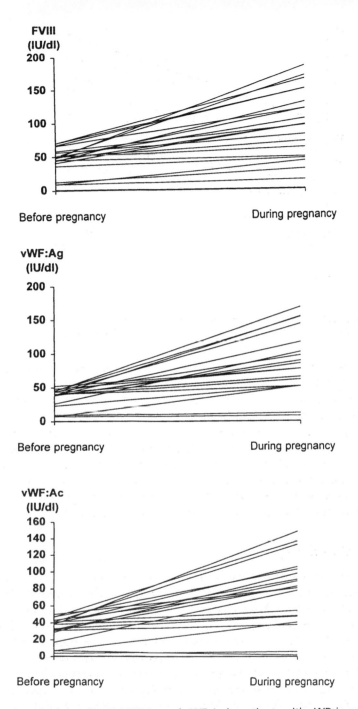

Fig. 5.3 Changes of FVIII, vWF:Ag and vWF:Ac in patients with vWD in pregnancy.

serious bleeding in normal vaginal delivery is small and that delivery of all fetuses known to be at risk of haemophilia by caesarean section is not expected to eliminate the risk. However, the use of vacuum extraction was shown in the same study to constitute a significant risk factor as 10 of 12 infants with

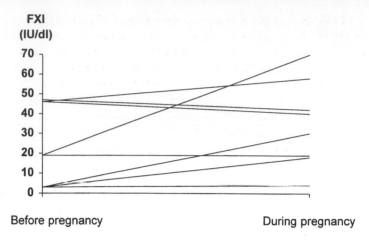

Fig. 5.4 Changes of FXI in FXI deficient patients in pregnancy.

subgaleal and cephalohaematoma were delivered by this instrument. Therefore, it is recommended that delivery should be achieved by the least traumatic method. Prolonged labour, especially prolonged second stage of labour, should be avoided and early recourse to caesarean section should be considered. Vacuum extraction and mid cavity forceps and forceps involving rotation of the head should be avoided. However, low forceps delivery may be considered less traumatic than caesarean section when the head is deeply engaged in the pelvis and delivery can be achieved as an easy outlet procedure and performed by an experienced obstetrician.

Knowledge of fetal gender is very valuable for management of labour in carriers of haemophilia who had not had specific prenatal diagnostic tests. In these situations, the risks of traumatic haemorrhage to a male fetus can be minimised by avoiding invasive monitoring techniques, vacuum extraction or difficult forceps deliveries. In addition, it has been shown that lack of prior knowledge of fetal gender influences the method of delivery resulting in unnecessary caesarean section.[33] The importance of this should be emphasised to the couple and the gender should be determined antenatally even if the mother declines prenatal diagnosis.

Analgesia

The use of regional analgesia/anaesthesia in labour and operative deliveries in patients with bleeding disorders has always been controversial because of the risk of spinal haematoma causing acute spinal cord compression and irreversible paraplegia. However, provided that the coagulation status is normal there should be no contra-indication to these procedures.[33,36,40] Each patient should be individually assessed by a consultant anaesthetist and haematologist and decision regarding these procedures should be made antenatally depending on the type of the disorder and factor levels. It is usually difficult to measure factor levels when patients present in advanced labour and provided that the levels were more than 50 IU/dl during the third trimester, it is then sufficient to assess platelet count, prothrombin time (PT) and activated partial thromboplastin time (APTT). However, it is particularly important to check factor levels prior to removal of the epidural catheter because the pregnancy induced rise in the coagulation factors may quickly reverse after birth and bleeding in the spinal canal may then arise. Regional block in these patients should be performed by an expert anaesthetist with the help of a specialised haematologist for assessment of coagulation status and arrangement of treatment when needed.

Third stage of labour and puerperium

The mother

There has been no report of increased risk of antepartum haemorrhage and it seems that the maternal bleeding complications are confined to the post-partum period.[33,35] The high incidence of primary post-partum haemorrhage (PPH) in vWD[34,35,41] and carriers of haemophilia[33,35,42] has been documented in several studies. The risk of primary PPH in patients with vWD and carriers of haemophilia has been found to be 22%[36] and 18.5%,[33] respectively, compared to 5%[43] in the general obstetric population. As the maternal clotting factor activity falls rapidly after delivery, the risk of secondary PPH is even higher, with reported incidence of 20–28%[35,36,41] in vWD and 11% in carriers of haemophilia,[33] compared with an incidence of 0.7% in a general obstetric population.[44] It has been suggested that childbirth in FXI-deficient patients is accompanied by relatively few problems;[12] however, in a recent study at our centre the incidence of primary and secondary post-partum haemorrhage was 16% and 24%, respectively.[36]

The risk of maternal haemorrhagic complications can be avoided by minimising maternal genital and perineal trauma at delivery and prophylactic treatment with desmopressin (DDAVP, 1-deamino-8-arginine vasopressin) or clotting factor concentrates when appropriate. Prophylactic infusion should start at the onset of labour aiming to raise factor levels to above 50 IU/dl, and maintaining this for 3–4 days after vaginal delivery and 4–5 days after caesarean section.[34] In case of haemorrhage, after initial assessment and restoration of circulatory volume, local causes should be excluded and replacement of the deficient clotting factor and monitoring of the levels should be performed in liaison with the haemophilia centre. It is also not uncommon for these patients to present with prolonged intermittent secondary PPH. In these situations, we recommend administration of tranexamic acid. Tranexamic acid is a fibrinolytic inhibitor which competitively inhibits the activation of plasminogen and non-competitively inhibits plasmin thus counteracting increased fibrinolysis in the uterus.[45] Its use in secondary PPH associated with coagulation defects has also been recommended by Bonnar et al.[45] Combined oral contraceptives are also useful to control this type of haemorrhage, especially in patients with vWD and carriers of haemophilia A.

The neonate

At the time of delivery, an anticoagulated sample of cord blood should be collected and sent to the haemophilia laboratory within 2 h of collection for investigation. When assessing the neonatal coagulation status and clotting factor levels, it should be appreciated that these tests correlate with gestational age and vary with the postnatal age of the infant and the near adult values are achieved for most components by 6 months of life.[46] At birth, APTT is prolonged and vitamin K-dependent factors (II, VII, IX and X) as well as FXI and FXII are lower, however, FVIII and vWF are elevated compared with the adult.[46] Thus, although severe forms of these disorders can be diagnosed at the time of birth, mild forms are not reliably diagnosed and the child should be screened later during the first year of life.

Intramuscular injections frequently cause bleeding in affected infants and should be avoided. Vitamin K should be given orally and the routine immunisations should be administered carefully intradermally or subcutaneously.[34] Hepatitis B immunisation should be considered in these infants. In the Jewish population, circumcision is performed soon after birth, the parents should be advised to postpone this procedure until the diagnosis of bleeding disorders has been confirmed or refuted in the neonate. Parents should be given follow-up counselling and affected babies should be registered with and reviewed regularly by the haemophilia centre.

DDAVP and plasma product therapy

Administration of DDAVP results in an increase in FVIII and vWF concentrations via V2 receptors. This rise lasts for more than 6 h and the biological half-life is only marginally shorter than that of exogenous FVIII and vWF from plasma concentrates.[47] It has also been shown to prevent bleeding in mild or moderate haemophilia and vWD. Some haematologists and obstetricians are reluctant to use it during pregnancy because, theoretically, DDAVP can cause uterine contractions and because of the possible harm to the fetus. However, DDAVP is very specific to V2 receptors but has little effect on smooth muscle V1 receptors and, consequently, does not cause uterine contraction.[48] There are several publications on the management of diabetes insipidus in pregnant women with no harm to the fetus.[49] While the theoretical risk of uterine contraction may be a contra-indication to use during pregnancy, this should not be a problem for a patient in labour, which is the usual time that DDAVP would be required. Carriers of haemophilia A, patients with type 1 vWD and some of patients with type 2A disease respond favourably to this treatment with no risk of viral transmission. However, patients with type 3 vWD do not respond to DDAVP and it is contra-indicated in patients with type 2B disease as it can precipitate thrombocytopenia.[50] DDAVP has also no effect on FIX levels and FIX concentrates would be required to cover any invasive procedures in carriers of haemophilia B with low levels. High-purity FIX concentrate should be used as FIX concentrate containing FII, FVII and FX is potentially thrombogenic.[51,52] For carriers of haemophilia, when administration of FVIII is indicated, recombinant FVIII should be used because plasma derived concentrates of FVIII at present carry a small risk of transmitting parvo virus B19.[53] This risk is of particular importance in pregnant women as it can cause severe fetal infection and hydrops fetalis. In patients with vWD, replacement therapy is by FVIII/vWF plasma concentrates. Prophylactic treatment with these blood products is seldom necessary in type 1 vWD, however, their use to cover labour and delivery has been advocated in patients with other types, especially type 3 vWD.[54]

In FXI deficiency, severely deficient individuals and heterozygotes with a clear history of abnormal bleeding and low FXI level usually require blood product support for labour, especially if delivery is operative. Fresh frozen plasma (FFP) provides adequate haemostatic cover for operative procedures but carries the risk of viral transmission. Because of this risk, FXI concentrate was introduced and its efficacy at preventing bleeding has been confirmed.[16] Recent data have shown that FXI concentrate is associated with thrombosis.[16,55] Therefore, careful consideration should be given to the use of FXI concentrate in pregnancy or the post-partum period.

ACQUIRED POST-PARTUM HAEMOPHILIA

Acquired post-partum haemophilia is induced by antibodies to FVIII (inhibitors), that partially or completely suppress FVIII procoagulant activity, in patients who previously had normal levels of FVIII. Although it is a rare condition, bleeding symptoms are usually very severe and associated with a high morbidity and mortality. Therefore, it is important that it is recognised early. Significant clues include unexplained excessive and/or prolonged vaginal bleeding or large soft tissue haematomas post-partum. Initial coagulation investigations show a prolonged APTT, but a normal PT. Due to the rarity of the disorder and the need for strict monitoring with FVIII assays and inhibitor levels, it is recommended that these patients are treated in a haemophilia centre by individuals specialised in the management of these disorders.[56] In the vast majority, complete remission (absence of inhibitors and normalisation of FVIII) is achieved spontaneously, within a few months. However, this can be extremely variable and in some cases inhibitors persist for years.

GYNAECOLOGICAL ASPECTS OF INHERITED BLEEDING DISORDERS

Menstrual disorders

Haemostasis during menstruation is a complex mechanism and not as fully understood as haemostasis elsewhere. However, haemostatic plug formation, fibrinolysis, prostaglandins and tissue regeneration and reepithelisation play an important role.[57] Therefore, any disorders of blood coagulation especially disorders of primary haemostasis (disorders of blood vessels, platelet abnormalities and vWD) may result in excessive menstrual loss.

In population studies, the prevalence of menorrhagia in the general population is calculated to be 9–11%.[58,59] Menorrhagia is frequent in sufferers of vWD, particularly in adolescent girls. Because the concentration of vWF tends to increase with age, bleeding manifestations become milder and less common.[60] Of women with mild vWD, 50% have been reported to suffer from profuse menstrual blood flow.[61] The first patient described to have vWD, originally called hereditary psuedohaemophilia by Dr Erik von Willebrand in 1926, died of uncontrollable menstrual bleeding at the age of 13 years.[62] The

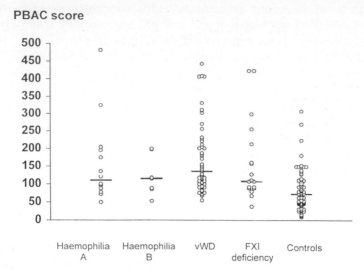

PBAC score

Fig. 5.5 Menstrual scores in carriers of haemophilia A, B, patients with vWD, FXI deficiency and controls. Short horizontal lines indicate mean score.

increased frequency of menorrhagia has also been reported in carriers of haemophilia[9] and FXI deficient patients.[63] Deficiencies of prothrombin, fibrinogen, FV, FVII and FX may also be associated with menorrhagia.

In our centre, objective assessment of menstrual loss, using a pictorial blood assessment chart,[64] in patients with inherited bleeding disorders showed that they not only suffer from heavy menstruation but also prolonged menstrual periods.[65] The prevalence of menorrhagia in patients with vWD, carriers of haemophilia and FXI deficiency was 73%, 57% and 59%, respectively (Fig. 5.5). We have also shown that menstruation has a negative effect on the quality of life, as 39% of women had to cut down on the time they spent on their work or other activities, 47% accomplished less than they would like, 38% were limited in the kind of work or other activities, and 40% experienced difficulties performing their work during the menstrual period.[66] Therefore, we recommend that these women should be asked regularly about their periods and an objective assessment of menstrual loss should be performed by PBAC in those who complain of excessive blood loss. Those with normal PBAC scores can be reassured and appropriate investigations, treatment and a gynaecological referral should be arranged for those with heavy loss.

Menorrhagia as a predictor for inherited bleeding disorders

Severe forms of inherited bleeding disorders are often easily suspected and diagnosed on the basis of clinical symptoms and pattern of inheritance. In contrast, the milder forms may go undiagnosed as they are often asymptomatic until subjected to a haemostatic challenge such as major trauma or invasive surgical procedures. In women, menorrhagia is not uncommon and can be the presenting symptom. However, the role of mild inherited bleeding disorders in the aetiology of menorrhagia is still underestimated and testing

Table 5.2 Patients with menorrhagia and normal pelvis examination screened for bleeding disorders at the Royal Free Hospital

Total	$n = 150$
Mild vWD	$n = 15$
Moderate vWD	$n = 3$
FXI deficiency	$n = 4$
vWD/FXI deficiency	$n = 1$
vWD/FXI/FX deficiency	$n = 1$
Carrier of haemophilia A	$n = 1$
Platelet dysfunction	$n = 1$

vWD, von Willebrand's disease; FXI, factor XI; FX, factor X.

for these disorders is not part of routine investigation for patients with menorrhagia.

We have recently demonstrated that undiagnosed inherited bleeding disorders, especially in their mild forms, can be a significant underlying factor in patients presenting with menorrhagia.[67] In 150 women with objectively confirmed menorrhagia and normal pelvic examination included in an ongoing study at our centre to date, the prevalence of inherited bleeding disorders was 17% (Table 5.2). Edlund et al[68] also showed that menorrhagia is a valuable predictor for bleeding disorders and can be a guideline in looking for mild forms of these disorders. In the same study,[68] 6 of 30 (20%) women with objectively verified menorrhagia were found to have mild vWD and in 2 of them menorrhagia was the only bleeding symptom. Therefore, we recommend that testing for these disorders, especially vWD, should be part of the routine work-up in patients with menorrhagia without any obvious pelvic pathology before embarking on any invasive procedures. Diagnosis of inherited bleeding disorders in these patients has several medical implications. Firstly, it enhances rapid and effective treatment of menorrhagia. Secondly, if any surgical intervention were to become necessary, the risk of bleeding complications can be prevented by appropriate pre-operative assessment and prophylactic treatment when indicated. Lastly, it has genetic implications and affects the management of any future pregnancies.

Treatment of menorrhagia

After exclusion of local causes for menorrhagia in patients with inherited bleeding disorders, treatment options are tranexamic acid, combined oral contraceptives or, more recently, intra-nasal DDAVP spray. Non-steroidal anti-inflammatory drugs are ineffective, and may increase the menstrual blood loss, in the treatment of menorrhagia in patients with underlying bleeding disorders.[69] Tranexamic acid is known to reduce significantly both plasminogen activator activity and plasmin activity in menstrual fluid of women with menorrhagia[70] and reduce bleeding in menorrhagia associated with inherited bleeding disorders.[45] The oral combined contraceptive pill is currently the most commonly used treatment of menorrhagia in these patients. An increase in FVIII activity (FVIII:Ac) in carriers of haemophilia taking the combined oral contraceptives has been reported.[71] An increase of FVIII/vWF-ristocetin cofactor activity and partial correction of prolonged bleeding time in women with vWD[72] by administration of oestrogen has also been reported. DDAVP administered intranasally as a spray has been shown to increase plasma levels of FVIII and vWF in patients with mild haemophilia A or vWD type 1.[73] It is effective when used prophylactically for minor procedures or for treatment of bleeding episodes in these patients.[73] Its effectiveness in the management of menorrhagia has also been described.[74] We are currently assessing this form of treatment in a double blind placebo controlled cross-over trial in patient with vWD, FXI deficiency or carriers of haemophilia A and menorrhagia.

Haemorrhagic complications following gynaecological operations

Gynaecological operations, like any other surgical procedures or injuries, can be complicated by haemorrhage in patients with inherited bleeding disorders. Even relatively minor operations, such as hysteroscopy and/or diagnostic curettage, have been reported to be associated with a significant haemorrhage in these patients.[65,75] Therefore, in all forms of surgery, good liaison between the local haemophilia centre and the surgical/anaesthetic team is essential. Patients' factor levels should be checked pre-operatively and adequate haemostatic cover provided. Any surgical intervention should be carried out by a senior gynaecologist, a technique with least risk of bleeding should be chosen and the use of surgical drains should be considered. It is also important to remember that excessive bleeding may be surgical rather than a result of failure of adequate replacement therapy. Monitoring postoperatively is continued depending on the nature of the operation and patient's factor levels. In contrast, unexplained operative and postoperative bleeding that does not respond to general measures should alert the gynaecologist to the possibility of an underlying bleeding disorder as a causative factor.

RARER INHERITED BLEEDING DISORDERS

These include prothrombin, fibrinogen, FV, FVII, FX and FXIII deficiency. Due to the rarity of these conditions, there is very limited experience in the management of obstetric and gynaecological problems in these patients. Therefore, they should be managed in a unit where the help of a haematologist experienced in haemophilia care and the laboratory facilities for monitoring factor levels and provision of blood products are readily available. Hereditary fibrinogenaemia has been reported to be associated with recurrent pregnancy loss and placental abruption. Recurrent spontaneous miscarriage has also been reported in FXIII deficiency.

CONCLUSIONS

Women with inherited bleeding disorders are at risk of excessive bleeding during menstruation, childbirth and after any surgical intervention. Increased awareness among obstetricians and gynaecologists, close collaboration with the local haemophilia centre and availability of management guidelines are essential to minimise these risks. On the other hand, inherited bleeding disorders – especially vWD – can be the underlying cause in patients with menorrhagia and testing for these disorders should be performed as part of the routine management of such patients. Lastly, unexplained post-partum, operative and postoperative haemorrhage that does not respond to general measures should alert obstetricians and gynaecologists to the possibility of bleeding disorders as a causative factor.

KEY POINTS FOR CLINICAL PRACTICE

- Prepregnancy counselling should be offered to all women with inherited bleeding disorders to discuss prenatal diagnosis and other aspects of pregnancy management

- Women with inherited bleeding disorders require special obstetric care with close liaison with the haemophilia centre; management guidelines should be followed by all professionals involved in pregnancy care

- Knowledge of fetal gender is very valuable for labour management in carriers of haemophilia and should be determined prior to labour

- The use of invasive fetal monitoring techniques and instrumental deliveries, specially vacuum extraction, should be avoided in at-risk fetuses

- The risk of post-partum haemorrhage can be reduced by minimising maternal genital and perineal trauma and appropriate prophylactic treatment for labour and post-partum period

- Menorrhagia is a common and major problem in patients with inherited bleeding disorders. Increased awareness among gynaecologists of the high prevalence of menorrhagia and the treatment options available is necessary for optimal management of these patients

- Screening for inherited bleeding disorders, especially vWD, should be part of the routine work-up in patients with menorrhagia without any obvious pelvic pathology before embarking on any invasive procedures

- The diagnosis of bleeding disorders in any unexplained post-partum, operative or postoperative haemorrhage should be considered.

REFERENCES

1 Rodeghiero F, Castaman G, Dini E. Epidemiological investigation of the prevalence of von Willebrand's disease. Blood 1987; 69: 454–459
2 Werner E J, Broxson E H, Tucker E L, Giroux D S, Shults J, Abshire T C. Prevalence of von Willebrand disease in children: a multiethnic study. J Pediatr 1993; 123: 893–898
3 Ruggeri Z M. Pathogenesis and classification of von Willebrand disease [Review]. Haemostasis 1994; 24: 265–275
4 Zimmerman T S, Ruggeri Z M. von Willebrand disease [Review]. Hum Pathol 1987; 18: 140–152

5 Ruggeri Z M, Pareti F I, Mannucci P M, Ciavarella N, Zimmerman T S. Heightened interaction between platelets and factor VIII/von Willebrand factor in a new subtype of von Willebrand's disease. N Engl J Med 1980; 302: 1047–1051

6 Forbes C D. Clinical aspects of the haemophilias. In: Ratnoff O D, Forbes C D. (eds) Disorders of haemostasis. New York: Grune & Stratton, 1984; 177–239

7 Rizza C R, Rhymes I L, Austen D E G, Kernoff P B A, Aroni S A. Detection of carriers of haemophilia: a 'blind' study. Br J Haematol 1975; 30: 447–456

8 Lyon M F. Sex chromatin and gene action in the mammalian X-chromosome. Am J Hum Genet 1962; 14: 135–148

9 Lusher J M, McMillan C W. Severe factor VIII and factor IX deficiency in females. Am J Med 1978; 65: 637–648

10 Graham J B, Barrow E S, Roberts H R et al. Dominant inheritance of hemophilia A in three generations of women. Blood 1975; 46: 175–188

11 Shpilberg O, Peretz H, Zivelin R et al. One of the two common mutations causing factor XI deficiency in Ashkenazi Jews (type II) is also prevalent in Iraqi Jews, who represent the ancient gene pool of Jews. Blood 1995; 85: 429–432

12 Bolton-Maggs P H B, Young Wan-Yin B, McCraw A H, Slack J, Kernoff P B A. Inheritance and bleeding in factor XI deficiency. Br J Haematol 1988; 69: 521–528

13 Leiba H, Ramot B, Many A. Heredity and coagulation studies in ten families with factor XI (plasma thromboplastin antecedent) deficiency. Br J Haematol 1965; 11: 654–665

14 Ragni M V, Sinha D, Seaman F, Lewis J H, Spero J A, Walsh P N. Comparison of bleeding tendency, factor XI coagulant activity, and factor XI antigen in 25 factor XI-deficient kindreds. Blood 1985; 65: 719–724

15 Brenner B, Lupo H, Laor A, Zivelin A, Lanir N, Seligsohn U. Predictors of bleeding in factor XI deficient patients. Thromb Haemost 1995; 73: 1441

16 Collins P W, Goldman E, Liley P, Pasi K J, Lee C A. Clinical experience of factor XI deficiency: the role of fresh frozen plasma and factor XI concentrate. Haemophilia 1995; 1: 227–231

17 Seligsohn U. Factor XI deficiency [Review]. Thromb Haemost 1993; 70: 68–71

18 Ginsburg D, Handin R I, Bonthron D T, Dolon T A, Bruns G A, Latt S A. Human von Willebrand Factor (vWF): isolation of complementary DNA (cDNA) clones and chromosomal localization. Science 1985; 228: 1401–1406

19 Verweij C L, deVries C J M, Distel B, van Zonneveld A J, van Kessel A G, van Mourik J A. Construction of cDNA coding for human von Willebrand factor using antibody probes for colony-screening and mapping of the chromosomal gene. Nucleic Acids Res 1985; 13: 4699–4717

20 Miller C H. Genetics of haemophilia and von Willebrand's disease. In: Hilgartner M W. (ed) Hemophilia in the child and adult. New York: Masson, 1982; 29–62

21 Antonarakis S E, Youssoufian H, Kazazian H H. Molecular genetics of hemophilia A in man (factor VIII deficiency) [Review]. Mol Biol Med 1987; 4: 81–94

22 Kato A, Asakai R, Davie E W, Aoki N. Factor XI gene (F11) is located on the distal end of the long arm of human chromosome 4. Cytogenet Cell Genet 1989; 52: 77–78

23 Asakai R, Chung D W, Ratnoff O D, Davie E W. Factor XI (plasma thromboplastin antecedent) deficiency in Ashkenazi Jews is a bleeding disorder that can result from three types of point mutations. Proc Natl Acad Sci USA 1989; 86: 7667–7671

24 Imanak Y, Mc Vey J H, Nishimura T. Identification and characterisation of mutations in factor XI gene of non-Jewish factor XI-deficient patients. Thromb Haemost 1993: 69: 752

25 Peretz U, Zivelin A, Usher S, Eichel R, Sligsohn U. Identification of a new mutation in factor XI gene of an Ashkenazi-Jew with severe factor XI deficiency. Blood 1993; 82 suppl 1: 66a

26 Pugh R E, McVey J H, Tuddenham E G D, Hancock J F. Six point mutations that cause factor XI deficiency. Blood 1995; 85: 1509–1516

27 Asakai R, Chung D W, Davie E W, Seligsohn U. Factor XI deficiency in Ashkenazi Jews in Israel. N Engl J Med 1991; 325: 153–158

28 Hancock J F, Wieland K, Pugh R E et al. A molecular genetic study of factor XI deficiency. Blood 1991; 77: 1942–1948

29 Koerper M A. Prenatal diagnosis of hemophilia in the United States. Prog Clin Biol Res 1990; 324: 13–17

30 Bronshtein M, Rottem S, Yoffe N, Blumenfeld Z, Brandes J M. Early determination of fetal sex using transvaginal sonography: technique and pitfalls. J Clin Ultrasound 1990; 18: 302–306

31 Miller C H, Hilgartner M W, Aledort L M. Reproductive choices in hemophilic men and carriers. Am J Med Genet 1987; 26: 591–598

32 Ranta S, Lehesjoki A E, Peippo M, Kaariainen H. Hemophilia A: experiences and attitudes of mothers, sisters, and daughters. Pediatr Hematol Oncol 1994; 11: 387–397

33 Kadir R A, Economides D L, Braithwaite J, Goldman E, Lee C A. The obstetric experience of carrier of haemophilia. Br J Obstet Gynaecol 1997; 104: 803–810

34 Greer I A, Lowe G D, Walker J J, Forbes C D. Haemorrhagic problems in obstetrics and gynaecology in patients with congenital coagulopathies. Br J Obstet Gynaecol 1991; 98: 909–918

35 Kadir R A, Lee C A, Sabin C A, Pollard D, Economides D L. Pregnancy in von Willebrand's disease or factor XI deficiency. Br J Obstet Gynaecol 1998; 105: 314–321

36 Briet E, Reisner H M, Blatt P M. Factor IX levels during pregnancy in a woman with hemophilia B. Haemostasis 1982; 11: 87–89

37 Rick M E, Williams S B, Sacher R A, McKeown L P. Thrombocytopenia associated with pregnancy in a patient with type IIB von Willebrand's disease. Blood 1987; 69: 786–789

38 Leko M, Sakurama S, Sagawa A et al. Effect of factor VIII concentrate on type IIB von Willebrand's disease-associated thrombocytopenia presenting during pregnancy in identical twin mothers. Am J Hematol 1990; 35: 26–31

39 Ljung R, Lindgren A C, Petrini P, Tengborn L. Normal vaginal delivery is to be recommended for haemophilia carrier gravidae. Acta Paediatr 1994; 83: 609–611

40 Walker I D, Walker J J, Colvin B T, Letsky E A, Rivers R, Stevens R (on behalf of the Haemostasis and Thrombosis Task Force). Investigation and management of haemorrhagic disorders in pregnancy [Review]. J Clin Pathol 1994; 47: 100–108

41 Ramsahoye B H, Davies S V, Dasani H, Pearson J F. Obstetric management in von Willebrand's disease: a report of 24 pregnancies and a review of the literature. Haemophilia 1995; 1: 140–144

42 Mauser Bunschoten M E, van Houwelingen J C, Sjamsoedin Visser E J et al. Bleeding symptoms in carriers of hemophilia A and B. Thromb Haemost 1988; 59: 349–352

43 Cunningham F G, MacDonald P C, Gant N F. Abnormalities of the third stage of labour. In: Cunningham F G, MacDonald P C, Gant N F. Williams (eds) Obstetrics, 18th edn. London: Prentice-Hall, 1989; 415–424

44 Lee C Y, Madrazo B, Drukker B H. Ultrasonic evaluation of the postpartum uterus in the management of postpartum bleeding. Obstet Gynecol 1981; 58: 227–232

45 Bonnar J, Guillebaud J, Kasonde J M, Sheppard B L. Clinical applications of fibrinolytic inhibition in gynaecology [Review]. J Clin Pathol 1980; 33 Suppl 14: 55–59

46 Andrew M, Paes B, Milner R et al. Development of the human coagulation system in the full-term infant. Blood 1987; 70: 165–172

47 Mannucci P M, Canciani M T, Rota L, Donovan B S. Response of factor VIII/von Willebrand factor to DDAVP in healthy subjects and patients with haemophilia A and Von Willebrand's disease. Br J Haematol 1981; 47: 283–293

48 Mannucci P M. Desmopressin: a nontransfusional form of treatment for congenital and acquired bleeding disorders [Review]. Blood 1988; 72: 1449–1455

49 Burrow G N, Wassenaar W, Robertson G L, Sehl H. DDAVP treatment of diabetes insipidus during pregnancy and the post-partum period. Acta Endocrinol (Copenh) 1981; 97: 23–25

50 Holmberg L, Nilsson I M, Borge L, Gunnarsson M, Sjorin E. Platelet aggregation induced by 1-desamino-8-D-arginine vasopressin (DDAVP) in type IIB von Willebrand's disease. N Engl J Med 1983; 309: 816–821

51 Magner A, Aronson D. Toxicity of factor IX concentrates in mice. Dev Biol Stand 1979; 44: 185–188

52 Lusher J M. Thrombogenicity associated with factor IX complex concentrates [Review]. Semin Hematol 1991; 28 (3 Suppl 6): 3–5

53 Santagostino E, Mannucci P M, Gringeri A, Azzi A, Morfini M. Eliminating parvovirus B19 from blood products [letter]. Lancet 1994; 343: 798

54 Mayne E E, Winter M, Bolton-Maggs P et al. Treatment and management of von Willebrand disease. Haemophilia 1997; 3 (Suppl 2): 4–8

55 Bolton-Maggs P H, Colvin B T, Satchi B T, Lee C A, Lucas G S. Thrombogenic potential of factor XI concentrate [letter]. Lancet 1994; 344: 748–749

56 Kadir R A, Koh M B, Lee C A, Pasi K J. Acquired haemophilia, an unusual cause of severe postpartum haemorrhage. Br J Obstet Gynaecol 1997; 104: 854–856

57 Christiaens G C, Sixma J J, Haspels A A. Hemostasis in menstrual endometrium: a review. Obstet Gynecol Surv 1982; 37: 281–303

58 Cole S K, Billewicz W Z, Thomson A M. Sources of variation in menstrual blood loss. J Obstet Gynaecol Br Commonw 1971; 78: 933–939

59 Hallberg L, Hogdahl A M, Nilsson L, Rybo G. Menstrual blood loss – a population study. Acta Obstet Gynecol Scand 1966; 45: 320–351

60 Zimmermann T S, Ruggeri Z M. von Willebrand disease. Hum Pathol 1987; 18: 140–152

61 Nilsson I M. Haemorrhagic and thrombotic diseases. London: Wiley, 1974; 97–98

62 Nilsson I M. Von Willebrand's disease – 50 years old. Acta Med Scand 1977; 201: 497–508

63 Bolton-Maggs P H B, Patterson D A, Wensley R T, Tuddenham E G. Definition of the bleeding tendency in factor XI-deficient kindreds: a clinical and laboratory study. Thromb Haemost 1995; 73: 194–202

64 Higham J M, O'Brien P M, Show R W. Assessment of menstrual blood loss using a pictorial chart. Br J Obstet Gynaecol 1990; 97: 734–739

65 Kadir R A, Lee C A, Sabin C A, Pollard D, Economides D L. Assessment of menstrual blood loss and gynaecological problems in patients with inherited bleeding disorders. Haemophilia 1998 (In press)

66 Kadir R A, Sabin C A, Pollard D, Lee C A, Economides D L. Quality of life during menstruation in patients with inherited bleeding disorders. Submitted

67 Kadir R A, Economides D L, Sabin C A, Owens D, Lee C A. Should patients with menorrhagia be investigated for inherited bleeding disorders? [abstract]. Br J Obstet Gynaecol 1997; 104: 860

68 Edlund M, Blomback M, von Schoultz B, Andersson O. On the value of menorrhagia as a predictor for coagulation disorders. Am J Hematol 1996; 53: 234–238

69 Mäkäräinen L, Ylikorkala O. Primary and myoma-associated menorrhagia: role of prostaglandins and effect of ibuprofen. Br J Obstet Gynaecol 1986; 93: 974–978

70 Dockeray C J, Sheppard B L, Daly L, Bonnar J. The fibrinolytic enzyme system in normal menstruation and excessive uterine bleeding and the effect of tranexamic acid. Eur J Obstet Gynecol Reprod Biol 1987; 24: 309–318

71 Schiffman S, Rapaport S I. Increased factor VIII levels in suspected carriers of hemophilia A taking contraceptives by mouth. N Engl J Med 1966; 275: 599

72 Alperin J B. Estrogens and surgery in women with von Willebrand's disease. Am J Med 1982; 73: 367–371

73 Rose E H, Aledort L M. Nasal spray desmopressin (DDAVP) for mild hemophilia A and von Willebrand disease. Ann Intern Med 1991; 114: 563–568

74 Lethagen S, Ragnarson Tennvall G. Self-treatment with desmopressin intranasal spray in patients with bleeding disorders: effect on bleeding symptoms and socioeconomic factors. Ann Hematol 1993; 66: 257–260

75 Purcell G J R, Nossel H L. Factor XI (PTA) deficiency. Surgical and obstetric aspects. Obstet Gynecol 1970; 35: 69–74

6

Jackie Tan   Michael de Swiet

Thromboembolism and thrombophilia in pregnancy and the puerperium

Thromboembolic disease has remained a major cause of maternal deaths in the UK over the past 2 decades.[1-6] Every year, an average of 10 women die from thromboembolic disease during pregnancy or the puerperium. In addition, non-fatal thromboembolic disease is associated with significant morbidity such as recurrent thromboembolism, the post-thrombotic syndrome or, more rarely, secondary pulmonary hypertension. There are also important implications in obstetrics in terms of thromboprophylaxis and fetal risks. This review will summarise recent advances in the investigation of thromboembolic disease and thrombophilia and their management.

PATHOPHYSIOLOGY

Physiological changes in the coagulation and vascular systems prime the pregnant woman to develop thromboembolic disease. This 6-fold increase in risk of thromboembolism is not only confined to pregnancy but extends into, and is clearly increased during the puerperium.[7] Increased levels of clotting factors (factors I, II, VII, VIII, IX and X) together with decreased fibrinolysis and reduced levels of the natural anticoagulant, protein S, contribute to this state of hypercoagulability during pregnancy.[8,9] Venous stasis resulting from pressure of the gravid uterus on the inferior vena cava and decreased venous tone are further predisposing factors present in all pregnant women. Other important risk factors include advanced maternal age (> 35 years), multiparity, obesity, operative or difficult instrumental delivery, prolonged bed rest, pre-eclampsia, previous thromboembolism and thrombophilia (Table 6.1).[1,3,5,10]

Dr Jackie Tan, Registrar, Institute of Obstetrics and Gynaecology, Queen Charlotte's and Chelsea Hospital, Goldhawk Road, London W6 0XG, UK

Dr Michael de Swiet, Academic Sub-Dean/Consultant Physician, Institute of Obstetrics and Gynaecology, Queen Charlotte's and Chelsea Hospital, Goldhawk Road, London W6 0XG, UK

Table 6.1 Risk factors for thromboembolism in pregnancy and the puerperium

Risk factors
Increased parity > 4
Advanced maternal age > 35 years
Obesity
Operative or difficult instrumental delivery
Prolonged immobility
Pre-eclampsia
Previous thromboembolism
Thrombophilia

Multiple risk factors are often present in women who develop thromboembolic disease during pregnancy or the puerperium and the risks are cumulative.

THROMBOPHILIA

Thrombophilia refers to any persistent and identifiable hypercoagulable state, either acquired or inherited, which is associated with an increased risk of thromboembolism (Table 6.2). The causes of acquired thrombophilia are varied and include conditions such as the antiphospholipid syndrome, myelo-proliferative disease, paroxysmal nocturnal haemoglobinuria, nephrotic syndrome and malignancy. Apart from the antiphospholipid syndrome, the other disorders are uncommon in pregnancy and, therefore, will not be discussed further in this review.

Inherited thrombophilias result from well-defined genetic defects such as protein C, protein S and antithrombin III deficiency, activated protein C resistance (due to factor V Leiden mutation), prothrombin gene G20210A variant and hyperhomocystinaemia. Although they were originally thought of as single gene disorders, a study of protein C deficiency among blood donors, as well as the recent discovery of the much more prevalent factor V Leiden, are beginning to change this concept. More studies are now emerging which

Table 6.2 Thrombophilic conditions

Inherited thrombophilia	Acquired thrombophilia
Protein C deficiency	Antiphospholipid syndrome
Protein S deficiency	Myeloproliferative disease
Anti-thrombin III deficiency	Malignancy
Activated protein C resistance	Paroxysmal nocturnal haemoglobinuria
(Leiden mutation)	Nephrotic syndrome
Prothrombin gene G20210A variant	
Homocystinuria	
Hyperhomocystinaemia	

support the view that familial thrombophilia is a multiple gene disease, with reports confirming the segregation of 2 or more defects within thrombophilic families and identifying individuals with multiple defects as those who are at greatest risk of thrombosis.[11-14] Clinical features suggestive of an inherited thrombophilia include a positive family history, recurrent thromboembolism, thrombosis in an unusual site and young age at presentation. Setting an age limit for thrombophilia screening, however, need not always apply because of the effect of increasing age on the clinical expression of these deficient states.

Inherited thrombophilia

Antithrombin III, protein C and protein S deficiency

Antithrombin III and proteins C and S are naturally occurring anticoagulants. Antithrombin III is a major inhibitor of thrombin and also inactivates other serine proteases (factors IXa, Xa and XIa). Protein C, together with its co-factor protein S, form an important natural anticoagulant mechanism. Activated protein C degrades factors VIIIa and Va in the presence of its co-factor protein S, thereby reducing thrombin generation. A deficiency in any of these factors, either quantitative or qualitative, results in a thrombotic tendency. Collectively, they account for about 5% of unselected patients presenting with objectively confirmed deep vein thrombosis. Among selected patients, the prevalence is higher (between 5–10%) (Table 6.3).[14,15]

The heterozygous deficiency states of these three conditions share clinical features except that antithrombin III deficiency appears to have a particularly high thrombotic risk. The first thrombotic event often occurs in early adulthood particularly within the first months of starting a combined oral contraceptive. The lifetime prevalence of thromboembolism in patients with a positive family history is over 50%. The commonest events are deep vein thromboses in the lower limbs and pulmonary embolism. A thrombotic episode in an unusual site, such as the axillary vein or the viscera, is another clue to an underlying deficient state or to acquired thrombophilia such as the

Table 6.3 Prevalence of inherited thrombophilia (%)

Thrombophilia	General population	Unselected patients with TED*	Selected patients with TED**
Antithrombin III deficiency	0.02	1	0.5–7
Protein C deficiency	0.2–0.4	3	1–9
Protein S deficiency	–	1–2	1–13
APC resistance	3-15	20	10–64
Prothrombin gene G20210A variant	1.2–2.3	5.5–6.2	18

APC = activated protein C; TED = thromboembolic disease.
*Consecutive patients with a first episode of TED.
**Patients with recurrent thrombosis, young age at presentation (< 45 years) or a positive family history.
Modified from Rosendaal[14] with the permission of the publisher.

antiphospholipid syndrome.[16] Thrombotic episodes may occur spontaneously or in association with other risk factors, such as surgery or pregnancy.

Activated protein C resistance

Activated protein C resistance due to factor V Leiden has recently been identified as the commonest inherited thrombophilia in the Caucasian population. It is at least 10 times more common than any of the other known genetic defects and has been found in 20–60% of women who developed thrombosis during pregnancy. Thrombotic risk increases with homozygosity and age; in addition to pregnancy, there is clearly interaction with other inherited thrombophilias as well as factors such as oral contraceptive use and surgery. The prevalence of the Leiden mutation varies in different populations – 15% in southern Sweden, up to 10% in Germany and Greece, 3–5% in the UK, The Netherlands and the US. It is rarely found in Asians and Africans.[13,17–20]

Under normal circumstances, activated protein C, together with its co-factor protein S, causes inactivation of factor Va and VIIIa thereby controlling the conversion of prothrombin to thrombin and factor X to Xa, respectively. In most cases (95%), activated protein C resistance is caused by factor V Leiden. This is a single point mutation in the gene coding for factor V which leads to the substitution of arginine by glutamine at position 506 (Arg 506 Gln), thereby altering the cleavage site which is responsible for factor Va inactivation. The resultant dysfunctional factor V molecule called factor V Leiden is resistant to inactivation by activated protein C.[21]

The screening test for activated protein C resistance (APCR) is based on measurement of the activated partial thromboplastin time (aPTT) in the presence and absence of activated protein C (APC); the results are then expressed as a ratio of aPTT with APC to aPTT without APC – the APC ratio. Resistance is defined when there is insufficient prolongation of the aPTT on addition of exogenous protein C (ratio < 2) and is usually confirmed by identifying the factor V Leiden mutation by polymerase chain reaction.[22] The APCR test, however, may be inaccurate in individuals with abnormal aPTTs such as those with the lupus anticoagulant, coagulation defects and patients who are receiving heparin or warfarin treatment.[19] In a small number of cases, activated protein C resistance is not associated with the presence of the Leiden mutation and thus appears to be acquired. One reason is the presence of antiphospholipid antibodies which may affect the actions of protein C.[23] Other conditions associated with activated protein C resistance include pregnancy and the use of the oral contraceptive pill. Reductions in the APC ratio have been observed in all stages of pregnancy when compared with the ratios at 8 weeks or more postpartum.[24,25] Similar changes have also been reported in women taking the combined oral contraceptive pill which normalised following discontinuation of the pill.[26] Results should always be interpreted carefully, taking into consideration circumstances under which testing was done. If necessary, the test can be repeated when confounding factors are no longer present.

The thrombotic risk associated with factor V Leiden is 6–8-fold for heterozygotes and 30–140-fold for homozygotes.[19] The commonest clinical presentation is deep vein thrombosis. The occurrence of thromboses in unusual sites is much less common than in antithrombin III, protein C, protein S deficiency or in the antiphospholipid syndrome (see below).

Prothrombin gene G20210A variant

The prothrombin gene G20210A variant is a very recently identified inherited thrombophilia. It is caused by a genetic variation resulting in a G to A nucleotide transition at position 20210 in the 3'-untranslated region of the prothrombin gene and is associated with elevated prothrombin levels. It has been found to increase the risk for venous thrombosis about 3–5-fold. Heterozygosity for the 20210 A allele has been identified in 5.5–6.2% of patients with thromboembolic disease and in 1.2–2.3% of healthy subjects.[27,28] At present, it is not included as part of most routine thrombophilia screening.

Hyperhomocystinaemia

Hyperhomocystinaemia may result from genetic defects affecting methionine homocysteine metabolism or from acquired factors such as deficiencies of vitamin B_6, folate, vitamin B_{12}, renal failure and the use of anti-folate drugs (methotrexate, anti-convulsants, inhaled nitrous oxide). Severe hyper-homocystinaemia (> 100 μmol/l) is classically caused by homocystinuria, an autosomal recessive condition which results from homozygous cystathionine synthase deficiency. It is associated with characteristic clinical features which include ectopia lentis, mental retardation, a Marfanoid habitus, premature atherosclerosis and venous thromboembolism. Mild (16–24 μmol/l) or moderate (25–100 μmol/l) hyperhomocystinaemia may result from the acquired conditions described above as well as genetic defects, such as heterozygous cystathionine synthase deficiency and homozygosity for the thermolabile mutant of methylene-tetrahydrofolate reductase. In contrast to homocystinuria, morphological abnormalities are usually not seen in these individuals. Hyperhomocystinaemia is, however, still associated with atherosclerotic vascular disease and a 2–3-fold increase in risk of venous thrombosis.[29,30] In a recent study by den Heijer et al, 10% of patients presenting with their first episode of deep vein thrombosis were found to have elevated homocysteine levels. This association appears to be stronger among women than men, suggesting that women are perhaps more susceptible to the pathologic effects of hyperhomocystinaemia.[30,31] It is still uncertain whether different causes of hyperhomocystinaemia carry the same risk of thrombosis. Diagnosis is based on either an elevated homocysteine level in the fasting state and/or after methionine loading. Postulated mechanisms include endothelial cell injury and inhibition of thrombomodulin expression and, hence, decreased protein C activation. Further studies are needed to clarify the clinical benefits of homocysteine lowering therapy with vitamin supplementation and to justify routine screening but in the absence of the more established risk factors, testing for hyperhomocystinaemia may be worth considering in the appropriate clinical setting.

Acquired thrombophilia

The antiphospholipid syndrome

The antiphospholipid syndrome is a multi-system disease associated with the presence of circulating antiphospholipid antibodies (anticardiolipin antibodies and lupus anticoagulant). The syndrome is 'primary' when there is no associated autoimmune disease and 'secondary' when it occurs in association with systemic lupus erythematosus. It has protean manifestations, the commoner of which include recurrent spontaneous abortions and a thrombophilic state with both venous and arterial thromboses.[22–34] Deep vein thromboses in the lower limbs and pulmonary embolism are the most frequent events but thrombosis can occur at almost any site. Thrombosis in the antiphospholipid syndrome tends to recur with rates of up to 70%. This justifies long-term anticoagulation and certainly throughout pregnancy and the puerperium in such patients.[35,36]

FETAL LOSS AND THROMBOPHILIA

There is now increasing evidence that maternal thrombophilia, particularly the presence of multiple defects, is associated with an increased risk of fetal loss.[37–40] Normal development of the utero-placental vascular system is crucial for a successful pregnancy outcome. An underlying thrombophilia may compromise pregnancy by causing thrombosis at the placental level. Such a relationship was first established in the antiphospholipid syndrome where utero-placental vascular thrombosis and placental infarction were noted in these patients. Animal studies have also suggested a direct link between these thrombogenic antibodies, placental thrombosis and recurrent pregnancy loss.[41] However, the heterogeneity of placental pathology in the antiphospholipid syndrome plus the fact that not all patients with antiphospholipid antibodies experience fetal loss suggest that other pathogenetic mechanisms may be involved as well.[42]

As a consequence of our increasing understanding of the pathophysiology of the antiphospholipid syndrome, various treatments including immunosuppresive therapy, antiplatelet agents and anticoagulants, have evolved to prevent fetal loss in these women. Initial studies with prednisone were encouraging but they were not without considerable side effects of steroid therapy.[43] Lockshin subsequently showed that steroid therapy did not prevent recurrent fetal loss.[44] In a randomised trial comparing aspirin and heparin versus prednisolone and aspirin, although fetal outcomes were similar in both treatment groups, there was greater maternal morbidity and higher frequency of pre-term delivery in the steroid group, suggesting that the former combination was a safer therapeutic option.[45] Since then, further trials have shown that heparin and aspirin are more effective than aspirin alone in preventing pregnancy losses.[46,47] As treatment with heparin is not without risks, our current policy is to confine its additional use in patients with antiphospholipid antibodies to those who also have a bad obstetric history or previous thromboembolism. Those who possess antibodies without any adverse clinical history receive only low dose aspirin and judicious monitoring of the pregnancy. Women with inherited thrombophilia are similarly managed.

DIAGNOSIS OF THROMBOEMBOLIC DISEASE

Clinically suspected thromboembolic disease should always be confirmed objectively because clinical assessment alone is inaccurate. Of patients with clinically suspected thromboembolic disease, 50–75% do not actually have the condition when objective tests are carried out.[48–50] Evaluation in pregnancy is particularly difficult because dyspnoea, leg swelling and discomfort are such common complaints. Accurate diagnosis is necessary because of the potential complications of unnecessary anticoagulation and the significant mortality associated with untreated pulmonary embolism.

Deep vein thrombosis

Non-invasive tests such as impedance plethysmography and Doppler ultrasound have gradually replaced venography in the diagnosis of deep vein thrombosis. Ultrasound is now the initial investigation of choice when evaluating deep vein thrombosis in pregnancy because it is non-invasive, allows serial testing to detect extension of calf vein thrombi and has high specificity and sensitivity (> 97%) for proximal thromboses.[51] It is not sensitive for asymptomatic thromboses. Although it is also less sensitive in diagnosing calf vein thrombosis, studies have shown that only 20% of these thrombi extend proximally and that calf vein thrombi are not threatening so long as they remain confined to the calf.[52] Venography remains the reference standard but it is invasive, painful and is associated with risks of provoking thrombosis and contrast reaction. The radiation risks to the fetus are small and certainly do not preclude its use in pregnancy, particularly when non-invasive testing is equivocal. Magnetic resonance imaging has recently been established to be a reliable method for diagnosing pelvic and lower extremity venous thromboses. It is at least as accurate as venography for proximal thromboses in the lower limb and possibly even more sensitive for pelvic vein thromboses. Obvious advantages in pregnancy include its non-invasiveness, lack of exposure to ionising radiation and excellent resolution of the inferior vena cava and the pelvic veins.[53]

Pulmonary embolism

The chest X-ray and arterial blood gas (taken with the patient sitting as pO_2 in the supine position may differ by up to 15 mmHg in the third trimester) remain important tests in the initial evaluation of pulmonary embolism. They are, however, non-specific and some form of diagnostic imaging is required. The electrocardiogram has too many non-specific changes related to pregnancy for it to be of significant help in the majority of cases. The next most frequently used test for suspected pulmonary embolism is the ventilation-perfusion scan. Its main limitation, however, is that a definitive diagnosis can only be made in 25% of patients as shown in the PIOPED study.[48] In general, the ventilation-perfusion scan is useful if it is normal, if there is low clinical suspicion and low scan probability or if there is high clinical suspicion combined with a high probability scan. The remaining patients with indeterminate findings require further investigation to confirm or exclude embolism. Pulmonary angiography remains the most sensitive and specific test for diagnosing pulmonary embolism; however, it is particularly underused during pregnancy because of concern about radiation exposure to the fetus and also because it is an invasive test. In fact, the amount of radiation a fetus is exposed to from a combination of chest X-ray, ventilation-perfusion scan and pulmonary angiography is less than 0.5 rad; most studies have shown that radiation exposure 10 times this amount, i.e. less than 5 rad, is not associated with significant fetal risk.[52,54]

Recent advances have led to the development of contrast-enhanced spiral CT angiography (SCTA) and gadolinium-enhanced magnetic resonance angiography (MRA) of the pulmonary arteries for diagnosing pulmonary embolism.[55,56] These new techniques have high sensitivity and specificity for clots in the central and segmental pulmonary arteries and have the additional advantages of being non-invasive, free from radiation (for magnetic resonance imaging though not from gadolinium) and providing images of the lungs, pleura and mediastinum. The main limitation of SCTA is its poor sensitivity in detecting emboli in the subsegmental vessels. In any case, the clinical significance of subsegmental emboli is uncertain and pulmonary angiography has similarly been shown to be less accurate in detecting such emboli.

MANAGEMENT OF THROMBOEMBOLIC DISEASE

Anticoagulants remain the mainstay of treatment of thromboembolic disease. Heparin has been well established as the safest anticoagulant during pregnancy; it does not cross the placenta and is not associated with teratogenicity or bleeding in the fetus. Warfarin, on the other hand, crosses the placenta readily and is associated with perhaps a 5% risk of embryopathy (including chondrodysplasia punctata) particularly if taken between the 6th and 12th weeks of pregnancy; it can also cause fetal and neonatal haemorrhage and for these reasons should be avoided during pregnancy unless specifically indicated. In addition, warfarin can cause major maternal bleeding and its action is not as easily reversed as that of heparin.

Treatment of antepartum thromboembolic disease

The initial treatment of acute thromboembolic disease in pregnancy is similar to that in the non-pregnant patient, i.e. with high dose intravenous heparin. A bolus dose of 5000 units is followed by a continuous infusion adjusted to maintain a 1.5–2.0-fold prolongation of the activated partial thromboplastin time or alternatively heparin levels of 0.4–0.7 U/ml (by anti-Xa assay). This is maintained for 5–10 days depending on the severity of the thromboembolic episode following which anticoagulation is continued using subcutaneous heparin in the chronic phase of therapy for the remainder of the pregnancy, aiming to maintain heparin levels not exceeding 0.2 U/ml (by anti-Xa assay).[57] In general, the dose of subcutaneous heparin which is required during pregnancy is about twice that of the non-pregnant patient, i.e. 10 000 units instead of 5000 units twice daily because of the increase in circulating blood volume and activation of the clotting system. The total duration of anticoagulation for an acute thromboembolic episode should extend till 6 weeks post-partum or for a period of 3 months, whichever is the longer. Postnatally, subcutaneous heparin may be substituted with warfarin if the patient prefers to discontinue injections; however, more frequent visits are then necessary to monitor the INR to ensure adequate anticoagulation. Neither drug is excreted in breast milk and both are compatible with breast-feeding though phenindione is not.

Complications of heparin treatment

One of the main problems associated with long-term heparin treatment is osteoporosis; this is particularly relevant to pregnancy because heparin treatment is frequently prolonged. In addition, pregnancy itself and breast-feeding have independent effects on bone demineralisation. Women who breast-feed for 6 months have been shown to demonstrate a 6% reduction of bone density in their lumbar spine.[58] The risk of symptomatic osteoporosis with prolonged heparin treatment is low (about 2%) but subclinical osteopaenia may occur in up to a third of women.[59,60] Fortunately, this effect appears to be at least partly reversible and bone density generally improves with discontinuation of heparin. All women who have completed 10 weeks or more of heparin therapy should therefore undergo post-partum bone densitometry if there is any question of further heparin treatment, say in another pregnancy.

Thrombocytopaenia is the other main problem associated with heparin treatment. It exists in 2 forms – an early benign form with mild thrombo-cytopaenia occurring after one to several days of treatment; and a delayed condition which occurs 6–10 days after commencing treatment; the latter is an immune-mediated reaction associated with severe thrombocytopaenia, paradoxical arterial or venous thromboses with significant morbidity and mortality and requires immediate withdrawal of heparin treatment. Patients on long-term heparin treatment should have their platelet counts checked 1 week after commencing treatment and monthly thereafter.

Low molecular weight heparins

An increasingly attractive alternative to subcutaneous heparin is the low molecular weight heparins which are fragments of conventional heparin produced by enzymatic or chemical breakdown; they have molecular weights of 4–6 kDa and, like heparin, do not cross the placenta. They are also not teratogenic. Conventional heparin is made up of polysaccharides with mean molecular weights of 12–14 kDa; it produces its effects by combining with antithrombin III, forming a complex which has roughly equivalent inhibitory action on factor Xa and IIa (thrombin). By virtue of their shorter and lighter structures – which contain the anti-thrombin III binding site but not the longer saccharide chains necessary for factor IIa inhibition – low molecular weight heparins produce a predominantly antithrombotic effect through their inhibition of factor Xa with little anticoagulant activity. Therefore, when used in prophylactic doses, their anticoagulant effects are predictable with minimal alteration in the thrombin time and activated partial thromboplastin time.[61] Theoretically, this translates into a lower risk of haemorrhagic complications and, indeed, in a recent study on the use of low molecular weight heparin in pregnancy by Nelson-Piercy et al, there was no detectable increased risk of bleeding. Neither were there any cases of epidural haematoma or other complications related to the use of regional anaesthesia in the presence of low molecular weight heparin.[62] Other advantages include a lower risk of heparin-induced thrombocytopaenia because they are less likely to activate resting platelets to release platelet factor 4 and also bind less well to platelet factor 4; their increased bioavailability (85–90% compared to 10% for conventional heparin) and longer half-life (3–18 h) permit once daily administration and this is clearly advantageous in pregnancy where treatment can sometimes extend up to 10 months. Although one study has suggested that bone density loss associated with the use of low molecular weight heparin is comparable to the physiological loss of pregnancy, there are as yet insufficient clinical data and further investigation is required.[63] Currently, use of low molecular weight heparins in pregnancy is mainly confined to the chronic phase of treatment and to thromboprophylaxis. In the future, low molecular weight heparins may be used in high dosage for the acute treatment of thromboembolism as has already been advocated for the non-pregnant state.

Other modalities of treatment

Inferior vena caval filters have been used safely in pregnancy to prevent pulmonary embolisation in women with extensive deep vein thrombosis.[54] Other situations in which their use may be indicated include the following: (i) patients in whom anticoagulation is contra-indicated; and (ii) those who develop serious complications from anticoagulation, such as heparin-induced thrombocytopaenia or bleeding or when there is recurrent pulmonary embolism despite adequate anticoagulation. Several trials on the use of thrombolytic therapy to treat pulmonary embolism in non-pregnant patients have demonstrated more rapid resolution of ventilation-perfusion scan abnormalities. Whether this translates to improved clinical outcome remains to be proven. There is even less experience with thrombolytic use during pregnancy particularly since it is associated with risks of premature labour and haemorrhage. At this time, its use should be restricted to patients with haemodynamically unstable and life-threatening pulmonary embolism. Other measures such as mechanical clot dispersion and surgical embolectomy are similarly reserved for severely compromised patients.[57]

Thromboprophylaxis

Patients who require obstetric thromboprophylaxis need to be assessed individually to determine their degree of risk of developing thromboembolism during pregnancy and, therefore, the appropriate type and duration of anticoagulation. In general, our policy is to categorise patients either as high or low risk according to the various risk factors shown in Table 6.4. High risk patients are considered to be at risk throughout the pregnancy and the puerperium and, therefore, receive antenatal, intrapartum and post-partum anticoagulation. Low risk patients are thought to be most vulnerable from the time of labour through the puerperium and anticoagulation is given to cover this period of greatest risk. The benefits of antepartum heparin prophylaxis in low risk patients are not sufficient to outweigh the risks of heparin-induced osteoporosis and we, therefore, advocate only the use of low dose aspirin antenatally.[65] Additional separate guidelines for short term thromboprophylaxis at the time of caesarean section have been published by the Royal College of Obstetricians and Gynaecologists.[66] All these recommendations need to be supported or refuted by large well designed clinical trials.

Table 6.4 Thromboprophylaxis for previous thromboembolism in pregnancy and the puerperium

Risk category	Risk factors	Prophylaxis

High risk	Previous TED + thrombophilia
	Previous TED +
	  antiphospholipid syndrome
	Previous TED +
	  family history of TED
	Recurrent TED
	TED in current pregnancy
		Antenatal: s/c UH or LMWH
		Intrapartum: s/c UH or LMWH
		Postpartum: s/c UH or LMWH
		for 3–7 days followed by UH or
		LMWH or warfarin for a total of
		6 weeks

Low risk	One previous episode of TED (no other risk factors)	*Antenatal*: aspirin 75 mg o.d. Intrapartum: s/c UH or LMWH Postpartum: as for high risk

TED = thromboembolic disease; UH = unfractionated heparin; LMWH = low molecular weight heparin; s/c = subcutaneous.

CONCLUSIONS

The importance of thromboembolic disease in pregnancy, its prevention and treatment cannot be overemphasised. Despite advances in diagnostic tests as well as treatment, it still remains the leading cause of maternal mortality in the UK. Perhaps increasing awareness of the problem, recognition of new inherited thrombophilias and the more widespread utilisation of appropriate thrombo-prophylaxis may lead to a positive change in maternal mortality trends.

KEY POINTS FOR CLINICAL PRACTICE

- Thromboembolism is a major cause of maternal mortality
- Pregnancy is a hypercoagulable state which is associated with a 6-fold increased risk of thromboembolism
- Thromboembolism occurring in pregnancy and the puerperium is frequently multifactorial. Risk factors relevant to obstetrics include underlying thrombophilia, pre-eclampsia, maternal age, caesarean section, obesity, multiparity and immobility
- Maternal thrombophilia is associated with an increased risk of fetal loss
- Clinically suspected thromboembolic disease should always be confirmed objectively
- Heparin is the safest anticoagulant to use during pregnancy; warfarin is teratogenic particularly if exposure occurs between the 6th and 12th weeks of pregnancy
- Thromboprophylaxis should be appropriate for the level of risk

REFERENCES

1 Department of Health and Social Security. Report on Confidential Enquiries into Maternal Deaths in England and Wales, 1973–1975. London: HMSO, 1979

2 Department of Health and Social Security. Report on Confidential Enquiries into Maternal Deaths in England and Wales, 1976–1978. London: HMSO, 1982

3 Department of Health and Social Security. Report on Confidential Enquiries into Maternal Deaths in England and Wales, 1979-1981. London: HMSO, 1986

4 Department of Health and Social Security. Report on Confidential Enquiries into Maternal Deaths in the United Kingdom, 1982–1984. London: HMSO, 1989

5 Department of Health and Social Security. Report on Confidential Enquiries into Maternal Deaths in the United Kingdom, 1985–1987. London: HMSO, 1991

6 Department of Health and Social Security. Report on Confidential Enquiries into Maternal Deaths in the United Kingdom, 1988–1990. London: HMSO, 1994

7 Royal College of General Practitioners. Oral contraception and thromboembolic disease. J R Coll Gen Pract 1967; 13: 367–369

8 Bonnar J. The blood coagulation and fibrinolytic systems in the newborn and the mother. Br J Obstet Gynaecol 1971; 78: 355–360

9 Warwick R, Hutton R A, Croff L, Letsky E, Heard M. Changes in protein C and free protein S during pregnancy and following hysterectomy. J R Soc Med 1989; 82: 591–594

10 Badaracco M A, Vessey M. Recurrence of venous thromboembolic disease and use of oral contraceptives. BMJ 1974; i: 215–217

11 Bertina R M. Introduction: hypercoagulable states. Semin Hematol 1997; 34: 167–170

12 Miletich J P, Sherman L, Broze G. Absence of thrombosis in subjects with heterozygous protein C deficiency. N Engl J Med 1987; 317: 991–996

13 Dahlback B, Carlsson M, Svensson P J. Familial thrombophilia due to a previously unrecognised mechanism characterised by poor anticoagulant response to activated protein C: prediction of a cofactor to activated protein C. Proc Natl Acad Sci USA 1993; 90: 1004–1008

14 Rosendaal F R. Risk factors for venous thrombosis – prevalence, risk and interaction. Semin Hematol 1997; 34: 171–187

15 Heijboer H, Brandjes D P M, Buller H R et al. Deficiency of coagulation inhibiting proteins and fibrinolytic proteins in outpatients with deep vein thrombosis. N Engl J Med 1990; 323: 1512–1516

16 Eby C S. A review of the hypercoagulable state. Hematol Oncol Clin North Am 1993; 7: 1121–1142

17 Koster T, Rosendaal F R, De Ronde H et al. Venous thrombosis due to a poor anticoagulant response to activated protein C : Leiden Thrombophilia Study. Lancet 1993; 342: 1503–1506

18 Rosendaal F R, Koster T, Vandenbroucke J P et al. High risk of thrombosis in patients homozygous for factor V Leiden (activated protein C resistance). Blood 1995; 85: 1504–1508

19 Dahlback B. Resistance to activated protein C as risk factor for thrombosis: molecular mechanisms, laboratory investigations and clinical management. Semin Hematol 1997; 34: 217–234

20 Rees D C, Cox M, Clegg J B. World distribution of factor V Leiden. Lancet 1995; 346: 1133–1134

21 Bertina R M, Koeleman R P C, Koster T et al. Mutation in blood coagulation factor V associated with resistance to activated protein C. Nature 1994; 369: 64–67

22 Perry D J, Pasi K J. Resistance to activated protein C and factor V Leiden. QJM 1997; 90: 379–385

23 Ehrenforth S, Radtke K P, Scharrer I. Acquired activated protein C resistance in patients with lupus anticoagulants. Thromb Haemost 1995; 74: 797–798

24 Cumming A M, Tait R C, Fildes S, Yoong A, Keeney S, Hay C R M. Development of resistance to activated protein C during pregnancy. Br J Haematol 1995; 90: 725–727

25 Peek M J, Nelson-Piercy C, Manning R A, de Swiet M, Letsky E A. Activated protein C resistance in normal pregnancy. Br J Obstet Gynaecol 1997; 104: 1084–1086

26 Olivieri O, Friso S, Manzato F et al. Resistance to activated protein C in healthy women taking oral contraceptives. Br J Haematol 1995; 91: 465–470

27 Poort S R, Rosendaal F R, Reitsma P H, Bertina R M. A common genetic variation in the 3′-untranslated region of the prothrombin gene is associated with elevated plasma prothrombin levels and an increase in venous thrombosis. Blood 1996; 88: 3698–3703

28 Cumming A M, Keeney S, Salden A, Bhavnani M, Shure K H, Hay C R M. The prothrombin gene G20210A variant: prevalence in a UK anticoagulant clinic population. Br J Haematol 1997; 98: 353–355

29 van den Berg M, Boers G H J. Homocystinuria: what about mild hyperhomocystinaemia? Postgrad Med J 1996; 72: 513–518

30 den Heijer M, Blom H J, Gerrits W B J et al. Is hyperhomocystinaemia a risk factor for recurrent venous thrombosis? Lancet 1995; 345: 882–885

31 den Heijer M, Koster T, Blom H J et al. Hyperhomocystinaemia as a risk factor for deep vein thrombosis. N Engl J Med 1996; 334: 759–762

32 Hughes G R V. Thrombosis, abortion, cerebral disease and lupus anticoagulant. BMJ 1983; 28: 1088–1089

33 Asherson R A, Khamashta M A, Ordi-Ros J et al. The 'primary' antiphospholipid syndrome: major clinical and serological features. Medicine (Baltimore) 1989; 68: 366–374

34 Lie J T. Vasculopathy in the antiphospholipid syndrome: thrombosis or vasculitis or both? J Rheumatol 1989; 16: 713–715

35 Rosove M H, Brewer P M C. Antiphospholipid thrombosis: clinical outcome after the first thrombotic event in 70 patients. Ann Intern Med 1992; 117: 303–308

36 Khamashta M A, Cuadrado M J, Mujic F, Taub N A, Hunt B J, Hughes G R V. The management of thrombosis in the antiphospholipid syndrome. N Engl J Med 1995; 332: 993–997

37 Preston F E, Rosendaal F R, Walker I D et al. Increased fetal loss in women with heritable thrombophilia. Lancet 1996; 348: 913–916

38 Rai R, Regan L, Hadley E, Dave M, Cohen H. Second-trimester pregnancy loss is associated with activated protein C resistance. Br J Haematol 1996; 92: 489–490

39 Sanson B J, Friederich P W, Simioni P et al. The risk of abortion and stillbirth in antithrombin, protein C and protein S deficient women. Thromb Haemost 1996; 75: 387–388

40 Wouters M G A J, Boers G H J, Blom J H et al. Hyperhomocystinaemia: a risk factor in women with unexplained recurrent early pregnancy loss. Fertil Steril 1993; 60: 820–825

41 Piona A, La Rosa L, Tincani A et al. Placental thrombosis and fetal loss after passive transfer of mouse monoclonal or human polyclonal anticardiolipin antibodies in pregnant naïve BALB/c mice. Scand J Immunol 1995; 41: 427–432

42 Salafia C M, Parke A L. Placental pathology in systemic lupus erythematosus and phospholipid antibody syndrome. Rheum Dis Clin North Am 1997; 23: 85–96

43 Lubbe W F, Palmer S J, Butler W S, Liggins G C. Fetal survival after prednisone suppression of maternal lupus anticoagulant. Lancet 1983; 1: 1361–1363

44 Lockshin M D, Druzin M L, Qamar T. Prednisone does not prevent recurrent fetal death in women with antiphospholipid antibody. Am J Obstet Gynecol 1989; 160: 439–443

45 Cowchock S, Reece E A, Balaban D, Branch D W, Plouffe L. Repeated fetal losses associated with antiphospholipid antibodies: a collaborative randomized trial comparing prednisone with low-dose heparin treatment. Am J Obstet Gynecol 1992; 166: 1318–1323

46 Kutteh W H. Antiphospholipid antibody associated recurrent pregnancy loss: treatment with heparin and low dose aspirin is superior to low dose aspirin alone. Am J Obstet Gynecol 1996; 174: 1584–1589

47 Rai R, Cohen H, Dave M, Regan L. Randomised controlled trial of aspirin versus aspirin plus heparin in pregnant women with recurrent miscarriage associated with phospholipid antibodies (or antiphospholipid antibodies). BMJ 1997; 314: 253–257

48 The PIOPED Investigators. Value of the ventilation-perfusion scan in acute pulmonary embolism. Results of the prospective investigation of pulmonary embolism diagnosis. JAMA 1990; 263: 2753–2759

49 Cranley J J, Canos A J, Sull W J. The diagnosis of deep venous thrombosis: fallibility of clinical symptoms and signs. Arch Surg 1976; 111: 34–36

50 Sandler D A, Duncan J S, Ward P et al. Diagnosis of deep vein thrombosis: comparison of clinical evaluation, ultrasound plethysmography and venoscan with X-ray venogram. Lancet 1984; ii: 716–719

51 Lensing A W, Prandoni P, Brandjes D et al. Detection of deep vein thrombosis by real-time B-mode ultrasonography. N Engl J Med 1989; 320: 342–345

52 Toglia M, Weg J G. Venous thromboembolism during pregnancy. N Engl J Med 1996; 335: 108–114

53 Spritzer C E, Evans A C, Kay H H. Magnetic resonance imaging of deep vein thrombosis in pregnant women with lower extremity edema. Obstet Gynecol 1995; 85: 603–607

54 Ginsberg J S, Hirsh J, Rainbow A J, Coates G. Risks to the fetus of radiologic procedures used in the diagnosis of maternal venous thromboembolic disease. Thromb Haemost 1989; 61: 189–196

55 Cross J J L, Kemp P M, Flower C D R. Diagnostic imaging in pulmonary embolic disease. Br J Hosp Med 1997; 58: 93–96

56 Meaney J F M, Weg J G, Chenevert T L, Stafford-Johnson D, Hamilton B H, Prince M R. Diagnosis of pulmonary embolism with magnetic resonance angiography. N Engl J Med 1997; 336: 1422–1427

57 de Swiet M. Thromboembolism. In: de Swiet M. (ed) Medical Disorders in Obstetric Practice,. 3rd edn. Oxford: Blackwell Science, 1995; 116–142

58 Black A J, Topping J, Farquharson R, Fraser W D. Bone metabolism in pregnancy: a review. Contemp Rev Obstet Gynaecol 1996; 8: 192–196

59 Dahlman T C. Osteoporotic fractures and the recurrence of thromboembolism during pregnancy and the puerperium in 184 women undergoing thromboprophylaxis with heparin. Am J Obstet Gynecol 1993; 168: 1265–1278

60 Ginsberg J S, Hirsh J. Use of antithrombotic agents during pregnancy. Chest 1995; 108: 305S–311S

61 Nelson-Piercy C. Low molecular weight heparin for obstetric thromboprophylaxis. Br J Obstet Gynaecol 1994; 101: 6–8

62 Nelson-Piercy C, Letsky E A, de Swiet M. Low molecular weight heparin for obstetric thromboprophylaxis: experience of sixty-nine pregnancies in sixty-one women at high risk. Am J Obstet Gynecol 1997; 176: 1062–1068

63 Shefras J, Farquharson R G. Bone density studies in pregnant women receiving heparin. Eur J Obstet Gynecol Reprod Biol 1996; 65: 171–174

64 Narayan H, Cullimore J, Krarup K, Thurston H, Macvicar J, Bolia A. Experience with the cardial inferior vena cava filter as prophylaxis against pulmonary embolism in pregnant women with extensive deep vein thrombosis [Erratum, Br J Obstet Gynaecol 1992; 99: 726]. Br J Obstet Gynaecol 1992; 99: 637–640

65 Nelson-Piercy C. Obstetric thromboprophylaxis. Br J Hosp Med 1996; 55: 404–408

66 Report of the RCOG Working Party on Prophylaxis against Thromboembolism in Gynaecology and Obstetrics. London: Chameleon; 1995

J. Guy Thorpe-Beeston

Management of breech presentation at term

When a thing ceases to be a subject of controversy it ceases to be a subject of interest

William Hazlitt (1778–1830)

The intense controversy that breech presentation has generated in obstetrics is drawing to an end. The frequent calls to establish a prospective randomised trial have been answered by the prospect of a large international randomised controlled trial, co-ordinated in Toronto.[1] However, some have estimated that a sample size of 18 000–26 000 will be required and, with an optimistic 50% participation rate, a background population of 900 000 term births may be needed.[2] A multicentre study of this magnitude will have to be of long duration introducing the possibility of significant bias. Those who advocate caesarean section for the delivery of the breech infant point out that if the hypothesis that caesarean section proves to be the safer option an excess of 22 infants will die.[2] In contrast, those who support vaginal delivery will point to the increased maternal morbidity and possibly mortality in those subjected to a caesarean section.

Whilst some obstetricians maintain that the only evidence available is retrospective and therefore invalid, many others involved in the counselling of women at term with a breech presentation are guided by the retrospective data or their own experience. However, in response to the increasing demands of various pressure groups not to increase further the caesarean section rate, obstetricians are frequently simply offering women the choice of elective delivery or a trial of vaginal delivery.

INCIDENCE AND AETIOLOGY

The incidence of breech presentation at term is 3–4%. The incidence in the preterm population is higher, 14% at 29–32 weeks.[3] In the majority of cases of

Mr J. Guy Thorpe-Beeston, Consultant Obstetrician, Chelsea and Westminster Hospital, 369 Fulham Road, London SW10 9NH, UK

Table 7.1 Aetiology of breech presentation

Prematurity
Fetal abnormality   Neural tube defects
Hydrocephalus
Growth retardation
Uterine abnormality
Bicornuate uterus
Fibroids
Placenta praevia
Short umbilical cord
Polyhydramnios/oligohydramnios
Multiple pregnancy
Smoking
Maternal diabetes

breech presentation no specific underlying cause will be found. With the widespread use of high quality ultrasound, many of the rare events that may predispose to breech presentation will already have been excluded by the gestation at which decisions regarding the mode of delivery will have to be taken. (Table 7.1)

Nonetheless, fetal abnormality, particularly of the central nervous system such as hydrocephalus and anencephaly,[4,5] uterine abnormality,[6] placenta and cord abnormalities,[7,8] oligohydramnios, polyhydramnios[9] and multiple pregnancy[10] should always be considered when breech presentation is suspected clinically. In a population based case control study of 3588 breech cases, low birth weight, prematurity, primiparity and increasing maternal age were associated with an excess risk of breech birth. In addition, after controlling for these factors, hydrocephalus, established maternal diabetes, congenital malformation, maternal smoking and late or no antenatal care were all associated with an increase in the relative risk of breech presentation.[11]

Fifty years ago it was proposed that fetal kicking helped the fetus establish a cephalic presentation and it has been hypothesised that abnormalities in limb strength due to hypotonia in the lower limbs or neurological defects affecting general movements of the fetus may contribute to some neuromuscular dysfunction and consequent breech presentation.[12,13] The association of breech presentation with maternal diabetes described by Rayl et al[11] is a logical link in view of the reports of decreased fetal movements and the increased risk of congenital malformations described in these pregnancies.

ASSESSMENT OF BREECH PRESENTATION AT TERM

One of the few areas of agreement between authors on breech presentation is that vaginal delivery should not be attempted in all cases and that some form of antenatal selection is preferable. The list of 'normal' criteria however is extensive (Table 7.2). Ultrasound of the fetus not only confirms the presentation, but should specifically document the site of the placenta, fetal

Table 7.2 Criteria for trial of labour

Estimated fetal weight 1.5–3.8 kg
Extended breech
Exclusion of footling presentation or hyperextended neck
Structurally normal fetus
Normal liquor
Normal placental site
Exclusion of significant fibroids
Normal clinical assessment of maternal pelvis
Exclusion of significant maternal disease. e.g. diabetes, hypertension, cardiac

Additional factors	? No induction of labour
	? No augmentation of labour

growth and estimated fetal weight as well as the type of breech including the presence of a hyperextended neck, liquor volume and finally it will exclude the majority of structural abnormalities.

Although having a reasonable specificity, the sensitivity of manual palpation is poor.[14] Ultrasound, if available, should be used, particularly if procedures such as external cephalic version or caesarean section are contemplated. Indeed there is now evidence that the presence of a breech presentation, determined by ultrasound after 25 weeks' gestation is associated with an increased incidence of term breech presentation.[15] The estimation of fetal weight is of considerable importance in helping to determine the mode of delivery. Most authors suggest an upper estimated weight of 3.8 kg. However, the limitations of ultrasound, particularly in the third trimester should be borne in mind. Even in the best hands an error of ± 15% should be allowed for. There is evidence that the error is increased in breech presentation.[16]

Three types of breech presentation are recognised. The extended or frank breech in which the legs are flexed at the hips and extended at the knee is the most favourable position and is found in two-thirds of cases. The flexed breech and the footling or incomplete breech are both associated with an increased incidence of cord prolapse. The significance of a hyperextended neck or 'star gazing' fetus is unclear. Historically, the finding has been apparent on lateral X-ray pelvimetry. The incidence in small studies is 1.4–7.4%.[17,18] In cases where the angle of extension is greater than 90 degrees, 8 of 11 vaginally delivered infants were found to have damaged cervical cords and, therefore, caesarean section may be the preferred route of delivery in such cases.[19]

EXTERNAL CEPHALIC VERSION

The use of external cephalic version (ECV) after 37 weeks' gestation will decrease the need for caesarean section in breech presentation. The technique has been clearly described.[20] The advantages of ECV at term are that most spontaneous versions will already have occurred, other pregnancy problems such as pre-eclampsia will be apparent and, in the event of a complication, the rapid delivery of a mature fetus can be undertaken. Furthermore, the incidence of complications at ECV is lower after 36 weeks.[21] The success rate is approximately 50% although in some centres ECV has been achieved in 77% of cases.[22] In a recent study, the success rate of ECV was 39% and it appeared that experience in the procedure was not a factor affecting the success rate.[23]

Meta-analysis of the six prospective randomised studies have demonstrated conclusively that the procedure will reduce the number of breech births and caesarean sections.[24] The odds ratio for the reduction in breech births was 0.13 and for the reduction in caesarean section was 0.36. The practical implication of these statistics is that for every 100 attempted ECVs, there will be 34 fewer vaginal breech deliveries and 14 fewer caesarean sections. A number of studies have advocated the use of tocolysis; however, because of limited enrolment in the studies, the statistical power is such that no benefit has been shown for the routine use of tocolysis during external cephalic version.[25] In a prospective, double blind, randomised study, 283 patients received either ritodrine or identical placebo by intravenous infusion for more than 20 min prior to ECV. A higher rate of success (52%) was achieved in the group receiving tocolysis, particularly in nulliparous women, in whom the success rate was doubled. It may, therefore, be prudent to consider the use of tocolysis in selected primiparous women, but in parous women no significant benefit has been described and it has been suggested that it should not be used for this group of women.[26]

ECV is safe and, although a number of adverse fetal outcomes have been documented, in a review of 979 cases of ECV at term when neither general anaesthesia or inhalational anaesthesia were used, no fetal losses occurred.[27] It would seem sensible to undertake these procedures on the labour ward, with the benefit of ultrasound and with easy access to fetal monitoring with cardiotocography and emergency delivery if required. A transient bradycardia is often noted after version has occurred, and the evidence for any long-term effects on the fetus is still awaited. The evidence for the potential beneficial effects of ECV is now compelling and the option of ECV should at least be discussed with women with a known breech presentation and a record of the discussion documented in the notes.

If ECV is successful, it would appear that the pregnancy remains at increased risk of obstetric intervention. In a study of 243 term pregnancies that underwent ECV, the successful version rate was 69.5%. However, the subsequent incidence of intrapartum caesarean section was 16.9%, 2.25 times higher than that of the control group. The large number of abdominal deliveries was attributed to a significantly higher incidence of fetal distress and dystocic labour.[28] In another series, the rate of caesarean section was even higher, with 31% of women who had had a successful version requiring a caesarean section in labour.[29] In a smaller series of 76 women who had undergone a successful version, no difference was noted in the caesarean section rate between women in whom a successful version had been performed and the control population.[30]

In women with a breech presentation, many women will be well informed about the options available to them before they attend the antenatal clinic. A variety of non-conventional forms of treatment have been advocated to increase the likelihood of version. Simple adoption of the knee-chest position with the buttocks higher than the trunk or abduction of the thighs in addition to elevation of the pelvis, coupled with breathing techniques have been suggested.[31] Other techniques have included the use of hypnosis and acupuncture. In a study of 100 pregnant women whose fetuses were in the breech position at 37–40 weeks' gestation, hypnosis was used with suggestions for general relaxation with release of fear and anxiety. ECV was also offered. In the intervention group, the conversion rate was 81% compared with 48% of those in the comparison group. The study concluded that motivated subjects can be influenced by a skilled hypnotherapist in such a manner that their fetuses have a higher incidence of conversion from breech to vertex presentation.[32] Acupuncture has also been suggested as a potentially useful technique and the results of a randomised prospective trial are awaited.[33]

MODE OF DELIVERY

Prospective evidence

The current gold standard of obstetric evidence is the Cochrane systematic review. A meta-analysis of the only prospective randomised trials found no significant difference between the two approaches in terms of perinatal mortality (malformations having been excluded) (typical OR 0.22 (95% CI 0.00–14.52)) and Apgar score at 5 min (OR 0.64 (95% CI 0.18–2.34)). Predictably, elective caesarean section was associated with higher rates of maternal morbidity (OR 1.63 (95% CI 1.03–2.57)).[34] In the study by Collea et al, those randomised to the trial of labour had a significantly higher rate of fetal morbidity (excluding low Apgar scores) than the caesarean group (14 of 115 [12.2%] versus three of 93 [3.2%], $P = 0.04$).[35]

In the two prospective studies, only 313 women were recruited and 75 (41%) of these were then excluded from attempting a trial of labour because of abnormal pelvimetry.[35,36] This suggests that either the population was abnormal or that the obstetricians had a very cautious interpretation of the pelvimetry. After excluding deaths from congenital malformations, one baby was lost following a vaginal delivery. The results of these studies and their meta-analysis do not suggest that caesarean section is a better option than vaginal delivery for the fetus. There are major limitations in the studies, principally in the small numbers recruited and thus the validity of any conclusions are questionable.

Retrospective evidence

The policy of delivering term breeches by elective caesarean section was based on a number of studies that reported a better neonatal outcome than that achieved following vaginal delivery. On the other hand, vaginal delivery for selected cases has been reported in a number of studies to result in perinatal outcome similar to those of abdominal delivery. Whilst accepting the limitations of retrospective studies, because of the paucity of prospective evidence, it is important to examine all the available data rather than completely disregard it.

In a painstaking systematic review, Cheng and Hannah searched the world literature from 1966 to 1992 and compared planned vaginal and elective caesarean deliveries with respect to perinatal mortality, low Apgar score at 5 min, neonatal morbidity, long term morbidity and mortality.[37] Inherent in such a study are several methodological problems, in particular the small sample sizes of most of the individual studies, incomplete or poorly defined outcome measures and the non-randomisation of cases to either trial of labour or no trial of labour. These limitations need to be born in mind when considering the results of the study, but in the absence of a randomised trial, observational data may be the only way of assessing the fetal risk. The corrected perinatal mortality rate was 9.7 per 1000 births (range 0–48) in the group of women allowed to labour and deliver vaginally and was higher than in the planned caesarean section group (0.5 per 1000 births, typical OR 3.86 (95% CI 2.22–6.69).

In a more recent meta-analysis of the retrospective studies that are available, it was estimated that the risk of any injury to the baby was 1% after a trial of labour and 0.09% after elective caesarean section. For any injury or death, the risk was 1.23% after a trial of labour and 0.09% after elective caesarean section. These findings suggest an increased risk of injury and injury or death for the baby after a trial of labour.[38]

In examining the retrospective data, other than the evidence presented in individual or hospital series, data have been emerging from a number of large databases comprising many thousands of deliveries. Undoubtedly the safe conduct of a trial of vaginal breech delivery is more likely if the individual obstetrician or institution has considerable experience of such cases. Such individual series continue to be published and the conclusions of these studies are that routine caesarean section for breech presentation is not warranted.[29,39] Unfortunately, the data from population studies conclude that vaginal breech delivery is more hazardous for the baby both in terms of morbidity and mortality,[40–44] except for one study.[45] This discrepancy is likely to be explained not by protocol violations, poor selection and inappropriate management as is often suggested, but by publication bias. Few individual practitioners or institutions will be keen to publicise their poor outcomes, but they will be picked up by large population studies.

PELVIC ASSESSMENT FOR TRIAL OF LABOUR

When attempting to 'select' suitable cases for a trial of vaginal delivery, considerable emphasis has been placed over recent years in assessment of the maternal pelvis. The clinical assessment of the sacral promontory, sacral curvature, ischial spines, sacrospinous ligaments and the intertuberous diameter is entirely subjective, but many would argue it remains the single most important form of maternal assessment and there are few substitutes for the clinical experience of the obstetrician. Maternal height is also a valuable guide to pelvic capacity.[46]

The value of X-ray pelvimetry in the assessment for vaginal breech delivery is controversial. Radiological information about the bony pelvis has been recommended by some authorities and an improved fetal outcome reported.[47,48] However fetal exposure to radiation increases the risk of subsequent malignancy before the age of 10 years and a linear dose-dependent relationship was described following obstetric X-ray examinations.[49,50] The other principal disadvantages are the varying quality of the images, the differing interpretation of the bony dimensions and the lack of information about soft tissue compliance.[51] It has been established that the bony diameters, in both the transverse and anterior posterior dimensions, may increase by as much as 28% in women between the supine and squatting positions.[52]

Undoubtedly the use of CT scanning will provide a more accurate and reproducible assessment of the pelvic size and anatomy, but it has never been compared to erect lateral X-ray pelvimetry and is performed lying down. The technique has the advantage of significantly reducing the radiation dose to which the fetus is exposed. It has been estimated that computed tomographic pelvimetry exposes the fetus to at least 82 mrad, in contrast to between 500 and 1100 mrad at the time of conventional X-ray pelvimetry.[53,54] In a study of 394 breech deliveries, 122 patients underwent computed tomographic pelvimetry. Eight-five (70%) of the patients fulfilled the criteria of adequate pelvimetry which was defined as: anteroposterior diameter of the inlet 10.0 cm, transverse diameter of inlet 11.5 cm, transverse (interspinous) diameter of midpelvis 9.5 cm, and posterior sagittal diameter of midpelvis 4.0 cm. Sixty nine (81%) of the study group had successful vaginal deliveries, with no difference in infant outcome between the group delivered vaginally and those delivered by caesarean section.[55] These results are excellent; however, the cost and availability of this facility may prevent its widespread application in many institutions. As with many of the trials purporting to resolve the dilemma of breech delivery, the numbers involved in the trials are very small.

INDUCTION OF LABOUR, AUGMENTATION & ANALGESIA

Assuming a trial of labour is the preferred option for the mother, two further issues are frequently raised in relation to breech delivery. Induction of labour and the use of oxytocin to augment labour remain controversies to which there are no answers to be found in the literature. Whilst many argue that a spontaneous onset of labour is an excellent predictor of a successful vaginal delivery, and that an induction may compound the potential problems of a breech, others suggest that induction may be appropriate to prevent the baby from becoming too big. With regard to the use of oxytocin, again some authors are keen to avoid its use for the fear of masking feto-maternal disproportion. Others assume that because oxytocin is used in many women to augment slow progress due to primary dysfunctional labour characteristic in primigravidae, then, if one is undertaking a trial of labour, it is appropriate to use oxytocin cautiously. The use of an intra-uterine pressure catheter under these circumstances might aid the judicious use of syntocinon and help to avoid hyperstimulation and forcing a baby that is too large into the pelvic cavity.

Epidural anaesthesia is often advocated for the labouring woman with a breech presentation. It is suggested that because of the significant risk that some form of assisted delivery will be required, either vaginally or abdominally, the early siting of an epidural is preferable to the emergency administration of either local or general anaesthesia. However, there is evidence that the use of epidural anaesthesia is associated with an increased incidence of caesarean delivery in both multiparous and primiparous women. In a retrospective study of 643 women (243 primparae and 370 multiparae) with a singleton breech presentation and spontaneous onset of labour, epidural anaesthesia was associated with a longer duration of labour in both the first and second stages, an increased use of oxytocin (37% and 39% in primiparae and multiparae using epidural anaesthesia) and a significantly higher caesarean section rate in the second stage in labour.[56] These findings indirectly support the argument that epidural anaesthesia may reduce the intensity of uterine activity. In addition, there is little doubt that women will push more effectively without the use of epidural anaesthesia. Therefore, provided the woman remains 'in control', it seems reasonable to discuss the use of epidural rather than to insist on its use. Clearly it is important that the woman remains co-operative during the second stage and the epidural is often advised in order that the obstetrician and the woman may retain control during any manipulations that may prove necessary during the second stage.

EMERGENCY MEASURES

Undiagnosed breech presentation will remain a feature of practical obstetrics. In a study of 305 singleton breech presentations, 79 (26%) were first diagnosed in labour.[57] Vaginal delivery was more common in those diagnosed intrapartum than in those delivered in the antenatal period and allowed to deliver vaginally (OR 1.68, 95% CI 1.0–3.0). The authors noted that women admitted with a cervical dilatation in labour of less than 3 cm were more likely to be delivered by caesarean section. Other than the degree of cervical dilatation the only significant assessment undertaken in the study was an estimate of the fetal weight. The authors emphasised that good perinatal outcome will heavily depend on close supervision of the labour and experienced medical staff.

A variety of emergency procedures have been described which may provide an escape from the obstetric nightmare of an obstructed aftercoming head. If the head fails to descend into the pelvis after the shoulders have delivered, attempts should be made using suprapubic pressure and increased flexion of the maternal hips and abduction of the thighs, gentle rotation of the body and insertion of a finger into the babies pharynx to bring the head into the maternal pelvis. Continued failure to do so may be an indication for undertaking a symphysiotomy, but the untrained practitioner should be wary of undertaking any procedure that he or she is not familiar with. Occasionally, the fetal body may be expelled through an incompletely dilated cervix. This is a particular problem in the preterm breech. In this case incision of the cervix at 4 o'clock and 8 o'clock will rapidly expedite delivery.

Intravenous nitroglycerine has been used in one case and it has been speculated that it acts by inducing uterine relaxation and may cause a change in the cervical architecture.[58]

In very rare cases of fetal head entrapment, abdominal rescue has been possible. However, this undoubtedly should remain an option of last resort in cases of head entrapment.[59]

SHORT-TERM OUTCOME

Not only are the studies examining short term outcome methodologically flawed, but the end points measuring fetal well-being are imprecise. Again, the retrospective data consist mainly of small studies which report no difference in short-term outcome for the fetus. However, despite the imperfect nature of the data overall, there is a consistently higher rate of neonatal traumatic morbidity in cases of planned vaginal delivery with typical OR of 3.96 (95% CI 2.76–5.67).[37] The types of birth injury include minor problems such as bruising and lacerations, but also a significant number of cases of skull fracture and intracranial haemorrhage. The incidence of brachial plexus injury is 8.5% and, whilst 70% of such cases resolve spontaneously, these figures suggest that over 1–2% infants delivered vaginally by the breech will suffer significant brachial plexus injury.[20,37] The protagonists of caesarean delivery can make a strong case for elective delivery on this point alone.

Jaundice, asphyxia, birth injury and sepsis occurs in 1–11.6% of all infants and a worse overall outcome is experienced with planned vaginal delivery.[37] These studies differ in their quality and measure different maternal and neonatal outcomes.

LONG-TERM OUTCOME

Conflicting reports concerning the long-term outcome of mature breech infants abound in the literature. Many studies have only reported on short-term outcome. A critical review of only three papers addressing long-term outcome concluded that infant morbidity seemed to occur more frequently among infants in the planned vaginal delivery groups, with a typical OR 2.88 (95% CI 1.04–7.97).[37,60–62] The three studies included 1068 vaginal breech deliveries and 272 infants delivered by caesarean section. In the vaginal delivery group, 16 of the 25 affected children had cerebral palsy. In contrast, only one infant delivered by caesarean section suffered subsequent cerebral palsy. However, in two of the studies only those with early signs of complication were followed,[60,61] whereas the third study compared two different methods of selection for vaginal delivery in two consecutive 4 year periods.[62] In this study, 5 infants were lost to follow-up and, therefore, under-reporting of adverse outcome is a possibility.

The methodological quality of these studies is questionable and Danielian et al examined the long-term morbidity (up to 4–5 years of age) of 1645 infants delivered in breech presentation between 1981–90 at term by a planned method of delivery.[63] Data for this study were obtained from maternity, health visitor, and school medical records and the handicap register. 1055 cases were intended vaginal deliveries and 590 (35.9%) underwent elective caesarean section. Handicap or other health problems were documented in 19.4% of the infants in whom it was possible to obtain medical records. There were no significant differences between the two groups in terms of severe handicap, developmental delay, neurological deficit or psychiatric referral. In only one of the 12 cases of handicap in the planned vaginal delivery group was the

Table 7.3 Antenatal consultation – points for discussion

Trial of vaginal delivery	Elective LSCS
External cephalic version	Maternal haemorrhage
	Maternal thrombosis/embolism
Risk of fetal mortality	Maternal infection
Risk of fetal morbidity	
Use of epidural	
Personnel present at delivery	
Place of delivery	
Description of vaginal breech delivery	
Success rate of trial of vaginal delivery	
Risk of emergency LSCS	

handicap attributable to the delivery. The very high rate of long-term disability among those delivered by the breech in this study, irrespective of the mode of delivery re-inforces the long held belief that there may be an inherent abnormality in such fetuses.

MAKING A DECISION

Despite strongly held views on both sides of the argument, many obstetricians feel that there is no 'right' or 'wrong' method of delivery. It should be the responsibility of the obstetrician to inform the mother, in the clearest terms possible of the evidence, imperfect though it may be, relating to perinatal morbidity and mortality. The risks of caesarean section, the nature of a trial of vaginal delivery, its success rate and the option of external cephalic version should all be clearly outlined and documented (Table 7.3). Many women may be encouraged to learn that, if they elect to have a caesarean section, over 80% of those allowed to labour in a second pregnancy will be able to achieve a vaginal delivery.[64]

Decision analysis has been used in an attempt to answer the question of the optimum mode of delivery. Thornton points out that it is not appropriate to compare the maternal risks of caesarean section with the fetal risks of vaginal delivery.[65] The decision is, in fact, between a trial of vaginal delivery (and its inherent failure rate) and an elective caesarean section. Assuming a very modest 20% rate of failed trial of labour, a policy of elective caesarean section would carry a lower maternal mortality than a trial of vaginal delivery. A policy of elective caesarean section would result in two maternal deaths per 100 000 procedures, but save 200 babies.

Cost and medicolegal concerns may often cloud the issues when difficult decisions are being contemplated and they are inseparable. A 'policy' of elective caesarean delivery may at first glance appear more expensive, but one surviving handicapped infant will rapidly exhaust any 'savings' an institution may consider it has made by opting for a policy of vaginal delivery. Undoubtedly, there are fewer instances of litigation following elective abdominal delivery, provided adequate counselling is undertaken and the options, including external cephalic version, discussed and appropriately noted.

Parents may ask what would be the personal choice of the clinician in such circumstances. In a structured anonymous postal survey of nearly 300 obstetricians, respondents where asked to answer if they or their partners were pregnant for the first time what their preferred mode of delivery would be assuming an otherwise uncomplicated breech presentation.[66] 57% opted for elective delivery rather than a trial of labour, a figure not dissimilar to the caesarean section rate in primparous women with a breech presentation in many hospitals across the UK and less than in many.

The issue of training and operator experience is not a new one and there is no substitute for experience. Obstetricians in training will have a far greater experience of caesarean delivery than vaginal breech delivery. The dilemma is how will obstetricians or, indeed, midwives in the Western world obtain the necessary experience of vaginal breech delivery? Any trial of vaginal breech delivery should be managed by the most senior member of the 'on-call' team. It is important that every opportunity is taken to ensure that junior obstetric staff are allowed to develop these skills, especially as 10–15% of breeches present late in labour. Obstetricians will always have to be able to deliver a breech baby vaginally.

CONCLUSIONS

The existing evidence regarding the optimal management is imperfect and, even if there was a prospective trial of significant magnitude, there remains an element of the equation to which it is impossible to assign a statistic or number, the individual woman's feelings. For some women labour is an integral and treasured experience of pregnancy, something to be looked forward to, and achieving a vaginal delivery a life event of enormous magnitude. For others, delivery is an unwelcome bridge that has to be crossed and the option of a caesarean section may appear to be the answer to quiet prayers. The answer must surely be to offer individual choice after appropriate consultation based on existing data, allowing time for reflection before arriving at a final decision.

REFERENCES

1 Hannah M, Hannah W. Caesarean section or vaginal birth for breech presentation at term. BMJ 1996; 312: 1433–1434
2 Krebs L, Langhoff-Roos J, Weber T. Breech at term – mode of delivery? A register study. Acta Obstet Gynecol Scand 1995; 74: 702–706
3 Haughey M J. Fetal position during pregnancy. Am J Obstet Gyncecol 1985; 153: 885–886
4 Mazor M, Hagay Z J, Leiberman J, Baile Y, Insler V. Fetal abnormalities associated with breech delivery. J Reprod Med 1985; 30: 884–886
5 Westgren L M, Ingemarsson I. Breech delivery and mental handicap. Ballières Clin Obstet Gynecol 1988; 2: 187–194
6 Ranney B. The gentle art of external cephalic version. Am J Obstet Gynecol 1973; 116: 239–248
7 Soernes T, Bakke T. The length of the human umbilical cord in vertex and breech presentations. Am J Obstet Gynecol 1986; 154: 1086–1087
8 Stevenson C S. The principal cause of breech presentation in single term pregnancies. Am J Obstet Gynecol 1950; 60: 41–53
9 Hall J E, Kohl S. Breech presentation. Am J Obstet Gynecol 1956; 72: 977–990

10 Kian L S. The role of placental site in the aetiology of breech presentation. J Obstet Gynecol 1963; 70: 795–797

11 Rayl J R, Gibson P J, Hickok D E. A population-based case-controlled study of risk factors for breech presentation. Am J Obstet Gynecol 1996; 174: 28–32

12 Dunn P M. Maternal and fetal aetiological factors to breech presentation. In: Rooth G, Bratteby L. E. (eds) Perinatal medicine: Fifth European congress of perinatal medicine. Stockholm: Almquist and Wiskell, 1976; 76–81

13 Sival D A. Studies on fetal motor behaviour in normal and complicated pregnancies. Early Hum Dev 1993; 34: 13–20

14 Thorp J M, Jenkins T, Watson W. Utility of Leopold manoeuvres in screening for malpresentation. Obstet Gynecol 1991; 78: 394–396

15 Tadmor O P, Habinowitz R, Alon L, Mostoslavsky V, Aboulafia Y, Diamant Y Z. Can breech presentation at birth be predicted from ultrasound examination during the second and third trimester? Int J Obstet Gynecol 1994; 46: 11–14

16 Chauhan S P, Magann E F, Naef 3rd R W, Martin Jr J N, Morrison J C. Sonographic assessment of birth weight among breech presentations. Ultrasound Obstet Gynecol 1995; 6: 54–57

17 Westgren M, Edvall H, Nordstrom E, Svalenius E. Spontaneous cephalic version of breech presentation in the last trimester. Br J Obstet Gynaecol 1985; 92: 19–22

18 Ophir E, Oettinger M, Yagoda A, Markovitis Y, Rojansky N, Shapiro H. Breech presentation after a caesarean section: always a section? Am J Obstet Gynecol 1989; 161: 25–28

19 Ballas S, Toaff R. Hyperextension of the fetal head in breech presentation: radiological evaluation and significance. Br J Obstet Gynaecol 1976; 83: 201–201

20 Penn Z J, Steer P J. Breech presentation. In: James D K, Steer P J, Weiner C P, Gonik B. (eds) High Risk Pregnancy Management Options. London: WB Saunders, 1994; 173–198

21 Saling E, Muller-Holve W. External cephalic version under tocolysis. J Perinat Med 1975; 3: 115–121

22 Zhang J, Bowes Jr W A, Fortney J A. Efficacy of external cephalic version: a review. Obstet Gynecol 1993; 82: 306–312

23 Healy M, Porter R, Galimberti A. Introducing external cephalic version at 36 or more in a district general hospital: a review and audit. Br J Obstet Gynaecol 1997; 104: 1073–1079

24 Hofmeyr G J. External cephalic version at term. In: Neilson J P, Crowther C A, Hodnett E D, Hofmeyr G J, Kierse M J N C. (eds) Pregnancy and Childbirth Module of The Cochrane Database of Systematic Reviews, [updated 03 June 1997]. Available in The Cochrane Library [database on disk and CDROM]. The Cochrane Collaboration; issue 3. Oxford: Update Software; 1997

25 Hofmeyr G J. Routine tocolysis for external cephalic version at term. In: Neilson J P, Crowther C A, Hodnett E D, Hofmeyr G J, Kierse M J N C. (eds) Pregnancy and Childbirth Module of The Cochrane Database of Systematic Reviews, [updated 03 June 1997]. Available in The Cochrane Library [database on disk and CDROM]. The Cochrane Collaboration; issue 3. Oxford: Update Software; 1997

26 Marquette G P, Boucher M, Theriault D, Rinfret D. Does the use of a tocolytic agent affect the success rate of external cephalic version? Am J Obstet Gynecol 1996; 175: 859–861

27 Hofmeyr G J. Breech presentation and abnormal lie in late pregnancy. In: Chalmers I, Enkin M W, Keirse M J N C. (eds) Effective Care in Pregnancy and Childbirth. Oxford: OUP, 1989; 653–665

28 Lau T K, Kit K W, Rogers M. Pregnancy outcome after successful external cephalic version for breech presentation at term. Am J Obstet Gynecol 1997; 176: 218–223

29 Laros Jr R K, Flanagan T A, Kilpatrick S J. Management of term breech presentation: a protocol of external cephalic version and selective trial of labor. Am J Obstet Gynecol 1995; 172: 1916–1923

30 Egge T, Schauberger C, Schaper A. Dysfunctional labor after external cephalic version. Obstet Gynecol 1994; 83: 771–773

31 Bung P, Huch R, Huch A. 1st die undische avendung der Beckenendelage frequenz. Geburtsh Frauenheild 1987; 47: 202–205

32 Mehl L E. Hypnosis and conversion of the breech to the vertex presentation. Arch Family Med 1994; 3: 881–887

33 Cardini F, Marcolongo A. Moxibustion for correction of breech presentation: a clinical study with retrospective control. Am J Chin Med 1993; 21: 133–138

34 Hofmeyr G J. Planned elective caesarean section for term breech presentation [revised 10 July 1995]. In: Kierse M J N C, Renfrew M J, Nielson J P, Crowther C, (eds) Pregnancy and childbirth module. In: The Cochrane database of systematic reviews. Issue 2, Oxford: Cochrane Collaboration, 1995

35 Collea J V, Chein C, Quilligan E J. The randomized management of term frank breech presentation: a study of 208 cases. Am J Obstet Gynecol 1980; 137: 235–244

36 Gimovsky M L, Wallace R L, Schifrin B S, Paul R H. Randomized management of the nonfrank breech presentation at term: a preliminary report. Am J Obstet Gynecol 1983; 146: 34–40

37 Cheng M, Hannah M. Breech delivery at term: a critical review of the literature. Obstet Gynecol 1993; 82: 605–618

38 Spelliscy Gifford D, Mortoon S C, Fiske M, Kahn K. A meta-analysis of infant outcomes after breech delivery. Obstet Gynecol 1995; 85: 1047–1054

39 Schiff E, Friedman S A, Mashiach S, Hart O, Barkai G, Sibai B. Maternal and neonatal outcome of 846 term singleton breech deliveries: seven-year experience at a single center. Am J Obstet Gynecol 1996; 175: 18–23

40 Sachs B P, McCarthy B J, Rubin G, Burton A, Terry J, Tyler C W. Cesarean section: risks and benefits for mother and fetus. JAMA 1983; 250: 2157–2159

41 Fortney J A, Higgins J E, Kennedy K I, Laufe L E, Wilkens L. Delivery type and neonatal mortality among 10 749 breeches. Am J Public Health 1986; 76: 980–985

42 Kiely J L. Mode of delivery and neonatal death in 17 587 infants presenting by the breech. Br J Obstet Gynaecol 1991; 98: 898–904

43 Thorpe-Beeston J G, Banfield P J, Saunders N J St G. Outcome of breech delivery at term. BMJ 1992; 305: 746–747

44 Krebs L, Langhoff-Roos J, Weber T. Breech at term – mode of delivery? A register-based study. Acta Obstet Gynecol Scand 1995; 74: 702–706

45 Schutte M F, van Hemel O J S, van de Berg C, van de Pol A. Perinatal mortality in breech presentation as compared to vertex presentations in singleton pregnancies: an analysis based upon 57 819 computer-registered pregnancies in The Netherlands. Eur J Obstet Gynecol Reprod Biol 1985; 19: 391–400

46 Todd W D, Steer C M. Term breech: review of 1006 term breech deliveries. Obstet Gynecol 1963; 22: 583–595

47 Joyce D N, Gime-Osagie F, Stevenson G W. Role of pelvimetry in active management of labour. BMJ 1975; 4: 505–507

48 Riddley J W, Jackson P, Stewart J H et al. Role of antenatal radiography in the management of breech delivery. Br J Obstet Gynaecol 1982; 89: 342–347

49 Redie D, Davidson J K. The radiation hazard in radiography of the female abdomen and pelvis. Br J Radiol 1967; 40: 489–492

50 Bithell J F, Stewart A M. Prenatal irradiation and childhood malignancy; a review of British data from the Oxford Survey. Br J Cancer 1975; 31: 271–287

51 Barton J J, Garbaciak J A, Laude D W. X-ray pelvimetry in clinical obstetrics. Obstet Gynecol 1980; 56: 296–300

52 Russell J G B. Moulding of the pelvic outlet. J Obstet Gynaecol Br Commonw 1969; 76: 817–820

53 Kitzmiller J L, Mall J C, Gin G D, Hendricks S K, Newman R B, Scheerer L. Measurement of fetal shoulder width with computed tomography in diabetic women. Obstet Gynecol 1987; 70: 941–945

54 Colcher A E, Sussman W. A practical technique for roentgen pelvimetry with a new positioning. Am J Roentgenol Radium Ther Nucl Med 1944; 51: 207–214

55 Christian S S, Brady K, Read J A, Kopelman J N. Vaginal breech delivery: a five-year prospective evaluation of a protocol using computed tomographic pelvimetry. Am J Obstet Gynecol 1990; 163: 848–855

56 Chadha Y C, Mahmood T A, Dick M J, Smith N C, Campbell D M, Templeton A. Breech delivery and epidural anaesthesia. Br J Obstet Gynaecol 1992; 99: 96–100

57 Nwosu E C, Walkinshaw S, Chia P, Manasse P R, Atlay R D. Undiagnosed breech. Br J Obstet Gynaecol 1993; 100: 531–535

58 Abouleish A, Corn S. Nitorglycerin for fetal head entrapment following vaginal breech delivery? Anesth Analg 1995; 81: 654–655

59 Sandberg E C. The Zavanelli maneuver extended: progression of a revolutionary concept. Am J Obstet Gynecol 1988; 158: 1347–1353

60 Bistoletti P, Nisell H, Palme C, Lagercrantz H. Term breech delivery: early and late complications. Act Obstet Gynecol Scand 1981; 60: 165–171

61 Ohlsen H. Outcome of term breech delivery in primigravidae. A feto-pelvic breech index. Act Obstet Gynecol Scand 1975; 54: 141–151

62 Svenningsen N W, Westgren M, Ingemarsson I. Modern strategy for the term breech delivery – a study with a 4-year follow-up of the infants. J Perinat Med 1985; 13: 117–126

63 Danielian P J, Wang J, Hall M H. Long term outcome by method of delivery of fetuses in breech presentation at term: population based follow up. BMJ 1996; 312: 1451–1453

64 Coltart T M, Davies J A, Katesmark M. Outcome of a second pregnancy after a previous caesarean section. Br J Obstet Gynaecol 1990; 97: 1140–1143

65 Thornton J G. Decision analysis. In: Cooke I E, Sackett D L. Ballière's Clin Obstet Gynaecol 1996; 10: 677–695

66 Al-Mufti R, McCarthy A, Fisk N M. Obstetricians' personal choice and mode of delivery. Lancet 1996; 347: 544

Robert D. Macdonald   Sanjay K. Vyas

Cervical incompetence

Cervical incompetence has long been recognised as a potential cause of pre-term delivery. The splendid description by Cole and Culpepper (1658) quoted by Adrian Grant in the *Effective Care of Pregnancy and Childbirth*,[1] although in unusual language, provides an elegant definition of cervical incompetence:

> ......*the orifice of the womb is so slack that it cannot rightly contract itself to keep in the seed; which is chiefly caused by abortion or hard labour and childbirth, whereby the fibres of the womb are broken in pieces one from another and they, and the inner orifice of the womb overmuch slackened.*

The phrase 'cervical incompetence' was first used in the mid 19th century, and consideration of possible treatment began in the early part of this century, with surgical 'repair' of the cervix being described in the 1930s and 1940s.[2] However, it was the description of surgical cervical cerclage, and the subsequent successful outcomes, initially by Shirodkar in India[3] and then McDonald in Australia[4] that provided the starting point for the present-day enthusiasm for cervical cerclage in cases of presumed cervical incompetence.

DEFINITION

The fundamental problem with the concept of cervical incompetence is the definition, or more precisely the lack of one. A diagnosis of cervical incompetence is usually made on the basis of the woman's past obstetric history. Classically, this consists of one or more late second trimester or early third trimester losses, characterised by a rapid, often relatively pain-free delivery, commonly following the rupture of membranes prior to labour and

Mr Sanjay K. Vyas MD MRCOG, Consultant Obstetrician and Gynaecologist, Department of Women's Health, Southmead Hospital, Westbury on Trym, Bristol BS10 5NB, UK

Dr Robert D. Macdonald MB ChB, Obstetric Research Fellow, Department of Women's Health, Southmead Hospital, Westbury on Trym, Bristol BS10 5NB, UK

in the absence of an obvious precipitating cause. This description of cervical incompetence is subjective (both on the part of the woman and the obstetrician) and also retrospective; a difficulty we will attempt to address later in the chapter.

INCIDENCE

The precise incidence of a condition with a subjective, retrospective diagnosis is difficult. Figures between 0.05–1% of all pregnancies have been suggested.[5] One method of obtaining an estimate of the incidence of cervical incompetence is to look at the cervical cerclage rate, i.e. the extent to which the usual treatment for the condition is used. Unfortunately, this also provides a wide variety of answers: cerclage rates vary from 30 per 1000 births (3%) in France to 5 per 1000 (0.5%) in Scotland, with an average of 0.8% in Britain as a whole.[1] This variation hides an even larger discrepancy between individual consultants, with cerclage rates of anything from 0–80 per 1000 births reported.[1] The implication is that neither the definition nor the treatment are standardised or totally accepted.

AETIOLOGY

The original description by Cole and Culpepper in the 17th century clearly implicated abortion or 'hard labour' in causing cervical incompetence, and an acquired cervical weakness due to forcible dilatation and subsequent damage is still considered to have a causative association. From epidemiological studies, up to two first trimester terminations of pregnancy are usually not considered a risk factor for a pre-term labour,[6,7] but three or more terminations or spontaneous miscarriages do carry a significant risk (12% or a relative risk of 5.6) of a subsequent pre-term delivery.[6,7] Significantly, a single second trimester abortion carries a 14% risk of a subsequent pre-term delivery.[7] Although there may be many related factors that contribute to these risks, most notably social factors and smoking, both of which are related to terminations of pregnancy, it is intriguing to note that the greater the surgical dilatation of the cervix (whether in terms of number of terminations or the degree of dilatation required for a late termination), the greater the subsequent risk of a pre-term delivery. Related to this issue, there is, however, no clear cut answer with regard to cervical surgery, cervical biopsies and pre-term labour; a large Danish study[8] found some increased risk of a pre-term delivery following cervical conisation, whilst a significant study in Aberdeen following women after a large loop excision of the transformation zone (LLETZ) showed no increased risk of a pre-term delivery.[9]

Evidence has also been reported for a possible congenital cause for some cases of cervical incompetence. Peterson et al[10] published results of histological investigation of women who had lost their first pregnancy as a result of what was thought to be cervical incompetence, with no history of previous cervical surgery. There were significant differences between the study group and the control group in terms of hydroxyproline concentration (a measure of cervical collagen concentration) and extractability (a measure of collagen stability) as well as marked differences between the pregnant and non-pregnant cervices. This final point has been demonstrated in previous studies,[11] where marked changes in the cervix, including loss of the structural integrity and loss of collagen (over 70%)[12] and the structurally important glycosaminoglycans (GAGs) occurs prior to, and during, labour. If these changes are required in the normal process of cervical effacement and dilatation, a congenitally structurally abnormal cervix, which at the outset of pregnancy has some of the features associated with cervical change (i.e. loss of collagen and cervical stability), would present a significant risk for recurrent pre-term delivery.

It must be remembered that the cervix is not simply a passive organ to be stretched and dilated in term (or pre-term) labour, but has an active role in maintaining competence. The cervical remodelling described above is a necessary step prior to the onset of labour, and the failure of this to occur (i.e. the absence of the collagen changes and reduction of elastin and muscle content) is shown in demonstrable cervical contractions during labour, and an increased possibility of a prolonged latent phase and slow progress in labour.[13] With regards to pre-term labour, one would assume the same process prior to or during labour is required to produce cervical effacement and dilatation, whilst in certain cases of threatened pre-term labour, where uterine contractions occur but without cervical effacement or dilatation, the necessary cervical remodelling has not occurred so labour does not progress.[14] This tends to imply that cervical competence is an active, not passive, phenomenon, and that cervical incompetence is a specific entity involving not just an abnormality or defect of cervical collagen as described by Peterson,[10] but is also due to either the absence of the usual cervical musculature in cases of congenital cervical incompetence, or injury or damage to the cervical musculature caused by previous trauma.

TREATMENT

Several avenues have been explored in an effort to arrive at successful treatment of cervical incompetence. Surgical repair of the cervix using a vaginal or abdominal approach has been examined in detail. Other alternatives that have been considered have included bed rest, for which no trial has been conducted and for which little evidence of effectiveness exists, and the use of vaginal pessaries to elevate and close the cervix. By far the most effort has been expended on surgical approaches to cervical incompetence, and this is, at present, the mainstay of treatment.

Lash and Lash[2] described techniques aimed at the repair of a specific anterior cervical structural defect. The cervical mucosa was opened anteriorly, the bladder reflected and the cervical defect repaired with interrupted transverse sutures before closing the vaginal mucosa. The initial descriptions of cervical cerclage for cervical incompetence came with Shirodkar and McDonald in the 1950s,[3,4] when both developed techniques for physical support for what was presumed to be a structurally weak cervix. Both initially started suturing with catgut, but Shirodkar turned to facia lata and McDonald to silk as they realised the importance of a permanent cervical support. One significant difference since then has been the present-day use of Mersilene tape as the suture material.

Many variants on the original operations have been described, but a vaginal approach to cervical cerclage essentially follows the original reports. Shirodkar, in an effort to place the suture as near the internal os as practical, described opening the anterior fornix and dissecting away the adjacent bladder, before placing the suture submucosally, tied anteriorly and the knot buried by suturing the anterior fornix mucosal opening. The original intention with the Shirodkar method was to leave the suture in place and aim for delivery by caesarean section. The McDonald technique requires no bladder dissection, and the cervix is closed using four or five bites with the needle to create a purse string around the cervix. The suture is then removed either electively or if labour ensues. Other methods of cervical suturing have been described (including the Wurm's procedure,[15] with two mattress sutures placed at right angles to each other), but present practice largely uses variants of McDonald's or Shirodkar's cerclage procedures.

One further development in the 1960s was the description of the transabdominal cerclage by Benson and Durfee in 1965,[16] a technique now largely used after the failure of vaginal cerclage procedures or in the presence of congenital anomalies, particularly those produced by diethylstilboestrol exposure.[17] In this method, a midline or Pfannenstiel abdominal incision allows access to the vesico-uterine fold of peritoneum, which is divided and the bladder reflected caudally. The uterine vessels are then identified and a Mersilene tape suture is passed through the broad ligament below the uterine vessels in the potential 'free space' between the uterine vessels and the ureter, with the suture tied anteriorly or posteriorly (anterior being reported as surgically easier) and the bladder replaced. The original intention with the transabdominal approach was that the suture was inserted between pregnancies or in early pregnancy, and left *in situ* for the rest of the woman's reproductive life, delivery being undertaken by caesarean section for each pregnancy.

On initial viewing, all these procedures appear to have impressive success. Shirodkar's first publication showed no specific outcome data, although Cousins' review of cervical cerclage in 1980[5] reported an improvement in outcome in terms of fetal survival from 21.8% to 82.5% following Shirodkar sutures in all published data. McDonald demonstrated a 94% success rate by 1971,[18] whilst the review in 1980 by Cousins also reported an improvement from a 27% to 74% successful pregnancy outcome in all published data. Two recent reports of single hospitals' experience of transabdominal cerclage[17,19] have reported successful outcomes of 93% and 85%, respectively. This was reported against a background of an 18% successful outcome rate prior to the abdominal cerclage in the study of Cammarano et al, and just 4 surviving babies out of the 167 pregnancies which continued beyond the first trimester prior to surgery in the 50 women in Gibb and Salaria's series. In a clinical situation of a persistently poor obstetric history and the failure of vaginal cerclage procedures, the transabdominal approach, although not without morbidity, does provide significant hope for success.

One area of treatment which has received little attention in recent years has been the use of vaginal pessaries as a treatment of cervical incompetence. The initial description came in 1961 from Vitsky,[20] who used a Smith-Hodge pessary to displace the cervix posteriorly and hence close the cervical canal, as well as probably elevate the fetal presenting part away from the internal os. The collection of reported cases in Cousin's review[5] compared very favourably with the surgical approach to cervical incompetence; an infant survival rate of 91% was reported, compared to successful pregnancy outcomes prior to treatment of just 22%. Despite these encouraging results, and the significant advantage of the absence of surgical risks, very little recent interest has been shown in this alternative treatment.

The results of all these forms of treatment, however, are muddied by the same complication; the lack of a precise (and objective) diagnosis or definition of what constitutes cervical incompetence, a difficulty which is likely to blur the results of any study by not distinguishing effectively between cervical incompetence and other causes of recurrent second trimester losses.

Trials of treatment

Several trials have endeavoured to study cervical cerclage using the 'gold standard' of a randomised controlled trial, with varying degrees of success. Rush et al[21] randomised 194 women felt to be at high risk of pre-term delivery to cerclage or control, whilst the MRC/RCOG trial[22] randomised 1292 women to cerclage or control. Dor et al[23] randomly allocated 50 women to cervical cerclage or control, but all were twin pregnancies so the results are not applicable to singleton pregnancies. Lazar et al[24] attempted a randomisation to treatment or control, but there appeared to be significant deviation from the randomisation allocation, and in France the background rate of cervical cerclage was high; furthermore the pre-term delivery rate of 6% implies that this was not a high risk population. Forster et al[25] ran a trial comparing cervical cerclage to vaginal pessaries in order to control cervical incompetence but without a control (none treatment) arm, and so cannot be compared to the randomised controlled trials.

Unfortunately, neither of the two randomised trials gives us the answer as to the success of cerclage procedures. The Rush trial showed no statistically significant improvement in terms of a change in gestation at delivery or neonatal outcome. The MRC/RCOG trial did show an improvement in neonatal outcome in terms of delivery after both 33 and 37 weeks' gestation in those women who had had a previous second trimester loss and who had a cervical cerclage in the index pregnancy. The intervention was associated with an increased incidence of puerperal pyrexia and medical intervention, particularly in the use of tocolytics and bed rest, and with some increased incidence of induction of labour and the use of caesarean section for delivery. The major criticism of the MRC/RCOG trial, however, was the entry criteria. Entry to the randomised trial was to be considered if the consultant in charge was uncertain whether a cervical suture was appropriate; an apparently deliberately vague entry criterion designed to encourage as many recruits as possible, but this criterion unfortunately excluded many women in whom cervical cerclage was being performed, and in whom the clearest results in terms of benefits and complications could have been demonstrated. In the group studied, there did appear to be a benefit of cervical cerclage; the reduction of the premature delivery rate was comparable to an improvement in outcome for 1 of every 25 women who received a cervical suture. However, this should be treated with some caution; the confidence intervals of between 1–12 to 1–300 suggests the potential benefit may be tenuous. Of particular importance was a point identified by the MRC/RCOG Working Party following the trial concerning identification of who would benefit from the probable benefit shown:

> It was disappointing .... that there is no evidence from this study that women are particularly likely to benefit if they have had a previous pregnancy judged to have been complicated by cervical incompetence or which ended with features typical of cervical incompetence.
> There is an urgent need for tests of cervical incompetence that are better predictors of early delivery than the indices currently used.[22]

The MRC/RCOG trial is promising in that benefit has been shown even in the marginal group studied, but the complete answer regarding cervical cerclage has not yet been found.

IMPROVEMENTS IN DIAGNOSIS

Any answers obtained from trials into cervical incompetence and its treatment will always be flawed until improvements in the diagnosis can be made. As has already been mentioned, the diagnosis is at present largely subjective and retrospective. If possible, an objective (i.e. measurable) diagnosis, made before pregnancy or in the early stages (first or early second trimester) would provide an accurate incidence of cervical incompetence, allow treatment to be targeted appropriately and also provide the basis for definitive trials of treatment.

Standard investigation of cervical incompetence has often relied on clinical acumen with regards to examination of the cervix, either digitally or by speculum. Digital cervical examination has not been shown to improve outcome,[26] whilst no study of regular speculum examinations has been published. Indeed, it would seem unlikely that much cervical change would be seen prior to the actual visualisation of the fetal membranes at the external os, by which stage significant cervical change has already occurred. Two main alternatives have been proposed and used, and both have shown promise.

Physical cervical assessment

The term cervical incompetence implies a physical weakness of the cervix, and several investigators have used various methods to measure cervical compliance. A cervical compliance score has been suggested[27] whilst several years earlier a similar Cervical Resistance Index (CRI) was suggested by Anthony.[28] Zlatnik and Burmeister[27] suggested the use of three scores to be measured at hysteroscopy; the canal-cannula ratio (the upper cervical canal width compared to the hysteroscope width on an X-ray film taken during hysteroscopy); the degree of difficulty of passing a No. 8 Hegar dilator, and the degree of traction required to pull a catheter out through the cervical canal with the balloon filled with 2 ml of saline (Table 8.1). The cervical scores

Table 8.1 Cervical compliance score (Zlatnik and Burmeister[27])

	Score 0	1	2
Canal/cannula ratio	< 1.5	1.5–1.9	> 1.9
No.8 Hegar	will not pass	moderate force	little or no force
Catheter traction	> 700 g	< 700 g	

obtained certainly appear to be relevant; of 102 pregnancies followed up, of those found to have a high cervical compliance score 24% delivered before 30 weeks' gestation ($n = 34$) compared to 9% of those with a low score ($n = 68$). However, this study was not observational, as those with a high cervical compliance score were recommended for, and largely received, a cervical suture. Interestingly, despite this intervention, the pregnancy outcome was still markedly worse in the 'high risk' group compared to those with low scores. This draws into question whether the findings at hysteroscopy before pregnancy do point towards cervical incompetence – although this does make the assumption that cervical cerclage is the definitive treatment.

Anthony et al designed a specific, simple strain gauge with which to measure the CRI.[29] The CRI in women who had previously had second trimester losses, those in whom the history was suggestive of cervical incompetence (not defined) was significantly lower than those with other causes for their second trimester loss or normal controls. A further report[30] described the CRI as a better predictor of outcome than obstetric history alone, and was useful in identifying those in whom a cervical cerclage may be beneficial.

The measurement of cervical resistance, cervical compliance and cervical strength is logical in the face of a presumed diagnosis of cervical weakness. However, there is a significant disadvantage in the reliance on hysteroscopically based investigation, in that no investigation or diagnosis can be done during pregnancy due to the invasive nature of the testing. Hence the test does still very much rely on past obstetric history before investigation can start.

Transvaginal ultrasound

Initial use of ultrasound to observe the cervix was transabdominal[31] but the necessity for a full bladder to visualise the cervix elongates the cervix to such a degree as to make objective, reproducible measurements difficult. The development of transvaginal scanning (TVS) allowed for accurate cervical measurements with an empty bladder and no distortion (Fig. 8.1).[32] Following this, large trials using TVS have shown a link between cervical length and an increased risk of pre-term delivery,[32,33] with a cervical length of less than 25 mm (the average normal cervical length being 38–42 mm) being associated with a 50% risk of a pre-term delivery (Macdonald, unpublished data). In contrast, several smaller studies and individual case reports have identified individual women (commonly those thought to be at high risk of a pre-term delivery) in whom the cervical appearances of TVS are markedly different from the norm.[34–36] The implication from these reports is that 'funnelling' or 'beaking' of

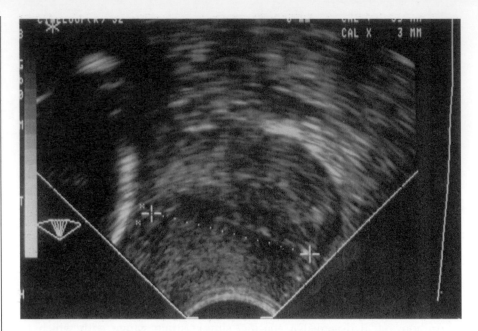

Fig. 8.1 Normal cervical appearance on transvaginal ultrasonography (TVS). +......+ indicates the length of the closed cervical canal (35 mm) (external os on the right, fetal head to the left); x......x shows position of the closed internal os, with no beaking (3 mm).

the internal cervical os, at rest or particularly in response to transabdominal pressure on the uterine fundus[35] is the ultrasonographic appearance of cervical incompetence (Fig. 8.2). This would, if proven, provide a significant advance in the diagnosis of cervical incompetence; an investigation that, in contrast to the hysteroscopic evaluation of the cervix, is non-invasive, repeatable over time and can be performed during pregnancy.

By implication, the term 'cervical incompetence' suggests cervical competence is either present or absent. This has been challenged by work in America,[36] in which the cervical length in the index pregnancy correlates to the gestation of a previous pre-term delivery, whilst a large multi-centre observational trial comparing cervical length to gestation at delivery showed a progressive increase in the relative risk of a pre-term delivery the shorter the cervix at 24 or 28 weeks' gestation.[33] The inference drawn from this work is cervical competence is graded, with incompetence being a relative not absolute concept. This corresponds with most medical conditions, where there are always degrees of severity. However, the appearance of a normally shaped, though short cervix (Fig. 8.2A) contrasts sharply with the appearance of a cervix with normal external dimensions, but amniotic membranes within the cervical canal (Fig. 8.2B). Guzman et al[35] amplified this in 1994 with a report of cervical change in response to fundal pressure; 31 women, who on past history had a clinical diagnosis of cervical incompetence, were scanned transvaginally between 8 and 25 weeks' gestation. Fourteen (45%) had cervical changes on TVS in response to firm pressure being placed on the uterine fundus. The original criticism of the work (93% of those with cervical changes received a cervical suture on demonstration of any cervical change) was countered in a

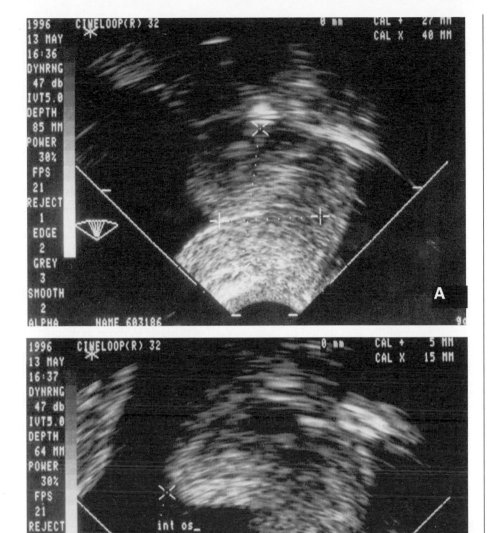

Fig. 8.2 TVS appearance of cervical incompetence. (**A**) +......+ length of closed cervical canal (27 mm); note there is no opening of the internal os at rest. (**B**) +......+ length of closed cervical canal (5 mm) after the application of pressure to the fundus of the uterus; x......x position of the internal os, now open (15 mm) with herniation of the amniotic membranes into the cervical canal.

later publication,[38] when an observational study of cervical changes in response to fundal pressure showed the cervical appearances originally described were not transitory but indeed were progressive. This observation is supported by our own work (Macdonald and Vyas, unpublished data) in

KEY POINTS FOR CLINICAL PRACTICE

- Cervical incompetence is rare but the actual incidence is unknown due to the difficulty in establishing an objective diagnosis

- A clinical diagnosis of cervical incompetence in a previous pregnancy does not necessarily indicate any benefit from a cervical suture in the present pregnancy; the implication is that either the treatment is ineffective or, most probably, the clinical diagnosis is subjective and of limited value

- A more accurate identification of cervical incompetence appears possible using either hysteroscopy and some measure of cervical resistance, or visualising the cervical canal using transvaginal ultrasonography, although neither has been proven in large scale trials

- Both the McDonald and Shirodkar cervical sutures are equally effective as a vaginal approach to cervical cerclage. By general consensus, the McDonald suture is generally easier to perform with no major difference in success

- The transabdominal cerclage, although more invasive, can be used successfully, and should be considered, particularly in those in whom the vaginal approach has previously failed

- Despite the large MRC/RCOG trial which showed cervical cerclage to be of likely benefit in specific circumstances, further investigation of cervical incompetence and the approaches towards an objective diagnosis is still needed

which progressive cervical changes resulted in visualisation of the amniotic membranes within the cervical canal or at the external os in 78% of those with cervical change in response to fundal pressure.

Transvaginal ultrasonography appears to hold significant promise in providing an accurate and objective diagnosis of cervical incompetence. Observational studies[37,38] have shown the relevance of the measurements to the risks of a pre-term delivery, and the specific appearance of amniotic membranes within the cervical canal, whether spontaneously or in response to fundal pressure suggests to us an ultrasound appearance of cervical incompetence.

CONCLUSION

Cervical incompetence remains a difficult and taxing problem for obstetricians, and a cause of great distress to those women unfortunate enough to have recurrent late pregnancy losses. Treatment appears to be effective and available in the form of surgical support for the cervix and, although its use is limited, available data suggest that a shelf pessary is also effective. However, the diagnosis of cervical incompetence continues to be difficult and, until objective indices such as cervical resistance or transvaginal ultrasound visualisation of the cervix have been tested on the level of the international MRC/RCOG trial of cervical cerclage, the veracity of the diagnosis and hence the treatment will remain unproven and the subject of debate.

REFERENCES

1 Grant A. Cervical cerclage to prolong pregnancy. In: Chalmers I, Enkin M, Kierse M J N C. (eds) Effective care in pregnancy and childbirth, Ch 40. Oxford: Oxford University Press, 1992; 633–646

2 Lash A F, Lash S R. Habitual abortion; the incompetent internal os of the cervix. Am J Obstet Gynecol 1950; 59: 68–76

3 Shirodkar V N. A new method of operative treatment for habitual abortions in the second trimester of pregnancy. Antiseptic 1955; 52: 299–300

4 McDonald I A. Suture of the cervix for inevitable miscarriage. J Obstet Gynaecol Br Commonw 1957; 64: 346–353

5 Cousins L. Cervical incompetence 1980; a time for reappraisal. Clin Obstet Gynecol 1980; 23: 467–479

6 Lumley J. The epidemiology of pre-term birth. Ballière's Clin Obstet Gynaecol 1993; 7: 477–498

7 Kristensen J, Langhoff-Roos J, Kristensen F B. Increased risk of preterm birth in women with cervical conization. Obstet Gynecol 1993; 81: 1005–1008

8 Cruickshank M E, Flannelly G, Campbell D M, Kitchener H C. Fertility and pregnancy outcome following large loop excision of the cervical transformation zone. Br J Obstet Gynaecol 1995; 102: 467–470

9 Holbrook R H, Laros R K, Creasy R K. Evaluation of a risk-scoring system for prediction of pre-term labour. Am J Perinatol 1989; 6: 62–68

10 Peterson L K, Uldbjerg N. Cervical collagen in non-pregnant women with previous cervical incompetence. Eur J Obstet Gynecol Reprod Biol 1996; 67: 41–45

11 Danforth D N, Veis A, Breen M et al. The effect of pregnancy and labour on the human cervix; changes in collagen, glycoproteins and glycosaminoglycans. Am J Obstet Gynecol 1974; 120: 641–649

12 Ekman G, Malmstrom A, Uldbjerg N. Cervical collagen: an important regulator of cervical function in term labour. Obstet Gynecol 1986; 67: 633–636

13 Olah K S, Gee H. The prevention of pre-term delivery – can we afford to continue to ignore the cervix? Br J Obstet Gynaecol 1992; 99: 278–280

14 Olah K S, Gee H. Cervical contractions: the response of the cervix to oxytocic stimulation in the latent phase of labour. Br J Obstet Gynaecol 1993; 100: 635–640

15 Hefner J D, Patow W E, Ludwig J M. The Wurm procedure: a new surgical procedure for the correction of the incompetent cervix during pregnancy. Obstet Gynecol 1961; 18: 616–620

16 Benson R, Durfee R. Transabdominal cervicouterine cerclage during pregnancy for the treatment of cervical incompetence. Obstet Gynecol 1965; 25: 145–155

17 Cammarano C L, Herron M A, Parer J T. Validity of indications for transabdominal cervicoisthmic cerclage for cervical incompetence. Am J Obstet Gynecol 1995; 172: 1871–1875

18 McDonald I A. Incompetence of the cervix. Aust N Z J Obstet Gynaecol 1978; 18: 34–37

19 Gibb D M F, Salaria D A. Transabdominal cervicoisthmic cerclage in the management of recurrent second trimester miscarriage and pre-term delivery. Br J Obstet Gynaecol 1995; 102: 802–806

20 Vitsky M. Simple treatment of the incompetent os. Am J Obstet Gynecol 1961; 81: 1194–1197

21 Rush R W, Issacs S, McPherson K, Jones L, Chalmers I, Grant A. A randomised controlled trial of cervical cerclage in women at high risk of pre-term delivery. Br J Obstet Gynaecol 1984; 91: 724–730

22 MRC/RCOG Working Party on cervical cerclage. Final report of the Medical Research Council/Royal College of Obstetricians and Gynaecologists multicentre randomised trial of cervical cerclage. Br J Obstet Gynaecol 1993; 100: 516–523

23 Dor J, Shalev, J, Mashiach G, Blankstein J, Serr D M. Elective cervical suture of twin pregnancies diagnosed following inducted ovulation. Gynaecol Obstet Invest 1982; 13: 55–60

24 Lazar P, Gueguen S, Dreyfus J, Renaud R, Pontonnier G, Papiernik E. Multicentred controlled trial of cervical cerclage in women at moderate risk of preterm delivery. Br J Obstet Gynaecol 1984; 91: 731–735

25 Von Forster F, During R, Schwarzlos G. Treatment of cervical incompetence – cerclage or pessary? Zentralbl Gynakol 1986; 108: 230–237

26 Buekens P, Alexander S, Houtsen M, Blondel B, Kaminski M, Reid M. Randomised controlled trial of routine cervical examinations in pregnancy. Lancet 1994; 144: 841–844

27 Zlatnik F J, Burmeister L F. Internal evaluation of the cervix for predicting pregnancy outcome and diagnosing cervical incompetence. J Reprod Med 1993; 38: 365–369

28 Anthony G S, Calder A A, McNaughton N C. Cervical resistance in patients with previous spontaneous mid-trimester abortion. Br J Obstet Gynaecol 1982; 89: 1046–1049

29 Fisher J, Anthony G S, McManus T J, Coutts J R T, Calder A A. Use of a force measuring instrument during cervical dilatation. J Med Tech Eng 1981; 5: 1940–1945

30 Anthony G S. Cervical incompetence – methods and results. Presentation at RCOG course on pre-term labour. 26–27th September 1996

31 Michaels W H, Montgomery C, Karo J, Temple J, Ager J, Olson J. Ultrasound differentiation of the competent from the incompetent cervix; prevention of pre-term delivery. Am J Obstet Gynecol 1986; 154: 537–546

32 Anderson H F, Nugent C E, Wanty S D, Hayashi R H. Prediction of risk of pre-term delivery by ultrasonographic measurement of cervical length. Am J Obstet Gynecol 1990; 163: 859–867

33 Iams J D Goldenberg R L, Meis P J et al. The length of the cervix and the risk of spontaneous premature delivery. N Engl J Med 1996; 334: 567–572

34 Joffe G M, Del Valle G O, Izquierdo L A et al. Diagnosis of cervical change in pregnancy by means of transvaginal ultrasonography. Am J Obstet Gynecol 1992; 166: 896–900

35 Guzman E R, Rosenberg J C, Houlihan C, Ivan J, Waldron R, Knuppel R. A new method using transfundal pressure to evaluate the asymptomatic incompetent cervix. Obstet Gynecol 1994; 83: 248–252

36 Fox R, James M, Tuohy J, Wardle P. Transvaginal ultrasound in the management of women with suspected cervical incompetence. Br J Obstet Gynaecol 1996; 103: 921–924

37 Iams J D, Johnson F F, Sonek J, Sachs L, Gebauer C, Samuels P. Cervical competence as a continuum; a study of ultrasonographic cervical length and obstetric performance. Am J Obstet Gynecol 1995; 172: 1097–1106

38 Guzman E R, Vintzileos A M, McLean D A, Martins M E, Benito C W, Hanley M L. The natural history of a positive response to transfundal pressure in women at risk of cervical incompetence. Am J Obstet Gynecol 1997; 176: 634–638

Catherine Bobrow   Rob Holmes   Peter W. Soothill

Aetiology of small for gestational age fetuses

Up to 10% of pregnancies result in a neonate that is small for gestational age (SGA). Being SGA is a major cause of fetal and neonatal mortality and long term morbidity so its effects are relevant not only to obstetricians and neonatologists but also to paediatricians. These children are at risk of impaired growth and neurodevelopment[1] and increased rates of cerebral palsy.[2] Furthermore, the implications of being SGA can be life-long, in that it appears to predispose to adult diseases, including maturity onset diabetes and cardiovascular disease.[3, 3a]

The prenatal definition of being SGA is an ultrasound scan measurement of the fetal abdominal circumference below an arbitrary percentile (usually between the 2.5th and 10th) on charts derived from a representative sample of fetuses. Within the SGA group of fetuses, only a minority will actually be small due to pathology. Indeed, by definition, 10% of the normal population have measurements below the 10th percentile of normal range charts. The skewed normal distribution of birthweight could be explained by two normal distributions, one appropriately grown fetuses the other growth restricted which overlap (Fig. 9.1).

Categorisation of decreased size by aetiology is very important as not every small fetus is at equal risk of adverse sequelae. Recent advances including serial ultrasound measurements (and so growth velocity), Doppler studies and cordocentesis have helped us to do this. Several different confusing terms have been used for types of SGA fetuses and so we propose the use of the following: (i) normal small fetuses (NSF) who have no structural abnormalities, normal umbilical artery Doppler's and normal liquor volume; (ii) abnormal small

Dr Catherine Bobrow, Research Fellow, Fetal Medicine Research Unit, University of Bristol, St Michael's Hospital, Southwell Street, Bristol BS2 8EG, UK

Mr Rob Holmes, Specialist Registrar, Fetal Medicine Research Unit, University of Bristol, St Michael's Hospital, Southwell Street, Bristol BS2 8EG, UK

Prof Peter W. Soothill, Professor of Maternal and Fetal Medicine, Fetal Medicine Research Unit, University of Bristol, St Michael's Hospital, Southwell Street, Bristol BS2 8EG, UK

fetuses (ASF), e.g those with chromosome abnormalities or structural malformations; or (iii) growth restricted fetuses (FGR) that have impaired placental function identified by abnormal Doppler's and reduced growth rate.

Ultrasound fetometry can define SGA fetuses as either symmetrical (where the abdominal circumference and the head circumference are both equally affected) or asymmetrical (where the head circumference is relatively spared). The aetiology of these two types of SGA fetus can be broadly divided into: (i) insults during organogenesis early in pregnancy, such as chromosomal abnormalities or infections causing symmetrically small fetuses; or (ii) placental dysfunction later in pregnancy being more likely to cause asymmetrically small fetuses.

Abnormal Doppler studies of umbilical arterial blood velocity are associated with FGR and nowadays increased resistance patterns in the umbilical artery are one of the criteria for the diagnosis of utero-placental insufficiency. Fetuses who are SGA with abnormal Doppler studies are likely to be growth restricted due to inadequate placental function. Cordocentesis allows us to karyotype, look at fetal acid–base status and screen for infection. With better investigation, it is becoming easier to identify the aetiology and assess the outcome of the SGA fetus. Furthermore, the management options for SGA fetuses vary depending on the aetiology. As yet, there are no effective intra-uterine therapies, so the mainstay of treatment remains limited to close observation, attempts to identify why the fetus is SGA and well-timed premature delivery where required. In this chapter, we will give an overview of the many aetiologies of SGA fetuses dividing them into maternal, placental and fetal causes.

MATERNAL CAUSES OF SGA

Chronic illness

Any debilitating disease in the mother increases the risk of having an SGA fetus. This may be because of deprivation of nutrients or oxygen available to

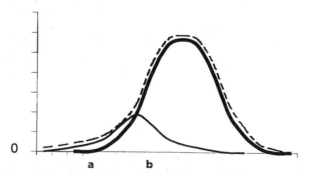

Fig. 9.1 A graph to show how two normal distributions that overlap could look like a single skewed normal distribution. The dark solid line represents appropriately grown fetuses, the light solid line growth retarded fetuses and the hashed line the skewed normal distribution when the two are combined. At point **a.** the fetus is much more likely to be growth restricted whereas at point **b.** it is more likely to be normal small.

the placenta or due to failure of normal maternal adaptation to pregnancy. As medical care improves, many women with disease (e.g. cystic fibrosis, congenital heart disease or renal failure after transplantation) who would previously not have conceived are now presenting in pregnancy.

With severe cardiorespiratory disease, such as partially corrected structural heart malformations, chronic maternal hypoxaemia may lead to growth restriction. Compromised haemodynamics may make the normal 30% increase in cardiac output during pregnancy impossible and so also contribute to reduced fetal growth.

Haemoglobinopathies, such as sickle cell disease, and collagen vascular disease, such as systemic lupus erythematosus, may cause localised placental hypoxia secondary to poor maternal perfusion. This can be due to placental microvascular changes that mirror those in other organs. Indeed, studies looking at pregnancies in women with antiphospholipid antibodies have a reported incidence of SGA fetuses of between 30–60%.[4] Placentas from these antiphospholipid positive patients have been found to have an atypical vasculopathy.[5]

Nutrition

The impact of nutritional deprivation on fetal growth depends on the stage of pregnancy at which it occurs and on its severity. Studies looking at the impact of nutrition on birthweight and subsequent growth in populations in The Netherlands during and after World War II found that significant effects were only seen at extremes of undernutrition.[6] Below a certain threshold, fertility was noted to decline, but if a woman conceived it seemed the fetus was usually protected against starvation. The fetus was relatively protected from the effects of nutritional deprivation in the first trimester because the requirements of the developing embryo are minimal. Growth restriction in the second trimester was rare and was likely to be symmetrical and in the third trimester it was usually asymmetrical.[6]

Anorexia nervosa and bulimia nervosa are eating disorders that cause malnutrition in women of childbearing age in the Western world. Fertility rates are often decreased in anorexics but not bulimics.[7] Little data are available on the effects these conditions have on pregnancy outcome, but a large series in Denmark found infants of anorexic mothers had twice the chance of having a birthweight of < 2500g.[7] A further study looking at women who had a body mass index < 19 at conception found that they had a 19% chance of delivering an infant weighing below the 10th percentile compared to 8% for normal weight mothers.[8]

Smoking

Smoking in pregnancy is a major cause of fetuses being SGA and it has recently been shown that the critical time of exposure is the third trimester.[9] Passive smoking can also reduce birthweight, as shown in a study of mothers with otherwise uncomplicated pregnancies delivered between 37–41 weeks' gestation classified as smokers, non-smokers who were exposed or non-smokers who were not exposed.[10] It demonstrated a weight deficit at birth of

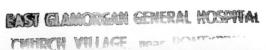

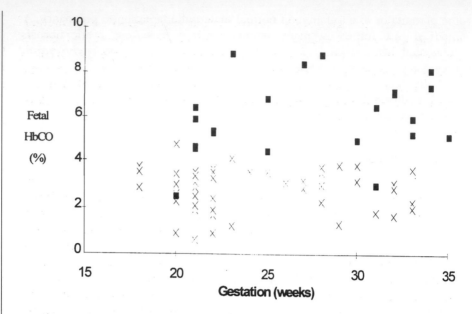

Fig. 9.2 Carboxyhaemoglobin levels in cord blood of smokers (dots) and non-smokers (crosses) adapted from Soothill et al.[11]

192 g in the infants of mothers exposed to passive smoking and of 458 g in infants of mothers who smoked. The authors explained the larger birthweight deficit in infants of smokers in their study compared with previous studies by commenting that previous research did not separate the mothers exposed to passive smoking from those who were not exposed at all.

The mechanism by which smoking causes reduced fetal growth is unclear. In a study of fetal blood samples taken by cordocentesis between 18–35 weeks' gestation, carbon monoxide was found to have crossed the placenta increasing fetal carboxyhaemoglobin concentration.[11] Carboxyhaemoglobin (HbCO) levels in fetal blood from pregnancies in which the mother smoked were almost double those of non-smokers (Fig. 9.2). They also noted a small increase in total fetal haemoglobin concentration associated with the rise in HbCO induced by fetal erythropoetin production in response to hypoxia induced by fetal erythropoeitin production (in response to hypoxia). Although carbon monoxide is trapped in the fetal circulation, this alone does not appear to explain fully the association between smoking and reduced fetal weight. Other possible factors include direct cell poisoning by the build up of toxic metabolites or blood flow disturbances in the fetal or uteroplacental circulation.

Alcohol

Damage to the fetus by alcohol is an important cause of being SGA and it is probably underdiagnosed in the UK. Studies in Sweden and France in the late 1970s suggested an incidence of alcohol related fetal damage of 1 in 300 deliveries,[12] but more recent studies have quoted an incidence of 1 in 2000.[13] Alcohol crosses the placental barrier freely in humans and, because the fetus has low alcohol dehydrogenase activity, the capacity to remove it is reduced which may lead to higher alcohol concentrations in the fetus than the mother. Both alcohol and its metabolite, acetaldehyde, are cytotoxic and act as teratogens in early pregnancy leading in severe cases to the fetal alcohol syndrome, one of the features of which is growth restriction. This tends to be symmetrical and Doppler studies of the umbilical artery are usually normal. Olegard et al[12] found that infants of alcoholics had a 12-fold increased risk of having a birthweight < −2 SDs.

Illegal drugs

Illegal drug taking is associated with both SGA fetuses and prematurity but the mechanisms are not fully understood. Studies have mainly looked at high risk individuals, relying on self reporting of exposure; but, because of other adverse factors often also present such as multiple substance abuse, they have often been hard to interpret. Cocaine is conventionally thought to be associated with being SGA. Its effects have previously been attributed to uterine vasoconstriction,[14] but specific transporter systems within the placenta may also be affected, leading to decreased transfer of essential nutrients to the fetus.[15] Amphetamines have been shown to produce adverse effects via similar mechanisms.[16] Interestingly, a recent large study in the US, where serum samples were taken in the mid-trimester and at delivery to identify objectively exposure to cocaine and marijuana, suggested neither drug was associated with preterm delivery or FGR after adjusting for confounding variables especially tobacco.[17]

Infection

Germain et al[18] reported an association between vaginal bacteria and the risk of having an SGA fetus and suggested a higher risk in women with certain pathological genital flora, especially *M. hominis, U. urealyticum, T. vaginalis* and the *Bacteroides* group. The risk was also proportional to the number of different microorganisms isolated, suggesting an additive or synergistic effect. Unidentified confounders may have explained this observation in women with multiple organisms especially as the mechanism by which microorganisms could cause a fetus to become SGA is unclear. However, the authors postulated that a chronic, low-grade infection could impair placental function.

Other evidence supports a role for certain maternal infections. In a large prospective study, the incidence of having an SGA fetus increased with the number of maternal protozoan and helminthic species detected. However, infected women were more likely to be poorly educated, living in less adequate conditions and nutritionally deprived making the results hard to interpret[19].

Endocrine

Severe maternal endocrine diseases tend to result in infertility, usually as a consequence of ovulatory dysfunction. If pregnancy occurs, the incidence of early loss is increased but among on-going pregnancies there is a low incidence of SGA. Maternal hormones do not cross the placenta in significant quantities, and so adverse growth in the fetus relates not to fetal hormone changes but to the more general consequences of a sick mother in whom nutrition is sub-optimal or in whom the physiological adaptations of pregnancy are defective.

In diabetes mellitus, excessive fetal growth due to fetal hyperinsulinaemia is more frequent than FGR but impaired growth may occur, usually in the presence of diabetic nephropathy. Birthweight is related inversely to maternal blood pressure and impaired creatinine clearance in the third trimester,[20] probably due to abnormalities of uteroplacental blood flow.[21] Uncontrolled maternal hyperthyroidism is associated with a high incidence of FGR[22] which can be largely prevented by aggressive maternal therapy. In contrast, maternal hypothyroidism is not associated with adverse effects upon fetal growth. FGR has been reported in Addison's disease,[23] possibly due to fetal hypoglycaemia either secondary to a fetal Addisonian state caused by transplacental passage of maternal antibodies or simply secondary to maternal hypoglycaemia.

FGR due to uteroplacental insufficiency is associated with low levels of placental GH,[24] a structurally distinct variant which forms the bulk of GH in the maternal circulation in the second half of pregnancy as the pituitary becomes down-regulated. Placental GH probably controls circulating maternal IGF-I and there are very low levels of maternal IGF-I in FGR.[25] Whether this is a cause or consequence of FGR is uncertain, but it may have adverse consequences for placental function because IGF-I is a potent mitogen in trophoblast culture[26] and leads to an uptake of amino acids.[27]

Maternal constraint

Maternal constraint is the term given to the process by which birthweight is controlled by maternal rather than paternal factors,[28] in contrast to the ultimate offspring size which relates to both maternal and paternal stature. Cross breeding studies of cattle, sheep and horses, have shown that birthweight of hybrid offspring closely matches the maternal breed.[29] In humans, there is a significant correlation between birthweights of half siblings with a common mother but not those with a common father.[30] The birthweight of donor egg assisted conceptions correlates with the recipient mother's weight but not with either the stature or birthweight of the donor.[31] Also, adult height is much more strongly correlated with length at 2 years than at birth[32] suggesting that genetic factors gain their prominent influence on growth in the postnatal period. The mechanisms by which the mother exerts constraint upon fetal growth have yet to be elucidated but may include limitations of utero-placental blood flow and/or placental transfer via endocrine or paracrine mechanisms.

PLACENTAL CAUSES OF SGA

To develop normally, a fetus requires an adequate supply of nutrients and oxygen across the placenta, via the uteroplacental and fetoplacental circulations. Abnormalities on either side of the placental circulation can cause insufficiency of supply and lead to FGR. The development of Doppler ultrasound scanning has allowed the study of both placental circulations non-invasively in normal and abnormal pregnancies and this has helped us to understand the pathology behind placental insufficiency.

Uteroplacental insufficiency

The maternal side of the placental circulation is formed by the action of endovascular trophoblast on the spiral arteries in the placental bed converting them to uteroplacental arteries. These extend back to the intervillous space and become unresponsive to vasomotor influences,[33] a conversion that appears to take place in two stages.[34] The first wave converts the decidual segments of the spiral arteries into uteroplacental arteries and occurs during the first and early second trimester. The second wave converts the myometrial segments by altering their musculoelastic architecture.

It has been proposed that the trigger for trophoblast invasion could be changes in oxygen concentration.[35] In the first trimester of pregnancy, a steep oxygen tension gradient exists between the high oxygen level in the maternal decidua and villous placenta and low level in the intervillous space. Hypoxia may cause proliferation of the cytotrophoblast but inhibit invasion.[36] However, towards the end of the first trimester, the oxygen gradient lessens and this change from relative hypoxia may stimulate the secondary wave of trophoblast invasion into the spiral arteries. In pregnancies affected by FGR and pre-eclampsia, there is sub-optimal trophoblast invasion of the spiral arteries leaving the myometrial segments unaltered.[37] It, therefore, seems that it is the secondary wave of trophoblast migration that fails in these pregnancies.

Cordocentesis from pregnancies affected by FGR has shown fetal blood to be hypoxic, acidotic and deficient of nutrients.[38] Until recently, the inadequate trophoblast invasion in the mid-trimester described above has been thought to cause uteroplacental ischaemia, placental villous hypoxia and so fetal hypoxia and acidosis. However, more recent studies have suggested that the villous space is not hypoxic but that the transfer of oxygen to the fetus is inadequate (see section on fetoplacental causes of SGA).

Fetoplacental insufficiency

Fetoplacental vascular anomalies such as a single umbilical artery, velamentous cord insertion or placental haemangioma may cause an SGA fetus through impaired fetoplacental circulation.

Studies of Doppler waveforms in the umbilical arteries of normal pregnancies have found that during the first trimester there is usually no end diastolic flow indicating a high level of vascular resistance.[39] By the early second trimester, end diastolic flow is usually present and increases steadily towards term.[40] These changes correlate with changes in the villous architecture and capillary network within them leading to a low impedance circulation by the mid-trimester. In pregnancies complicated by FGR, abnormalities of the Doppler waveforms in the umbilical arteries with reversed or absent end diastolic flow are often found, suggesting increased vascular impedance in the fetoplacental circulation. This may be due to an obliterative process with platelet aggregation causing a reduction in the numbers of small stem villous vessels,[41-43] but no direct evidence of arteriolar obstruction or thrombosis in vessels has been demonstrated.[44]

Ultrastructural and immunochemical studies of the terminal villi of FGR placentas where oxygen and nutrient transport takes place[45,46] have shown a reduction in the diameter of terminal villi as well as a reduced number of villi per unit placenta. The terminal villi were also abnormal, with decreased cytotrophoblast nuclei and syncytial nuclei arranged in 'syncytial knots' which are usually seen in term placentas and are thought to be a mechanism for removing old nuclei from the syncytium. Both of these findings suggest a reduction in both cytotrophoblast proliferation and syncytial regeneration. Stromal deposition of collagens was increased and the trophoblast surface was thickened with fibrin plaques. Capillary loops were sparse with fewer branches and coils suggesting that villous angiogenesis was changed. These findings indicate that the fetal terminal villous compartment of the placenta also develops abnormals in pregnancies with uteroplacental insufficiency. This could be why there is increased vascular impedance in the fetal circulation as well as impaired transport of gases and nutrients.

FETAL CAUSES OF SGA

Normal small fetuses

Of the normal population, 2.5–10% can be identified as 'small' using standardised charts to plot fetal size and growth. NSF cases will be symmetrically small and their growth velocity will be parallel to the standard curves both prenatally and postnatally.[47] Doppler studies of their umbilical arteries are normal. In multiple pregnancies, the mean gestation adjusted birthweight decreases with increasing number of fetuses, especially in monochorionic pregnancies. This is not fully explained by prematurity and so there may also be an element of relative placental insufficiency or maternal constraint but the majority of these fetuses are NSF. It is vital that obstetricians are aware that the majority of 'small' fetuses have no pathology in order to avoid unnecessary admission and intervention with concomitant risk of iatrogenic damage and parental anxiety.

Infection

Infections of the fetus should be considered when severe early growth restriction is noted in the presence of normal chromosome and Doppler studies. Examples include cytomegalovirus, rubella, syphilis and toxoplasmosis which can all cause reduced fetal growth by direct action on cell division and growth. The apparent incidence of these infections in the developed world is currently so low that they have minimal impact on the mean birthweight but in some places, such as Africa, syphilis, malaria and possibly the human immunodeficiency virus remain major causes of SGA fetuses.[48] The presence of the malarial parasite in placental and umbilical cord blood is significantly associated with SGA and the use of antimalarial drugs in pregnancy reduces this incidence.[49]

Fetal abnormality

Chromosomal
Low birth weight is a common feature of chromosomally abnormal neonates. Because many fetuses with chromosomal abnormalities abort spontaneously

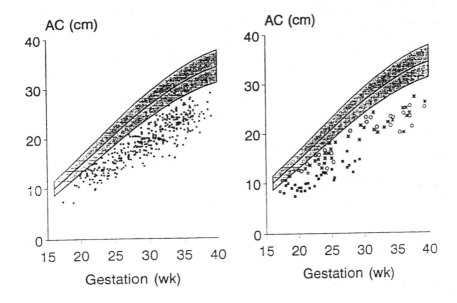

Fig. 9.3 Abdominal circumference (AC) of chromosomally normal (left) and abnormal (right) growth-retarded fetuses plotted on appropriate reference range (mean 95th and 5th percentiles) for gestation. Open squares, triploidy with molar placenta; solid squares, triploidy without molar placenta; stars, trisomy 18; open circles, other. Reproduced with kind permission from Snijders et al.[50]

or are stillborn, the incidence of chromosomal abnormality in fetuses who are SGA is gestation dependent. In the second trimester, the incidence of abnormal karyotype in SGA cases can be as high as 19%,[50] but in the third trimester SGA neonate this drops to 1–2%.[51] Not only is the incidence of chromosomal abnormalities higher with earlier presentation, but the type of defect also varies with gestation. Overall, the most commonly seen chromosome abnormalities in SGA fetuses are the trisomies 13, 18 and 21, deletions or triploidy but at less than 26 weeks the commonest is triploidy whereas after 26 weeks it is trisomy 18.[50] Therefore, the gestation at which the growth retardation presents is important (Fig. 9.3).

Ultrasound findings which increase the chance of chromosomal abnormality in a severely growth retarded fetus are structural malformations, normal or increased volume of amniotic fluid and no evidence of impaired fetoplacental or uteroplacental perfusion.[50] Fetuses diagnosed with trisomy before 30 weeks' gestation are usually symmetrically small whereas those diagnosed after 30 weeks tend to be asymmetrically small. However, those with triploidy (which is much more common in fetal than neonatal medicine) are markedly asymmetrical, even at less than 30 weeks.[50]

The aetiology of SGA in fetuses with chromosomal abnormalities may be due to several factors. Cell hyperplasia and hypertrophy may be deficient both in the placenta and the fetus. Disordered organogenesis may have adverse consequences such as abnormal haemodynamics if there is a cardiac abnormality.

Structural malformations

Low birthweight is a common feature in fetuses with non-chromosomal structural abnormalities ranging from Russell Silver syndrome to gastroschisis. Khoury et al[51] used a population based birth defects surveillance system to identify all infants born with serious structural defects diagnosed during the first year of life and looked at the incidence of being SGA (< 10th percentile) in these infants. They defined major malformations as those that interfered with the child's survival, required substantial medical care or resulted in marked physical or psychological handicap. They found a 2.6-fold increase in the risk of being SGA in fetuses with major structural defects. Almost all structural defects were associated with reduced growth and the frequency of SGA fetuses increased with increasing number of defects, so that a fetus with a syndrome was more at risk than one with an isolated defect.

The aetiology of growth restriction in chromosomally normal fetuses with structural abnormalities will depend upon the organs involved and, for certain malformations, a causal link seems clear. For example, major cardiac defects can alter the haemodynamics through the placenta. In a recent study in our unit looking at infants with gastroschisis, patent bowel cases were more growth restricted than those with atresia perhaps because of less leakage of nutrients from the fetal intestine into the amniotic fluid.[52] Other malformations with no obvious mechanism to cause reduced growth, for example anencephaly, micro-ophthalmia, limb defects or cleft palate, may be the result of the same underlying mechanism that causes the fetus to be SGA. To support this, there are several environmental events that can cause both reduced growth and malformations, e.g. prenatal infection with rubella or the fetal alcohol syndrome. There are many dysmorphic syndromes suspected of having a genetic aetiology but in which no genetic defect has yet been characterised. This is partly because conventional cytogenetic techniques are not sensitive enough to identify the smaller aberrations. Currently, it is not feasible to use the FISH based (fluorescent in situ hybridization) techniques to check all the chromosomes of every case with a suspected genetic disease. Furthermore, the probes are expensive and many are not commercially available. New molecular techniques may allow the detection of chromosome abnormalities that might not have been identified using standard cytogenetic techniques.[53]

Endocrinology

In postnatal life, growth is directed along genetically influenced pathways by central endocrine controls involving growth hormone (GH), thyroid hormones, glucocorticoids and insulin. With the exception of insulin, these hormones do not have a major role in controlling fetal growth and so fetal endocrine disease is not a significant cause of growth restriction. For example, children with a congenital deficiency of GH have only a slight reduction in birth length but normal birthweight[54] and Laron dwarfs who lack GH receptors are also normally grown *in utero*.[55] A significant role for other pituitary hormones, such as prolactin, is very unlikely because pituitary agenesis does not affect fetal growth although interpretation is confounded by the presence in the circulation of hormones of placental origin. Congenital agenesis of the thyroid leads only to delayed bone maturation with no reduction in body size, although thyroxine production from ectopic sites might provide essential baseline secretion. Cortisol has little, if any, effect upon overall growth but it is important for maturation of several organs including lung, liver and adrenal.

The major role of insulin in fetal growth is shown by the somatic overgrowth which results from hyperinsulinism secondary to increased glucose from a diabetic mother and the growth restriction caused by insulin deficiency from pancreatic agenesis or insulin resistance.[56] Insulin promotes growth by increasing the rate of glucose uptake and utilisation and increases amino acids tissue accretion.[57] Disruption of the IGF genes, either *Igf1* or *Igf2*, leads to profound fetal growth restriction with a reduction in size at birth[58,59] providing evidence for a key role of the fetal IGF system in fetal growth.

Umbilical venous blood IGF-1 is low and IGFBP-1 (which is inhibitory to the growth promoting actions of the IGFs in vitro) is high both *in utero* and at delivery when a fetus is growth restricted due to limitations of substrate supply as a consequence of uteroplacental insufficiency.[60,61] However, similar changes in the fetal IGF system have not been observed in SGA fetuses with normal placental function,[25] suggesting that low IGF-1 is not a primary cause of SGA. However, a child with impaired growth who was also small at birth has recently been reported to have low levels of IGF-1 as a consequence of being homozygous for an IGF-1 gene deletion.[62] It is, therefore, possible that gene defects in the IGF-1 system may be a small but important group of SGA cases.

CONCLUSION

Studies of fetuses that are SGA have in the past often been poorly defined with many using size as the only criteria for inclusion. Even with a very small cut off such as −2 SD this results in many healthy fetuses being included and decreases the power of the studies. With the increased availability of detailed ultrasound scanning, Doppler waveforms of the maternal and fetal circulation and cordocentesis it has become possible to subdivide broadly the group of SGA fetuses by aetiology into NSF, ASF and FGR small fetuses. Improved classification facilitates better definition of study populations and their outcomes. This will not only improve our knowledge of the aetiology of SGA fetuses but may also lead to more effective and logical management strategies and the development of novel therapies.

REFERENCES

1 Soothill P W, Ajayi R A, Campbell S, Ross E M, Nicolaides K H. Fetal oxygenation at cordocentesis, maternal smoking and childhood neurodevelopment. Eur J Obstet Gynaecol Reprod Biol 1995; 59: 21–24
2 Blair E, Stanley F. Intrauterine growth retardation and spastic cerebral palsy. II. The association with morphology at birth. Early Hum Dev 1992; 28: 91–96
3 Barker D J P, Gluckman P D, Godfrey K M, Harding J E, Owens J A, Robinson J S. Fetal nutrition and cardiovascular disease in adult life. Lancet 1993; 341: 938–941

3a Barker D J P, Mothers, babies and diseases in later life. London: BMJ Publishing, 1994

4 Polzin W J, Kopelman J M, Robinson R D, Read J A, Brady K. The association of antiphospholipid antibodies with pregnancies complicated by fetal growth restriction. Obstet Gynecol 1991; 78: 1108–1111

5 Lockshin M D. Pregnancy and systemic autoimmune disease. Semin Clin Immunol 1993; 5: 5–11

6 Stein Z, Susser M, Saenger G et al. Famine and human development: the Dutch hunger winter of 1944–1945. New York: Oxford University Press, 1975

7 Brinch M, Isager T, Tolstrup K. Anorexia nervosa and motherhood: reproductional pattern and mothering behaviour of 50 women. Acta Psychiatr Scand 1988; 77: 98–104

8 Van den Spuy Z M, Steer P J, McCusker M, Steele S J, Jacobs H S. Outcome of pregnancy in underweight women after spontaneous and induced ovulation. BMJ 1988; 296: 962–965

9 Lieberman E, Gremy I, Lang J M, Cohen A P. Low birthweight at term and the timing of fetal exposure to maternal smoking. Am J Public Health 1994; 84: 1127–1131

10 Roquer J M, Figueras J, Botet F, Jimenez R. Influence on fetal growth of exposure to tobacco smoke during pregnancy. Acta Paediatr 1995; 84: 118–121

11 Soothill P W, Morafa W, Ayida G A, Rodeck C H. Maternal smoking and fetal carboxyhaemoglobin and blood gas levels. Br J Obstet Gynaecol 1996; 103: 78–82

12 Olegard R, Sabel K G, Aronsson M et al. Effect on the child of alcohol abuse during pregnancy. Retrospective and prospective studies. Acta Paediatr Scand Suppl 1979; 275: 112–121

13 Coles C D. Impact of prenatal alcohol exposure on the newborn and the child. Clin Obstet Gynecol 1993; 36: 255–266

14 Plessinger M A, Woods J R. Maternal, placental and fetal pathophysiology of cocaine exposure during pregnancy. Clin Obstet Gynecol 1993; 36: 267–278

15 Ganapathy V, Leibach F H. Human placenta: a direct target for cocaine action. Placenta 1994; 15: 785–795

16 Ramamoorthy J D, Ramamoorthy S, Leibach F H, Ganapathy V. Human placental monoamine transporters as targets for amphetamines. Am J Obstet Gynecol 1995; 173: 1782–1787

17 Shiono P H, Klebanhoff M A, Nugent R P et al. The impact of cocaine and marijuana use on low birthweight and preterm birth: a multicenter study. Am J Obstet Gynecol 1995; 172: 19–27

18 Germain M, Krohn S L, Eschenbach D A. Genital flora in pregnancy and its association with intrauterine growth retardation. J Clin Microbiol 1994; 32: 2162–2168

19 Villar J, Klebanoff M, Kestler E. The effect on fetal growth of protozoan and helminthic infection during pregnancy. Obstet Gynecol 1989; 74: 915–920

20 Kitzmiller J L, Brown E R, Phillippe M et al. Diabetic nephropathy and perinatal outcome. Am J Obstet Gynecol 1981; 141: 741–751

21 Madsen H. Fetal oxygenation in diabetic pregnancy. Dan Med Bull 1986; 33: 64–74

22 Sugrue D, Drury M I. Hyperthyroidism complicating pregnancy: results of treatment by antithyroid drugs in 77 pregnancies. Br J Obstet Gynaecol 1980; 87: 970–975

23 Osler M. Addison's disease and pregnancy. Acta Endocrinol 1962; 4: 67–70

24 Mirlesse V, Frankenne F, Alsat E, Poncelet M, Hennen G, Evain-Brion D. Placental growth hormone levels in normal pregnancy and in pregnancies with intrauterine growth retardation. Pediatr Res 1993; 34: 439–442

25 Holmes R, Montemagno R, Jones J, Preece M, Rodeck C, Soothill P. Fetal and maternal insulin like growth factors and binding proteins in pregnancies with appropriate or retarded fetal growth. Early Hum Dev 1997; 49: 7–17

26 Fant M, Munro H, Moses A C. An autocrine/paracrine role for insulin-like growth factors in the regulation of human placental growth. J Clin Endocrinol Metab 1986; 63: 499–505

27 Kniss D A, Shubert P J, Zimmerman P D, Landon M B, Gabbe S G. Insulin-like growth factors. Their regulation of glucose and amino acid transport in placental trophoblasts isolated from first trimester chorionic villi. J Reprod Med 1994; 39: 249–256

28 Ounsted M K. Maternal constraint on foetal growth. Dev Med Child Neurol 1965; 7: 479–491

29 Walton A, Hammond J. The maternal effects on growth and confirmation in the Shire horse–Shetland pony crosses. Proc R Soc Biol 1938; 125: 311–335

30 Robson E B. Principles and prenatal growth. In: Faulkner F, Tanner J M. (eds) Human growth. New York: Plenum, 1978; 285–297

31 Brooks A A, Johnson M R, Steer P J, Pawson M E, Abdalla H I. Birthweight: nature or nurture? Early Hum Dev 1995; 42: 29–35

32 Tanner J M. Growth at adolescence, 2nd edn. Oxford: Blackwell, 1962

33 Boyd J D, Hamilton WJ. The human placenta. Cambridge: Heffer and Sons, 1970

34 Pijnenborg R, Bland J M, Robertson W B, Brosens I. Uteroplacental arterial changes related to interstitial trophoblast migration in early human pregnancy. Placenta 1983; 4: 387–414

35 Ahmed A, Kilby M. Hypoxia or hyperoxia in placental insufficiency? Lancet 1997; 350: 826–827

36 Genbacev O, Joslin R, Damsky C H, Pollitti B M, Fischer S J. Hypoxia alters early gestation human cytotrophoblast differentiation/invasion in-vitro and models the placental defects that occur in pre-eclampsia. J Clin Invest 1996; 97; 540–550

37 Khong T Y, De Wolf F, Robertson W B, Brosens I. Inadequate maternal vascular response to placentation in pregnancies complicated by pre-eclampsia and by small-for-gestational age infants. Br J Obstet Gynaecol 1986; 93: 1049–1059

38 Soothill P W, Nicolaides K H, Campbell S. Prenatal asphyxia, hyperlacticaemia and erythroblastosis in growth retarded fetuses. BMJ 1987; 297: 1051–1053

39 Fisk N M, MacLachlan N, Ellis C, Tannirandorn Y, Tonge H M, Rodeck C H. Absent end diastolic flow in first trimester umbilical artery. Lancet 1988; 2: 1256–1257

40 Hendricks S K, Sorensen T K, Wang K Y, Bushnell J M, Seguin E M, Zingheim R W. Doppler umbilical artery waveform indices-normal values from fourteen to forty-two weeks. Am J Obstet Gynecol 1989; 161: 761–765

41 Giles W B, Trudinger B J, Baird P J. Fetal umbilical artery flow velocity waveforms and placental resistance: pathological correlation. Br J Obstet Gynaecol 1985; 92: 31–38

42 Van den Hof M C, Nicolaides K H. Platelet count in normal, small and anemic fetuses. Am J Obstet Gynecol 1990; 162: 735–739

43 Wilcox G R, Trudinger B J. Fetal platelet consumption: a feature of platelet insufficiency. Obstet Gynecol 1991; 77: 616–620

44 Macara L, Kingdom J C P, Kohnen G, Bowman A W, Greer I A, Kaufmann P. Elaboration of stem villous vessels in growth restricted pregnancies with abnormal umbilical artery Doppler waveforms. Br J Obstet Gynaecol 1995; 102: 807–812

45 Macara L, Kingdom J C P, Kaufmann P et al. Structural analysis of placental terminal villi from growth restricted pregnancies with abnormal umbilical artery Doppler waveforms. Placenta 1996; 17: 37–48

46 Krebs C, Macara L M, Leiser R, Bowman A W, Greer I A, Kingdom J C P. Intrauterine growth restriction with absent end diastolic flow velocity in the umbilical artery is associated with maldevelopment of the placental terminal villous tree. Am J Obstet Gynecol 1996; 175: 1534–1542

47 Bates J A, Evans J A, Mason G. Differentiation of growth retarded from normally grown fetuses and prediction of intra-uterine growth retardation using Doppler ultrasound. Br J Obstet Gynaecol 1986; 103: 670–675

48 Taha T E, Dallabetta G A, Canner J K et al. The effect of human immunodeficiency virus infection on birthweight, and infant and child mortality in urban Malawi. Int J Epidemiol 1995; 24: 1022–1029

49 Steketee R W, Wirima J J, Hightower A W, Slutsker L, Heyman D L, Breman J G. The effect of malaria and malaria prevention in pregnancy on offspring birthweight, prematurity, and intrauterine growth retardation in rural Malawi. Am J Trop Med Hygiene 1996; 55 (Suppl 1): 33–41

50 Snijders R J M, Sherrod C, Gosden C M, Nicolaides K H. Severe fetal growth retardation: associated malformations and chromosomal abnormalities. Am J Obstet Gynecol 1993; 168: 547–555

51 Khoury M J, Erickson J D, Cordero J F, McCarthy B J. Congenital malformations and intrauterine growth retardation: a population study. Pediatrics 1988; 82: 83–90

52 Dixon J, Penman D M, Soothill P W. The influence of atresia on fetal distress in labour and birthweight in cases of gastroschisis. J Obstet Gynaecol 1998; 18(Suppl 1); 18

53 Thein A T A, Charles A, Reid T, Soothill P W. Comparative genomic hybridisation to detect underlying genetic causes in dysmorphic fetuses. J Obstet Gynaecol 1998; 18(Suppl 1):54–55

54 Gluckman P D, Gunn A J, Wray A et al. Congenital idiopathic growth hormone deficiency is associated with prenatal and early postnatal growth failure. J Pediatr 1992; 121: 920–923

55 Laron Z, Peutzelan A, Karp M, Kowaldo-Silbergeld A, Daughaday W H. Administration of growth hormone to patients with familial dwarfism with high plasma immunoreactive growth hormone measurement of sulfation factor. Metabolic and linear growth responses. J Clin Endocrinol Metab 1971; 33: 332–342

56 Hill D J, Milner R D. Insulin as a growth factor. Pediatr Res 1985; 19: 879–886

57 Fowden A L. The role of insulin in fetal growth. Adv Perinat Med 1992; 29(1–3): 177–181

58 DeChiara T M, Efstradiadis A, Robertson E J. A growth deficiency phenotype in heterozygous mice carrying an insulin-like growth factor II gene disrupted by targeting. Nature 1990; 345: 78–80

59 Liu J-P, Baker J, Perkins A S, Robertson E J, Efstratiadis A. Mice carrying null mutations of the genes encoding insulin-like growth factor 1 (IGF-1) and Type 1 receptor (IGF-1R). Cell 1993; 75: 59–72

60 Lassarre C, Hardouin S, Daffos F, Forestier F, Frankenne F, Binoux M. Serum insulin-like growth factors and insulin-like growth factor binding proteins in the human fetus. Relationships with growth in normal subjects and in subjects with intrauterine growth retardation. Pediatr Res 1991; 29: 219–225

61 Langford K, Blum W, Nicolaides K H, Jones J, McGregor A, Miell J. The pathophysiology of the insulin-like growth factor axis in fetal growth failure: a basis for programming by undernutrition. Eur J Clin Invest 1994; 24: 851–856

62 Woods K A, Camacho-Hubner C, Savage M O, Clark A J. Intrauterine growth retardation and postnatal growth failure associated with deletion of the IGF-I gene. N Engl J Med 1996; 335: 1363–1367

Deborah C. M. Boyle   J. Richard Smith

Persistent vaginal discharge

The presence of a heavy or persistent vaginal discharge is a highly subjective phenomenon. Some women may be very troubled by a discharge which is not profuse whilst others may have a much heavier discharge and consider this to be quite normal. It may also be the presenting symptom of a woman who has an underlying psychosexual problem. There are a number of causes of heavy and/or persistent vaginal discharge which should be considered when a woman complains of this symptom. This chapter aims to review the causes and basic management of this condition.

PHYSIOLOGICAL

There are a number of physiological influences on the production of vaginal discharge. Hormonal changes during the menstrual cycle are reflected by the production of mucus by the cervix. At the time of ovulation, cervical mucus becomes thinner and clearer and is often produced in greater quantities than at other times during the cycle. Cervical mucus production may also be influenced by the administration of exogenous hormones either in the form of contraceptives or hormone replacement therapy and by pregnancy, again mediated by hormonal influences. An increase in the circulating level of oestrogen may produce cervical ectopy which, in turn, enhances the production of thin clear mucus. In some women, this may become so profuse as to be troublesome and cryotherapy to ablate the area may be recommended. Sexual arousal also increases the amount of vaginal fluid which is rich in

Dr Deborah C. M. Boyle, Research Fellow, Academic Department of Obstetrics and Gynaecology, Charing Cross and Westminster Medical School, Chelsea and Westminster Hospital, 369 Fulham Road, London SW10 9NH, UK

Mr J. Richard Smith, Senior Lecturer/Consultant, Academic Department of Obstetrics and Gynaecology, Charing Cross and Westminster Medical School, Chelsea and Westminster Hospital, 369 Fulham Road, London SW10 9NH, UK

glycoproteins. These substances facilitate penetrative sex and also reduce that ability of organisms to adhere to vaginal cells thus reducing the risk of infection. Physiological discharge may be sufficiently heavy to produce irritation, but this does not always indicate infection. If the amount of discharge has become more pronounced in the recent past, especially if there is accompanying irritation, infection is likely. A bloodstained discharge is suspicious and warrants investigation.

PATHOLOGICAL

Infection

This is the commonest cause of vaginal discharge. Infections mainly involve the lower genital tract but may also extend to the upper genital tract and urological system.

Candida

A very common condition which may or may not give rise to symptoms. It is estimated that 75% of women will experience an episode at some point, most commonly following a course of antibiotics or a pregnancy.[1] Although not a sexually transmitted infection as such, the infection may be passed to male partners who may act as reservoirs of infection or develop balanitis. The commonest species of *Candida* is *C. albicans*. Other *Candida* species which may be isolated include *C. glabrata*, *C. krusei* and *C. tropicalis*. Additionally, non-Candidal yeast species such as *Torulopsis glabrata* and *Trichophyton* species may also be responsible for symptoms. Although organisms other than *C. albicans* account for less than 10% of cases,[1] they are often refractory to standard treatment regimens used to treat vulvovaginal candidiasis. Consequently, identification of the species of yeast is important in women who appear to have refractory infection.

Infection with *Candida* requires a disturbance of the local or systemic immunity. Normal vaginal flora are dominated by *Lactobacilli* of which a proportion will produce hydrogen peroxide and bacteriocins which inhibit the overgrowth of other organisms in the vagina. The balance of vaginal flora and hence local immunity may be disturbed by administration of broad-spectrum antibiotics, trauma to the skin following intercourse, allergens causing skin sensitisation or the presence of other vaginal infections producing inflammation or a change in the microbiological environment. Any pathological cause of immunosuppression will predispose to candidiasis as will the reduced cellular immunity of late pregnancy. Candidiasis is also more common in endocrine abnormalities such as diabetes mellitus and diseases of the thyroid, parathyroid and adrenal glands. It has been hypothesised that recurrent candidiasis may be due to an endometrial reservoir of *C. albicans* but this has been demonstrated not to be the case.[2]

Classically, *Candida* causes vulval and vaginal itching. The itching may be intense and is usually worse at night and with warmth and moisture. Some women will complain of superficial dyspareunia. The discharge is most often described as thick, white and having the appearance of 'cottage cheese'. This is not, however, universal and the discharge may be thin and mucopurulent. Symptoms vary widely and range from nil to extremely distressing itch and irritation which may have caused pronounced excoriation from scratching, often whilst asleep. Symptoms do not necessarily correlate well with signs and, whilst some women with pronounced symptoms may have little to see on examination, others may have more obvious infection but be little troubled by symptoms.

Findings in vaginal candidiasis are typically of an adherent white discharge in patches with erythema of the tissues. Vulvar candidiasis may produce erythema and oedema as well as satellite lesions.

Gonorrhoea

Neisseria gonorrhoea or *Gonococcus* is a Gram-negative intracellular diplococcus which may infect the cervix, urethra, rectum or pharynx depending on the sites have been exposed. It is easily transmitted by direct sexual contact but may also be transmitted by mutual masturbation. The highly infectious nature of gonorrhoea is reflected in the estimates of a 60–90% chance of infection from a single exposure.[3] As well as having the potential to cause complications, such as ascending pelvic and disseminated infection, gonorrhoea has been demonstrated to be an independent co-factor in the acquisition of HIV.[4] Complications may result in partners if a woman has an untreated infection with gonorrhoea and has unprotected sex. For all of the above reasons, it is vital that gonorrhoea be identified early, treated appropriately and advice given regarding partners of infected patients.

Gonorrhoea in women frequently causes few symptoms and examination may be unremarkable.[5] Vaginal and/or urethral discharge, dysuria and pelvic pain may suggest infection with gonorrhoea but, as these may be the presenting symptoms of other infections, it makes clinical diagnosis unreliable. In the majority of women the endocervix is infected and although urethral colonisation occurs in 70–90% of women, it is not usually the only site of infection.[3]

Trichomonas vaginalis

Trichomonas vaginalis is another sexually transmitted infection caused by a flagellate protozoan. Patients characteristically present with malodorous vaginal discharge and itching or irritation. Women infected with TV may have no symptoms. Up to 50% of infected women will be asymptomatic. However, 30% of women will develop symptoms if followed without treatment for 6 months.[6] The most common symptom, vaginal discharge, is found in more than half of symptomatic cases.[7] *T. vaginalis* frequently co-exists with bacterial vaginosis because *T. vaginalis* alters the vaginal flora creating an anaerobic environment.[8]

Examination of the patient may reveal vulvar and vaginal erythema, vaginal discharge and colpitis macularis ('strawberry cervix'). The reported frequency of symptoms and clinical signs is highly variable: for example, the frequency with which 'strawberry cervix' is reported varies between 2 and 92%,[9–11] making clinical diagnosis alone unreliable. In the genito-urinary medicine (GUM) clinic, TV is diagnosed either by seeing motile protozoans on a wet mount of vaginal discharge or by culturing the organism. Some infections will also be diagnosed by cervical cytology. The diagnosis of TV is impaired by all methods of diagnosis individually having relatively low sensitivities. Quoted rates of sensitivities for diagnostic methods are as follows: wet mount 40–75%,[6,7,12] and culture 86–97%.[8,13] Trichomonads diagnosed by cervical smears may be confused with inflammatory cells or cell fragments as they lack characteristic motility[14] and sensitivity rates for this method of diagnosis are quoted between 33–79%.[15]

Chlamydia

Chlamydia trachomatis is a sexually transmissible bacterium which may infect the cervix or urethra and is now the commonest STD in the UK.[16] Prevalence rates vary according to the population under study. Prevalence in GUM clinics is 5–15%,[17] in community clinics 7.1%,[18] in women presenting for termination of pregnancy 8%[19,20] and up to 12% in asymptomatic women attending for smear tests at their general practitioner.[21] *C. trachomatis* may cause ascending infection leading to pelvic inflammatory disease and damage to the uterine tubes which, in turn, may produce infertility, chronic pelvic pain and an increased incidence of ectopic pregnancy.[22]

Women infected with *C. trachomatis* may be asymptomatic or may present with non-specific symptoms such as dysuria, vaginal discharge, lower abdominal pain or urinary frequency. Clinical findings may be entirely normal or there may be evidence of inflammation on the cervix and a mucopurulent discharge.

There are a number of diagnostic tools for the detection of *C. trachomatis*. The most commonly used methods are enzyme immunoassay (EIA) or direct immunofluorescence (DFA) performed on a sample from an endocervical swab. Newer methods of detection are based on molecular biological techniques. Polymerase chain reaction (PCR) has been developed to test endocervical swabs. Ligase chain reaction (LCR) has been demonstrated to have high sensitivity and specificity values for the testing of urine specimens. *Chlamydiae* are isolated almost as often from the urethra as the cervix although in smaller numbers[23] requiring that urine be tested by only the most sensitive method.[24] The ideal is to test an endocervical specimen using the most sensitive test available. If the only test that is available for testing cervical specimens is the relatively insensitive EIA, then a urine sample could be tested instead as there is little to choose between them with regard to sensitivity. Otherwise, urine testing should be considered as an adjunct to cervical testing.[25] An argument can be made for the use of urine testing when a speculum would not otherwise need to be passed, but this is not the case with a woman presenting to the gynaecology outpatient clinic with the complaint of persistent vaginal discharge.

Treatment is with tetracyclines or macrolide antibiotics. Standard treatment is doxycycline 100 mg twice daily for 7 days,[26] although many prefer to treat for 10–14 days. Other tetracyclines may be used, e.g. oxytetracycline 250 mg four times daily for 7 days but the selection of treatment may impair compliance and this should be borne in mind. Erythromycin may be used at a dose of 500 mg four times daily for 7 days or twice daily for 14 days but gastrointestinal side-effects are common and this may also affect compliance. This regimen is suitable for pregnant or lactating mothers. Newer drug treatments are azalide macrolide antibiotics, including azithromycin which has been shown to be as effective in a single dose of 1 g orally to be as effective as doxycycline 100 mg twice daily for 7 days,[27–30] although is considerably more expensive and should, therefore, be reserved for women in whom compliance is likely to be a problem.

It is crucial, as with all sexually transmitted agents that any sexual partners are seen and treated.

Herpes simplex virus

Herpes simplex virus (HSV) infection of the genital area is usually attributable to HSV type 2, however, HSV type 1 may also cause genital infection if a woman has had oral-genital contact with a partner who has active HSV 1 lesions around the mouth. HSV infection of the cervix may cause a profuse mucopurulent vaginal discharge. This is more common with a primary episode of the infection which tends to be more severe than any subsequent episodes. HSV may also affect the vulval and peri-anal areas. Although a potential cause of vaginal discharge, HSV is unlikely to be the cause of a persistent problem.

Bacterial vaginosis

Bacterial vaginosis produces a disturbance of the normal vaginal flora. It is held to be the commonest cause of vaginal discharge and accounted for 55 539 new female attendances in genito-urinary medicine clinics throughout the UK in 1995.[31] The normally predominant *Lactobacilli* are reduced and replaced by a number of organisms including *Gardnerella*, *Mobiluncus*, *Ureaplasma*, *Bacteroides* and other anaerobes. Classically, bacterial vaginosis presents with a white or grey fishy smelling vaginal discharge. The pH of the vagina rises to between 4.5 and 7.0. Bacterial vaginosis may have a relapsing and remitting course in some women. The exact aetiology of bacterial vaginosis is unknown, although a rise in vaginal pH either following exposure to semen during unprotected intercourse or following menstruation has been associated with the development of bacterial vaginosis. Whether menstruation or intercourse can be regarded as aetiological factors or whether they simply make a woman more aware of the smell because of the rise in pH is the subject of discussion. At least one study has demonstrated that unprotected heterosexual intercourse was associated with resolution of bacterial vaginosis,[32] which conflicts with findings of other workers who consider unprotected intercourse to be a precipitant. A further lack of association with semen together with evidence for possible sexual transmission was demonstrated in the high concordance rates in lesbian couples with and without bacterial vaginosis.[33] Hydrogen peroxide producing *Lactobacilli* appear to be protective as women with *Lactobacilli* were less likely to develop bacterial vaginosis than those without. A change in sexual partner and douching cause these hydrogen peroxide producing *Lactobacilli* to disappear and, therefore, increase the likelihood of developing bacterial vaginosis. For women with recurrent bacterial vaginosis, the condition most often arises at the time of menstruation and disappears spontaneously in the mid-cycle.[32] Episodes of candidiasis may be followed by bacterial vaginosis in women who have recurrent bacterial vaginosis as a reflection of alteration in the *Lactobacilli* status of the vagina. For other women, there seems to be no obvious reason for their recurring symptoms. Although there is clearly an alteration in the vaginal microflora with a reduction in *Lactobacilli* which produce hydrogen peroxide and bacteriocins which inhibit the overgrowth of bacteria in the vagina, it is not clear what precipitates this.

Patients should be advised to avoid douching and the use of soaps, bubble baths and shower gels in the genital area as all may alter vaginal pH and eradicate *Lactobacilli* thus predisposing to bacterial vaginosis. In women with frequent recurrences of candida and bacterial vaginosis, a once monthly treatment regimen has been suggested,[32] although this has not yet been trialled.

Streptococcus agalactiae

Streptococcus agalactiae or Group B *Streptococcus* (GBS) is a vaginal commensal which has known obstetric complications, but is not usually regarded as a cause of any gynaecological pathology. In one study,[34] in which women with vaginal symptoms were studied, GBS was isolated in 10% of samples in which a leucocyte count of greater than 10 per high power field on microscopy was taken to be an indicator of active infection. Of these 10%, GBS was the only pathogen in 83% of cases. Furthermore, the relative risk of GBS infection was 2.38 in patients with purulent vaginal discharge. A case report[35] of a woman whose symptoms appeared to be entirely attributable to GBS and which disappeared on treatment provides further evidence that, in symptomatic women with GBS, in the absence of pathogens, treatment should be instigated.

Mucopurulent cervicitis

The diagnosis of mucopurulent cervicitis is based on the presence of a mucopurulent (yellow) discharge and more than 10 polymorphonuclear leucocytes (PMNL) per high power field on microscopy of the cervical secretions. Clinically, cervicitis may be diagnosed as the presence of erythema or oedema within the columnar cell epithelium which will only be visible on speculum examination if there is an ectopy. Mucopurulent cervicitis has been described as the equivalent in women of non-gonococcal urethritis in men[36] and has been associated with *Chlamydia* in one study[36] *Ureaplasma urealyticum*, *T. vaginalis* and bacterial vaginosis in another study.[37] In a further study,[38] all women who had yellow discharge had 10 PMNLs per high power field on microscopy and all had clinical evidence of cervicitis as described above. There were significant associations of mucopurulent cervicitis with gonorrhoea, *Chlamydia* and bacterial vaginosis. This demonstrates that the finding of yellow discharge alone is a good indication for treatment and that treatment should be effective against all associated infections especially in the absence of full diagnostic facilities, i.e. erythromycin and metronidazole. Male contacts of women diagnosed with mucopurulent discharge should be advised to attend the GUM clinic for screening and epidemiological treatment.

Other pathological conditions

Tumours

Although the commonest presenting complaint of both carcinoma of the cervix and endometrium is abnormal bleeding, these conditions may also present with vaginal discharge which may be foul-smelling as a result of sloughing of necrotic tissue. A woman who is post-menopausal and presents with abnormal discharge should certainly have an ultrasound scan of the uterus and endometrial biopsy as a minimum. She may also require full STD screening but this should be guided by the history. Discharge in a post-menopausal woman caused by a pyometra will reveal a carcinoma in about 50% of cases.[39]

PSYCHOLOGICAL

Whether subjective or objective measures are used, many women experience psychological morbidity in relation to the presence of vaginal discharge. In a study of women attending their GP conducted to compare those who complained of vaginal discharge with those who did not,[40] it was found that 65% of women with complaints and 27% of those without were bothered by their usual secretion. 20% of women with complaints had a normal examination and 14% of those without complaint had abnormal vaginal secretions. Most women with complaints had an external locus of control in relation to their symptoms (i.e. believed that the cause was something extraneous) but had an internal locus of control in relation to their health in general (i.e. believed that their health is something under their own control). Fear of having something seriously wrong or of an STD being present was the reason for the consultation in 58% of cases. This study strongly demonstrates the need to establish what the patient believes to be normal and what she thinks may be wrong with her as well as information relating to possible biological causes.

MANAGEMENT

History

A full history should be taken and include a detailed gynaecological and sexual history. It is important to ask all relevant questions in an open and confident manner and to try to avoid too many presumptions. The taking of a sexual history involves intimate questioning, but the details may be highly relevant to the diagnosis or at least in guiding the practitioner in their investigations. It is, therefore, important to become comfortable in asking such questions whilst remaining sensitive to the patient. A suggested line of questioning is: when did you last have sex ? Was this with a regular partner or a new/casual partner? When did you last have sex with another partner?

Examination

The mainstay of examination in a woman who has persistent vaginal discharge is the speculum examination although no aspect of the gynaecological examination should be omitted.

Investigations

These will be guided to an extent by the history and are summarised in Table 10.1. Where the word 'swab' appears under an investigation category, this

Table 10.1 Investigations performed in an average gynaecology department to diagnose the majority of vaginal infections

1 High vaginal swab (HVS) taken from the posterior fornix for culture. This will diagnose the presence of Group B *Streptococcus*, *C. albicans* and some cases of *T. vaginalis* and bacterial vaginosis.

2 Vaginal pH measured by placing HVS onto narrow range pH paper prior to placing swab into transport medium.

Vaginal pH	Presumptive diagnosis
< 4.5	Normal
4.0–4.5	*C. albicans*
5.0–6.0	Bacterial vaginosis/*T. vaginalis*
> 6.0	Atrophic vaginitis

3 Endocervical swab for the diagnosis of gonorrhoea.

4 Endocervical swab placed in appropriate transport medium for the diagnosis of *Chlamydia*.

5 Cervical cytology. Although a woman may have had previously normal smears and be up-to-date in the screening programme, a smear may be performed on the basis of the higher rates of smear abnormalities associated with STDs. Certainly, if there is any clinical suspicion regarding the appearance of the cervix, a smear should be performed as a minimum and colposcopy considered.

6 In the presence of dysuria and other urinary symptoms, a urethral swab placed in appropriate transport medium for the diagnosis of *Chlamydia* and a midstream urine specimen for the exclusion of urinary tract pathogens should be taken.

should be taken to mean a swab placed in universal transport medium unless otherwise stipulated. Although in some cases this does not represent the investigation of greatest diagnostic sensitivity or specificity and other investigations will also not be those which are ideal, the list describes investigations which can be carried out in the average gynaecology outpatient clinic and which will adequately diagnose the majority of infections.

Diagnosis and treatment by organism

Candida

It is important not to rely solely on clinical examination for diagnosis as even the most experienced physicians may be mistaken. This is particularly important in women for whom a previous diagnosis of *Candida* has been made and who appear to have a recurrence. Diagnosis may be made by microscopic examination of the vaginal discharge. Saline or potassium hydroxide wet mount or a Gram-stained preparation are accurate and rapid methods of diagnosis. These facilities are not usually available in a gynaecology clinic and, in this case, the culture of a high vaginal swab will give accurate, if delayed, results. Determination of the vaginal pH using narrow range pH paper can also be usefully employed in the gynaecology clinic. A pH within the normal range (3.5–4.5) greatly reduces the likelihood of symptoms being due to *Trichomonas* or bacterial vaginosis. *Candida* occurs at all pH values but the vast majority occur at normal pH.[41] Thus use of pH paper allows accurate determination of the vaginal pH and assists in outpatient diagnosis of vaginitis.[42]

Underlying causes should be identified and treated if possible. Treatment of *Candida* is usually with pessaries or cream containing drugs of the imidazole group such as clotrimazole, miconazole or econazole. These drugs are not generally associated with adverse reactions and yeast resistance is very rare. Systemic treatments are also available and are more acceptable to some patients as they require a single oral dose and do not appear to be associated with serious adverse reactions. They are, however, significantly more expensive than topical treatments.

Chronic recurrent candidiasis may require other treatment regimens. Prolonged courses of imidazole pessaries or combinations of treatments such as the use of pessaries and oral treatment concurrently have been used with some success. Longer courses of oral treatments such as ketoconazole or itraconazole may also be used for highly resistant cases but require adequate monitoring of liver function as they can be hepatotoxic.

Accurate diagnosis is the key to good management of women with candidiasis. Co-existent infections, for example with *Trichomonas* or bacterial vaginosis, must be identified and treated appropriately and it should be remembered that although *Candida* may be identified, that this may not be the cause of symptoms. It has been demonstrated that *C. albicans* may be encountered in the vaginas of 3.8% of healthy asymptomatic women.[43] Conversely, there may be women who have symptoms highly suggestive of candidiasis but who in fact have an allergy to detergents used in washing powder or soaps used in the genital area or the latex of condoms. Another scenario which should be avoided is the presumptive treatment on several occasions without re-establishment of the diagnosis of a woman who has been previously demonstrated to have candidiasis. If physical examination and diagnostic tests are all normal, the patient would be far better served by the reassurance that her vaginal discharge which is of normal volume, smell, colour and pH and which grows no pathogens harbours no infection.

Gonorrhoea

Diagnosis depends on detection of *Neisseria gonorrhoea*. This may be done by microscopy of a Gram-stained preparation, culture or by use of ELISA (enzyme-linked immunoabsorbent assay) or other diagnostic techniques using nucleic acid hybridisation. The gold standard method of diagnosis is culture as it not only allows specificity of 100% but also enables antibiotic sensitivity testing to be performed. From the gynaecologist's viewpoint, the number of women presenting to the outpatient clinic with a persistent vaginal discharge attributable to gonorrhoea is likely to be very small. This does not mean that it should be disregarded as a potential cause of symptoms, but rather that a single endocervical swab sent in regular transport medium, although not as sensitive a method of diagnosis as direct plating onto appropriate medium or as quick as examination of a Gram stained film in clinic, is a reasonable investigation in a low prevalence population.

N. gonorrhoeae may be treated with a penicillin for example ampicillin/ amoxycillin 2–3 g plus 1 g probenicid. Alternatively, drugs with activity against penicillinase-producing *N. gonorrhoea* (PPNG) for example ciprofloxacin 250–500 mg may be used depending on the sensitivity of the organism. Cure rates are estimated at 94–98% for the penicillin plus probenicid regimen[44–46] and in excess of 95% for ciprofloxacin.[47]

Any woman who has been diagnosed with gonorrhoea in the gynaecology clinic should be referred to the GUM clinic as there are a number of issues which require to be addressed. The first is that she is adequately treated and that at least one test of cure is performed at least 48 h post treatment to ensure that the infection has been eradicated. Secondly, it is crucial that her sexual partner(s) is/are also seen at the GUM clinic, screened and treated. The issue of safer sex may also be addressed at the GUM clinic visit during discussion with a health adviser.

T. vaginalis

Given the lack of availability of wet mount and culture facilities in the gynaecology outpatients clinic, a different approach is required to diagnose women in whom *T. vaginalis* may be a cause of symptoms. There are a number of other conditions which share some of the clinical features of *T. vaginalis*. Purulent discharge is significantly and independently associated with gonorrhoea, *C. trachomatis* and herpes simplex virus as well as *T.vaginalis*.[48] However, a rise in vaginal pH above normal is not usually seen with conditions other than trichomoniasis and bacterial vaginosis, with *T. vaginalis* commonly producing pH values of 6.0 or above. Both *T. vaginalis* and bacterial vaginosis are treated similarly although, as only *T. vaginalis* currently has implications for the treatment of partners of patients, it is important to use whatever facilities are available to diagnose it. Although the sensitivity of Papanicoloau smears is quoted variably, it is the only method of potential diagnosis, other than clinical findings, open to the gynaecologist routinely. It could be reasonably argued that, given the higher rate of smear abnormalities amongst women with STDs,[48] that a smear is justified in all women attending a clinic with a complaint of persistent vaginal discharge. This would not only allow the clinician to check that cytology is normal but would then provide a method of diagnosing at least a percentage of *T. vaginalis*.

Treatment is with either metronidazole by mouth or intravaginally. The symptoms of *T. vaginalis* may also be relieved by the use of clotrimazole, but it should be noted that this treatment is far less effective than oral metronidazole at actually killing the organisms.[6] Clotrimazole has generally been reserved for use in the first trimester of pregnancy as oral metronidazole crosses the placenta to achieve similar fetal levels to those of the mother[49] and has, therefore, been thought to be best avoided, although the evidence for teratogenicity is small and inadvertent administration to women during the first trimester has not produced reports of adverse effects.

Sexual partners of women diagnosed as having *T. vaginalis* should be seen and treated epidemiologically at the GUM clinic.

Herpes simplex virus

Diagnosis is primarily clinical but may also be made by culturing the virus. Treatment of HSV is by acyclovir or a related compound although this will only ameliorate an episode rather than effect a cure. In women who have frequently recurring episodes of HSV, long term treatment with acyclovir may be beneficial. Also under trial for long term prophylaxis is the use of echinacea which is a natural product with immunostimulant properties.

Group B Streptococcus

Diagnosis is made on a high vaginal swab. Treatment is with a penicillin or erythromycin in pencillin-allergic patients.

Bacterial vaginosis

Diagnosis may be made by microscopy of a Gram-stained film of vaginal secretions taken from the posterior fornix. The presence of 'clue' cells (vaginal epithelial cells obscured by bacterial vaginosis organisms) in the absence of *Lactobacilli* is diagnostic. Vaginal pH is raised from its normal value of 4.5 and the addition of potassium hydroxide to a sample of vaginal secretions produces a characteristic fishy odour (amine test). bacterial vaginosis organisms may also be cultured from a high vaginal swab.

Treatment is either by metronidazole in the form of tablets (400 mg twice daily for 5 days or a 2 g single dose, although this may be associated with a higher rate of recurrence/relapse) or 0.75% vaginal gel (5 g per night for 5 nights) or intravaginal clindamycin 2% cream (5 g per night for 7 days).

Infections requiring epidemiological treatment

Infections that are definitively sexually transmissible require that any partners of the patient are screened for sexually transmitted diseases and treated for the infection that has been identified in the patient. This is best achieved by referring any partners to the nearest GUM clinic. The taking of an accurate sexual history from the patient is of paramount importance in allowing identification of those partners who may be at risk.

To facilitate further the correct ongoing management of the patient, ensure adequate follow-up and treatment of partners, the patient herself can be referred to the GUM clinic.

Infections that require such action are: *Chlamydia*, gonorrhoea and *Trichomonas*. Any woman identified as having HSV may also benefit from being seen in the GUM clinic.

CONCLUSIONS

Persistent vaginal discharge is a common, and often distressing, complaint. It is hoped that this chapter will provide a basic framework for its investigation and management. We also hope that the chapter amply demonstrates that whilst gynaecologists do not have quite the facilities of the genitourinary medicine physicians that they come reasonably close to optimal management with the judicious use of standard swabs and a roll of narrow range pH paper.

REFERENCES

1 Kinghorn G R, Priestley C J F. Sexually transmitted diseases. In: Shaw R W, Soutter W P, Stanton S L (eds) Gynaecology. London: Churchill Livingstone, 1997; 825–843

2   Smith J R, Wells C, Jolly M et al. Is endometrial infection with *Candida albicans* a cause of recurrent vaginal thrush? BMJ 1993; 69: 295–296

3   Hook E W, Handsfield H H. Gonococcal infection in the adult. In: Holmes K K, Mardh P-A, Sparling P F et al. (eds) Sexually transmitted diseases. New York: McGraw Hill, 1990; 149-165

4   Laga M, Nzila A, Goeman J. The interrelationship of sexually transmitted diseases and HIV infection; implications for the control of both epidemics in Africa. AIDS 1991; 5 (Suppl 1): S55–S63

5   Barlow D, Phillips I. Gonorrhoea in women – diagnostic, clinical and therapeutic aspects. Lancet 1978; i: 761–764

6   Rein M F, Muller M. Trichomonas vaginalis. In: Holmes K K, Mardh P-A, Sparling P F et al. (eds) Sexually transmitted diseases. New York: McGraw Hill, 1990; 525–536

7   Thomason J L, Gelbart S M. *Trichomonas vaginalis*. Obstet Gynecol 1989; 74: 536–541

8   Thomason J L, Gelbart S M, Sobun J F et al. Comparison of four methods to detect *Trichomonas vaginalis*. J Clin Microbiol 1988; 26: 1869–1870

9   Fouts A C, Kraus S J. *Trichomonas vaginalis*: re-evaluation of its clinical presentation and laboratory diagnosis. J Infect Dis 1980; 141: 137–143

10 Lang W R, Ludmir A. A pathogenomonic colposcopic sign of *Trichomonas vaginalis* vaginitis. Acta Cytol 1961; 5: 390–392

11 Borton M, Friedman E A. Duration of colposcopic changes associated with *Trichomonas vaginitis*. Obstet Gynecol 1978; 51: 111–113

12 Krieger J N. Urologic aspects of trichomoniasis. Invest Urol 1981; 18: 411–417

13 Lossick J G. The diagnosis of vaginal trichomoniasis. JAMA 1988; 259: 1230

14 Werness B A. Cytopathology of sexually transmitted diseases. In: Judson F N (ed) Clinics in laboratory medicine. Philadelphia: WB Saunders, 1989

15 Roongpisuthipong A, Grimes D A, Hadgu A. Is the Papanicolaou smear useful for diagnosing sexually transmitted diseases? Obstet Gynecol 1987; 69: 820–824

16 Robinson A J, Ridgway G L. Modern diagnosis and management of genital *Chlamydia trachomatis* infection. Br J Hosp Med 1996; 55: 388–393

17 Zelin J M, Robinson A J, Ridgway G L et al. Chlamydial urethritis in heterosexual men attending a genitourinary medicine clinic: prevalence, symptoms, condom usage and partner change. Int J STDs AIDS 1995; 6: 27–30

18 Hopwood J, Mallinson H. Chlamydia testing in community clinics – a focus for accurate sexual health care. Br J Family Planning 1995; 21: 87–90

19 Blackwell A I, Thomas P D, Wareham K, Emery S J. Health gains from screening for infection of the lower genital tract in women attending for termination of pregnancy. Lancet 1993; 342: 206–210

20 Smith N, Nelson M R, Hammond J, Purkayastha S, Barton S J. Screening for lower genital tract infections in women attending for termination of pregnancy. Int J STDs AIDS 1994; 5: 212–213

21 Smith J R, Murdoch J, Carrington D et al. The prevalence of *Chlamydia trachomatis* infection in women having cervical smear tests. BMJ 1991; 302: 82–84

22 Buchan H, Vessey M, Goldacre M, Fairweather J. Morbidity following pelvic inflammatory disease. Br J Obstet Gynaecol 1993; 100: 558–562

23 Hay P E, Thomas B J, Horner P J, MacLeod E J, Renton A M, Taylor-Robinson D. *Chlamydia trachomatis* in women: the more you look, the more you find. Genitourin Med 1994; 70: 97–100

24 Lee H H, Chernesky M A, Schacter J et al. Diagnosis of *Chlamydia trachomatis* genitourinary infection in women by ligase chain reaction assay of urine. Lancet 1995; 345: 213–216

25 Taylor-Robinson D. Tests for infection with *Chlamydia trachomatis*. Int J STDs AIDS 1996; 7: 19–26

26 Morbidity and Mortality Weekly Report. Recommendations for the prevention and management of *Chlamydia trachomatis* infections. MMWR 1993; 42 RR-12

27 Martin D H, Mroczkowski T F, Dula Z A et al. A controlled trial of single dose azithromycin for the treatment of chlamydial urethritis and cervicitis. N Engl J Med 1992; 327: 921–925

28 Ossewarde J M, Plantema F H F, Rieffe M et al. Efficacy of single dose azithromycin versus doxycycline in the treatment of cervical infections caused by *Chlamydia trachomatis*. Eur J Clin Microbiol Infect Dis 1992; 11: 693–697

29 Lister P, Balachandran T, Ridgway G L, Robinson A J. Comparison of azithromycin and doxycycline in the treatment of non-gonococcal urethritis. J Antimicrob Chemother 1993; 31 (Suppl e): 185–192

30 Stamm W E, Hick C B, Martin D H et al. Azithromycin for empirical treatment of the non-gonococcal urethritis syndrome in men. JAMA 1995; 274: 545–549

31 Department of Health. New cases seen at NHS genitourinary medicine clinics 1994. Annual figures. Summary information from KC60. London: DOH, 1995

32 Hay P E, Ugwumadu A, Chowns J. Sex, thrush and bacterial vaginosis. Int J STDs AIDS 1997; 8: 603–608

33 Skinner C J, Stokes J, Kerlew Y, Kavanagh J, Forster G E. A case-controlled study of the sexual health needs of lesbians. Genitourin Med 1996; 72: 277–280

34 Maniatis A N, Palermos J, Kantzanou M et al. *Streptococcus agalactiae*: a vaginal pathogen? J Med Microbiol 1996; 44: 199–202

35 Boyle D C M, Smith J R Group B Streptococcal vulvovaginitis J R Soc Med 1997; 90: 298–299

36 Brunham R C, Paavonen J, Stevens C E et al. Mucopurulent cervicitis – the ignored counterpart in women of urethritis in men. N Engl J Med 1984; 311: 1–6

37 Paavonen J, Critchlow C W, Rouen T et al. The etiology of cervical inflammation. Am J Obstet Gynecol 1986; 154: 556–564

38 Willmott F E. Mucopurulent cervicitis: a clinical entity? Genitourin Med 1988; 64: 169–171

39 Quinn M A, Anderson M C, Coulter A E, Soutter W P. Malignant disease of the uterus. In: Shaw R W, Soutter W P, Stanton S L. (eds) Gynaecology. London: Churchill Livingstone, 1997; 585–604

40 Bro F. Vaginal discharge in general practice – women's perceptions, beliefs and behaviour. Scand J Prim Health Care 1993; 11: 281–287

41 Kaufman R H. Establishing a correct diagnosis of vulvovaginal infection. Am J Obstet Gynecol 1988; 158: 986–988

42 Friedrich E G. Vaginitis. Pract Ther 1983; 28: 238–242

43 Merkos J M W, Bisscop J M, Stolte L M. The proper nature of vaginal candidosis and the problem of recurrence. Obstet Gynecol Survey 1985; 40: 493–504

44 Waugh M A, Cooke E M, Nehaul B B G, Brayson J. Comparison of minocycline and ampicillin in gonococcal urethritis. Br J Vener Dis 1979; 55: 411–414

45 Thin R N, Symonds M A E, Shaw E W et al A double blind trial of amoxycillin in the treatment of gonorrhoea. Br J Vener Dis 1977; 53: 118–120

46 Sherrard J, Barlow D. PPNG at St Thomas' Hospital – a changing provenance. Int J STDs AIDS 1993; 4: 330–332

47 Balachandran T, Roberts A P, Evans B A, Azadian B S. Single-dose therapy of anogenital and pharyngeal gonorrhoea with ciprofloxacin. Int J STDs AIDS 1992; 3: 49–51

48 Wolner-Hanssen P, Krieger J N, Stevens C E et al. Clinical manifestations of vaginal trichomoniasis. JAMA 1989; 261: 571–576

49 Amon I, Amon K. Placental transfer and fetal distribution of metronidazole in early human pregnancy. Int J Biol Res Pregnancy 1980; 1: 61–64

R. F. Lamont   B. M. Chin

The use of antibiotics in the prevention of preterm birth

Preterm birth is the major cause of perinatal mortality and morbidity in the developed world and accounts for 8–10% of all births.[1] Whether due to preterm labour or preterm prelabour rupture of the membranes (PPROM), spontaneous preterm birth accounts for 60–75% of preterm deliveries, with variations in frequency depending on socio-economic status[2] and other factors. In recent years, many systems have been suggested to identify the risk of preterm birth, yet efforts to predict and prevent delivery remain unsuccessful. Bed rest is not consistently effective, and methods, such as home uterine monitoring, have been controversial in their ability to reduce preterm labour and delivery.[3,4] Many different oral tocolytic agents have been tried but have been found to be ineffective in preventing preterm labour[5] and can only prolong labour when administered parenterally.[6–8]

Preterm birth itself is a heterogeneous condition which is affected by many factors, such as faulty placentation and immune response, cervical incompetence, trauma, and fetal anomalies.[9] In recent years, an increasingly closer causal relationship has been found between intra-uterine infection and preterm labour and delivery. Infection by certain organisms has been found to lead to preterm delivery as the result of activation of the preterm labour process.[1,10–14] As a result of this, to assess the potential for prolongation of pregnancy, many studies have examined the effect of antimicrobial therapy either used prophylactically or following the onset of preterm labour or PPROM in addition to the effect on reducing perinatal infectious morbidity. This paper attempts to review the present literature and to assess the role of antimicrobial therapy in preventing preterm labour and delivery and in reducing maternal and neonatal morbidity and mortality.

Mr R. F. Lamont, Consultant in Obstetrics and Gynaecology, Northwick Park Hospital, Harrow, Middlesex HA1 3UJ, UK

Mr B. M. Chin, Visiting Research Fellow, Department of Biology, University of Richmond, Virginia, USA

INFECTION AS A CAUSE OF PRETERM LABOUR

To assess the effectiveness of antimicrobial therapy on the prevention of preterm labour and delivery, it is important to appreciate the association between abnormal bacterial colonisation and preterm labour. Bacteria or their products can cause abortion or labour when administered to animals.[15,16] The ability of systemic maternal infections to cause the onset of labour, together with the frequent association of intra-uterine infection with preterm labour and delivery,[1,10–14] has led to the current acceptance of intra-uterine infection as one of the causal agents of preterm birth. The route of intra-uterine colonisation is most likely to be through ascending infection.[17] This is supported by a number of different factors. Histological chorioamnionitis is more common and severe at the site of membrane rupture than at other locations.[18] Virtually all cases of congenital pneumonia are accompanied by inflammation of the chorioamniotic membranes. The flora associated with congenital infections is similar to the flora of the lower genital tract. Twin studies have shown that the presenting sac of twin I is always infected first and with a greater inoculum size than twin II.[19] These findings have led to a proposed mechanism for infection in which there is an overgrowth of organisms in the vagina or cervix (e.g. bacterial vaginosis), ascending colonisation of the decidua (e.g. deciduitis and chorionitis), invasion of the fetal membranes, passage through the amnion to the liquor amnii, and colonisation of the fetus through aspiration or seeding through other sites into the fetal circulation. The role and mechanism of infection as a possible cause of preterm labour is strongly suggested and supported. There are three ways in which the use of antibiotics might prevent preterm delivery: (i) used prophylactically; (ii) used therapeutically in preterm labour; or (iii) used in the presence of PPROM.

ANTIBIOTIC PROPHYLAXIS OF WOMEN AT RISK FOR PRETERM DELIVERY

Since 66% of neonatal deaths occur in babies delivered before 29 weeks' gestation, the role of prophylactic antibiotics may be important. Certain infections or abnormal states of colonisation have been found to be associated with a greater risk of preterm delivery, e.g. bacterial vaginosis, asymptomatic bacteriuria, and carriage of group B *Streptococcus* (GBS).

Bacterial vaginosis

Bacterial vaginosis has been linked to perinatal morbidity, prematurity, and preterm labour.[20] By definition, bacterial vaginosis is a polymicrobial condition in which there is a significant reduction of *Lactobacilli* spp. in the vagina which is replaced by a 1000-fold increase in other organisms, such as anaerobes and *Mycoplasma hominis*. Since *Lactobacilli* spp. normally produce H_2O_2 which is toxic to bacteria, a reduction in the number and quality of *Lactobacilli* spp. results in an increase in the colonisation of potential pathogens with very little host response.[21]

As an infection, bacterial vaginosis is a risk factor for preterm labour because many of the organisms associated with the condition are commonly found in association with preterm labour and delivery.[22-24] Gravett et al[25] found that amniotic fluid colonised with bacterial vaginosis was associated with significantly shorter latency periods, a decreased success rate for tocolytic therapy, and an increased rate of intrapartum chorioamnionitis, and they cited a 3.8-fold increased risk of preterm labour if bacterial vaginosis was present. Kurki et al[26] found that women with bacterial vaginosis between 8 and 17 weeks' gestation had a 2–6-fold increased risk of preterm birth, and Hillier et al[20] found bacterial vaginosis to be associated with preterm delivery and low birthweight infants, independent of other recognised risk factors. Meis et al[27] found that women with bacterial vaginosis at 28 weeks' gestation had an increased risk of spontaneous preterm birth, and Holst et al[28] found that the presence of bacterial vaginosis was associated with a 2.1-fold increased risk for preterm birth and a greater chance of low birthweight. Using multiple logistic regression analysis, bacterial vaginosis was found to be associated with a 5-fold increased risk of late miscarriage and preterm delivery when this was detected before 16 weeks' gestation irrespective of recognised risk factors such as black race, smoking or previous preterm delivery.[29] Bacterial vaginosis appears to be associated with preterm labour and its complications, but whether it is a problem in itself or is just a marker for another, specific infection remains unclear.

Even though the role of bacterial vaginosis has yet to be decided, recent studies have been performed to determine whether treating bacterial vaginosis would decrease the incidence of preterm delivery and its complications. Oral metronidazole is an effective way of treating bacterial vaginosis.[30] Morales et al[31] gave women with a history of bacterial vaginosis and preterm delivery oral metronidazole and found a significant reduction in the incidence of preterm labour, preterm delivery, low birthweight and PPROM. McGregor et al[32] used oral clindamycin to treat women with bacterial vaginosis and continued treatment to 32 weeks' gestation. They found that this reduced bacterial vaginosis-linked preterm birth or PPROM by 50%.

Subsequent studies found conflicting results about the effectiveness of antibiotics. McGregor et al[33] gave 2% clindamycin vaginal cream to women with bacterial vaginosis and found that antibiotic administration only temporarily reduced mucinase and sialidase activity, which are enzymes that allow microbial penetration of the cervical mucous plug, but that it did not reduce perinatal morbidity. In a similar multicentre randomised trial with 2% clindamycin vaginal cream, Joesoef et al[34] found a 85% cure rate of bacterial vaginosis, but no reduction in morbidity with antibiotic treatment. They concluded that systemic therapy might be required to reduce the incidence of preterm delivery through the eradication of organisms which had already gained access to the upper genital tract. Hauth et al[35] treated women with bacterial vaginosis and a history of preterm delivery with either metronidazole and erythromycin or a placebo and found a marked reduction in the incidence of preterm delivery. An association between vaginal colonisation with bacterial vaginosis and preterm delivery has been suggested, particularly in women with a past history of preterm birth, and systemic treatment of the condition appears to decrease the incidence of preterm delivery and its complications. The studies are summarised in Table 11.1.

Table 11.1 Prophylactic antibiotics for the treatment of bacterial vaginosis and the risk of preterm labour

Study	Year	Org.	Antibiotic regimen	Maternal/neonatal results
Morales et al[31]	1994	BV	Oral metronidazole	Reduction in preterm labor, preterm delivery, low birth weight, and premature rupture of the membranes
McGregor et al[33]	1994	BV	2% clindamycin cream	Decrease in BV symptomatology, but no reduction in preterm delivery or low birth weight
McGregor et al[32]	1995	BV	Oral clindamycin	A 50% reduction in BV related preterm birth or PPROM
Joesoef et al[34]	1995	BV	2% clindamycin cream	No reduction in preterm delivery or low birthweight
Hauth et al[35]	1995	BV	Oral metronidazole and erythromycin	Reduction in preterm delivery

BV = Bacterial vaginosis
Org. = Organisms or groups of organisms

The most successful antibiotic regimen would appear to be systemic clindamycin or metronidazole, since these agents are known to be active against bacterial vaginosis-related organisms, in contrast to ampicillin and erythromycin which have lower activity against anaerobes or *Mycoplasma hominis*. Local antimicrobial therapy is helpful due to the high concentrations of antibiotics required to treat bacterial vaginosis-related organisms. Systemic therapy may be better to ensure eradication of organisms, which have already gained access to the decidua.

Asymptomatic bacteriuria

In 1962, the association between urinary tract infections and perinatal morbidity was first suggested by Kass.[36] Conflicting reports followed with respect to the association between asymptomatic bacteriuria and preterm labour and its complications. In a randomised, double-blinded, placebo-controlled study, Kincaid-Smith and Bullen[37] found a significantly higher morbidity associated with bacteriuria but could find no reduction in morbidity with antibiotic therapy, and this was confirmed by Little.[38] Conversely, Robertson et al[39] found a significant reduction in prematurity and low birthweight with treatment of bacteriuric patients. Schieve et al[40] studied 25 746 women with antepartum urinary tract colonisation and found an increased risk of fetal morbidity from bacteriuria but no significant decrease after treatment. Romero et al[41] carried out a meta-analysis of prospective trials and found that women with asymptomatic bacteriuria who were untreated had a higher risk of preterm delivery and low birth weight. In addition, they found antibiotic therapy led to a highly significant reduction in the incidence of low birth weight, but no effect on the preterm delivery rate.

Group B *Streptococcus* (GBS)

GBS has been linked to prelabour rupture of the membranes (PROM)[42,43] and PPROM.[44] Katz[45] found an increase rate of PROM and preterm labour in association with GBS, and implied a relationship between gestational age at time of positive culture and the risk of preterm labour. Women with positive GBS urine cultures after 28 weeks' gestation had a higher incidence of preterm labour.

A number of studies have examined the effects of antibiotics on GBS carriage and the effects on morbidity and mortality associated with preterm birth. The Vaginal Infections and Prematurity Study group[46] examined the effects of antibiotic treatment on perinatal morbidity, and even though they found a preterm delivery rate of approximately 12% for GBS carriers, no reduction in preterm delivery was found with antibiotic treatment by erythromycin. They did, however, admit certain deficiencies that might have influenced their results, such as too small a sample size, the use of non-trial antibiotics, and the lack of a specified density of colonisation. McGregor et al[47] found that the use of either erythromycin or clindamycin was effective and provided cover for GBS colonisation. In summary, existing studies suggest that maternal GBS is a potential marker for preterm delivery, but data are inadequate to suggest that treatment of carriers remote from delivery will improve pregnancy outcome.

ANTIBIOTIC THERAPY FOR WOMEN IN PRETERM LABOUR

Given the strong correlation between intra-uterine infection and prematurity, many investigators have considered the possibility that antibiotics used therapeutically in women in preterm labour might prolong pregnancy and, therefore, reduce perinatal morbidity. Two randomised trials of adjunctive antibiotic therapy in women in preterm labour have been carried out.[48,49] In the first trial they found a significant mean increase in latency, the incidence of term birth, and mean birthweight with the use of oral erythromycin administered to women in preterm labour. In the second study which used intravenous clindamycin, pregnancy was prolonged in treated women with bacterial vaginosis, but no increase in term delivery or mean birthweight was found. Morales et al[50] used ampicillin or erythromycin, or no antibiotics, together with parenteral tocolytics and prophylactic oral therapy with terbutaline. They found significantly longer latency periods with the use of either ampicillin or erythromycin and a decrease in preterm delivery with ampicillin therapy, but, no increase in mean birthweight.

Winkler et al[51] randomised women receiving fenoterol to either erythromycin or placebo and found that women colonised with *Ureaplasma urealyticum* who were treated with erythromycin had a prolonged latency period and an increased mean birthweight. No benefit was obtained by women who were not colonised by the organism. There is also a case report of eradication of *U. urealyticum* for the amniotic fluid of women in preterm labour at 32 weeks' gestation using 10 days of oral erythromycin.[52] Oral ampicillin when given to women in the latent-phase of preterm labour increased gestational age and birthweight and significantly reduced the incidence of intra-uterine growth retardation, as well as histological chorioamnionitis, and puerperal endometritis.[53] Intravenous ampicillin given to women in similar circumstances produced a significant reduction in the incidence of neonatal infection, as well as histological chorioamnionitis, and puerperal endometritis.[54] Women in active preterm labour were randomised to receive either intravenous ampicillin with oral metronidazole or a placebo. Pregnancy was significantly prolonged in the antibiotic group, particularly for those women between 26 and 34 weeks' gestation, although this was not statistically significant. The neonates of the control group who received no antibiotics developed significantly more cases of necrotising enterocolitis.[93] A recent study[97] from Scandinavia found that treatment with ampicillin and metronidazole significantly prolonged gestation.

Some studies have failed to demonstrate any significant improvement with antibiotic treatment. Newton et al[55] gave women at risk of preterm labour ampicillin followed by erythromycin but were unable to find any significant improvement in neonatal and maternal mortality and morbidity. They repeated the study using ampicillin with sulbactam or a matching placebo, but again no significant improvement was seen with antibiotics.[56] However, women with positive amniotic fluid cultures were eliminated and so it is not surprising that antibiotics were of no benefit since these were discontinued if an infection was present. Cox et al[57] found no significant increase in gestational age and birthweight or any reduction in neonatal morbidity and perinatal death when they administered ampicillin and sulbactam and amoxicillin-clavulanic acid to women in preterm labour between 24 and 34 weeks' gestation. In a large NICHD-funded multicentre trial, Romero et al[58] gave women in preterm labour either intravenous ampicillin and erythromycin followed by oral therapy with an amoxicillin/erythromycin base or a matching placebo, but they were unable to demonstrate an improvement in latency or reduction in maternal or neonatal morbidity with antibiotic treatment. The results may be due to the fact that only 60% of the women completed all the study medications and that over 2000 women would have had to have been recruited to assess accurately the impact of antibiotics.

McCaul et al[59] gave women in preterm labour or with PPROM ampicillin or placebo and found a significant prolongation in latency for women with PPROM but no change in women with intact membranes. McDonald et al found no benefit from metronidazole but based the diagnosis of bacterial vaginosis on culture of *Gardnerella vaginalis* which is not specific for bacterial vaginosis and not sensitive to this particular antibiotic.[98]

Though there is undeniable evidence to link intra-uterine infection and preterm labour, no consistent benefit has been found between antibiotic treatment and pregnancy prolongation or reduction of perinatal mortality or morbidity. However, many of the trials suffered from a high incidence of post-randomisation exclusion and, consequently, are unable to address adequately the outcome criteria. The lack of consistent benefit may also be explained by the different types of antibiotics used. Agents such as clindamycin and

Table 11.2 Studies of antibiotics in preterm labour which showed latency

Authors	Year	Numbers	Antibiotics	Results and comments
McGregor et al[48]	1986	58	Erythromycin (p.o.)	Increased pregnancy prolongation Increased birthweight
Morales et al[50]	1988	205	Ampicillin (p.o.) or Erythromycin (p.o.)	Increased pregnancy prolongation with ampicillin only Women also received tocolytics
Winkler et al[51]	1988	43	Erythromycin	Increased pregnancy prolongation if colonised by U. urealyticum
McGregor et al[49]	1991	117	Clindamycin (i.v.)	Increased pregnancy prolongation if colonised by bacterial vaginosis. Trend rather than statistically significant (P = 0.07)
Norman et al[93]	1994	82	Ampicil in (i.v) and metronidazole (p.o.)	Increased pregnancy prolongation Decrease in necrotising enterocolitis
McGregor et al[47]	1996	(Review)	Clindamycin	Reduction in bacterial vaginosis linked preterm birth and PPROM
Nadisauskiene et al[53]	1996	110	Ampicillin (p.o.)	Used in women in latent phase of labour Increased pregnancy prolongation Increased birthweight Decreased histological chorioamnionitis
Nadisauskiene et al[54]	1996	102	Ampicillin (i.v.)	Used in women in active phase of labour Reduced neonatal infection Reduced histological chorioamnionitis Reduced puerperal endometritis
Svare et al[97]	1997	112	Ampicillin and metronidazole (p.o.)	Significantly prolonged gestation No increase in maternal or neonatal sepsis

metronidazole, are active against bacterial vaginosis related organisms, in contrast to ampicillin and erythromycin which do not have as great activity against anaerobes or *Mycoplasma hominis*. While erythromycin may be partially active against bacterial vaginosis associated organisms, it cannot be fully activated in the vaginal fluid. It is interesting to speculate on the different antibiotic regimens used in those studies which showed latency and those that did not. Of those nine studies which showed latency, eight studies used single agent antibiotics or agents such as metronidazole which are known to be active against bacterial vaginosis or related organisms. This is in contrast to only one of five of those studies which failed to show latency. The choice of combined therapy raises the question of bacterostatic and bactericidal antibiotics cancelling out each other's efficacy by their mode of action together with the problems of trying to carry out large multicentre studies.[94]

It is still recommended that intrapartum prophylaxis against GBS in the form of penicillin (i.v.) four hourly should be given to women delivering preterm who are known carriers of GBS or who have a history of perinatal morbidity due to this organism. The use of antibiotics for intrapartum chemoprophylaxis against early onset neonatal GBS infection is important but

Table 11.3 Studies of antibiotics in preterm labour which showed no latency

Authors	Year	Numbers	Antibiotic	Results and comments
Newton et al[55]	1989	103	Ampicillin (i.v.) then erythromycin (p.o.)	No increase in pregnancy prolongation. Tocolytics discontinued after positive amniotic fluid cultures
Newton et al[56]	1991	91	Ampicillin and sulbactam (i.v.)	No increase in pregnancy prolongation. Indomethacin given to antibiotic group Tocolytics discontinued after positive amniotic fluid culture
McCaul et al[59]	1992	75	Ampicillin (i.v. then p.o.)	No increase in pregnancy prolongation
Romero et al[58]	1993	277	Ampicillin and erythromycin (i.v.) Amoxicillin and erythromycin (p.o.)	Multicentre study; only 60% completed medication No increase in pregnancy prolongation. Power calculations required 2000 women
Cox et al[57]	1996	86	Ampicillin and sulbactam (i.v.) then ampicillin and clavulanic acid (p.o.)	No increase in pregnancy prolongation
McDonald et al[98]	1997	879	Metronidazole (p.o.)	No reduction in preterm birth rate Reduced risk of preterm birth in women with previous preterm birth Diagnosis of bacterial vaginosis based on culture of *Gardnerella vaginalis*

not pertinent to this review. The revised guidelines by the American Academy of Pediatrics, the Centers for Disease Control and the American College of Obstetricians and Gynecologists discuss the options and form an essential template for any discussion between obstetrician and paediatrician about a protocol for the management of GBS in pregnancy.[99] The studies pertaining to the use of antibiotics for delay of preterm birth and their outcomes are summarised in Tables 11.2 and 11.3.

ANTIBIOTIC THERAPY FOR PPROM

PPROM is found in approximately 30% of all preterm deliveries in the US, and it is responsible for up to 10% of all perinatal deaths.[60] The correlation between PPROM and positive amniotic fluid cultures, placental cultures, clinical and histological chorioamnionitis, and maternal cytokine response to intra-uterine infections has been well documented[61–63] and amniotic fluid cultures are positive in 14–37% of patients after PPROM.[64–66] Cultures obtained from the amniotic fluid and decidua after PPROM have many types of Gram-positive and Gram-negative aerobic and anaerobic bacteria as well as genital mycoplasmas, and similar organisms have been found in placental cultures after preterm birth.[67–69] The maternal consequences of PPROM are infection with a 8–28% risk of chorioamnionitis and an increased risk of 7–17% of endometritis. The rate of abruption and caesarean section is also increased.[70,71] The fetal consequences of PPROM are prematurity, infection, positional deformities, and an increased mortality rate. Immaturity is the most frequent cause of perinatal mortality, and respiratory distress syndrome due to hyaline membrane disease is the most common complication following preterm birth.[72,73]

Prevention of PPROM

Since PPROM plays such a major role in maternal and fetal morbidity and mortality, the role of antibiotics in the management of PPROM has been investigated. McGregor et al[74] examined the benefit of erythromycin and clindamycin in preventing the bacterial protease-induced weakening of the amniochorion, and they found that used together, erythromycin and clindamycin prevented bacteria cell growth and the release of their proteases, which characteristically cause membrane damage. In this way, antibiotic treatment may have a role in the prevention of PPROM. This is supported by the fact that antibiotics given to women with PPROM will significantly prolong the interval from membrane rupture to delivery and result in an improved neonatal outcome.[75]

Prophylaxis against infection after PPROM

Most studies focus on the use of antibiotics after membrane rupture to treat subclinical deciduitis and amniotic fluid colonisation or to prevent ascending infection. A number of randomised prospective clinical trials have been performed to evaluate the use of systemic antibiotic therapy in managing PPROM remote from term and its effect on the maternal and infant morbidity associated with PPROM.[47,59,76–88,91,92] The studies have different designs, antimicrobial agents, routes of therapy, duration of therapy, treatment of GBS, use of corticosteroids for fetal pulmonary maturation, and tocolytic therapy, and the results are summarised in Table 11.4.

One of the areas examined was latency. Nine out of seventeen studies[76,78,81–83,85,86,91,92] found an increase in the number of women still undelivered after 7 days. In one study by Blanco et al[85] the control group had a median latency of 11.4 days, but this was in a low risk population. Two peer-review meta-analyses[89,90] found that antibiotics increased the chance of prolonging the pregnancy by 7 days. However, a majority of women will deliver in this time regardless of antibiotic therapy, and it is estimated that only 15% of women are likely to accrue benefit from treatment.

Antibiotics also appear to be of benefit in reducing maternal morbidity. Nine trials[59,76,79–81,84,87,88,91] found a reduction in chorioamnionitis with antibiotic treatment, and this was confirmed by meta-analyses.[89,90] In only one out of nine studies was a reduction found in the incidence of endometritis following PPROM.[81] The incidence of caesarean section was not changed by antibiotic treatment. Mercer et al[76] found that the administration of erythromycin instead of a placebo prolonged pregnancy and delayed the onset of symptoms in women who would subsequently develop chorioamnionitis. The overall incidence of chorioamnionitis was not decreased and seemed to indicate that only aggressive antibiotic regimens will actually reduce clinical amnionitis.

The purpose of antibiotics is to reduce the perinatal mortality and morbidity related to intra-uterine infection and prematurity. Despite this, none of the quoted studies have found a reduction in stillbirth, neonatal death, or improvement in overall infant survival, which was high (92–93%) irrespective of whether or not antibiotic treatment was used. The mean gestation age in the evaluated trials was 30 weeks, which is far enough in gestation for the majority of PPROM patients to survive without antibiotic treatment.

In contrast, antibiotics can still be of some use, since the commonest cause of perinatal morbidity following PPROM is respiratory distress syndrome (RDS), which complicates 39% of preterm births. No published studies have found that antibiotics reduce this morbidity, but this might be due to the large range of gestation ages included within the trials. When only those gestations beyond 32 weeks were studied, the risk of RDS was too low for any observed benefit. Conversely, many of the studies were conducted as gestations as low as 20 or 23 weeks which is so close to the limit of viability that it is unlikely that it would be possible to reduce the occurrence of RDS.[76,78,81–85] A large NICHD-funded multicentre trial of intravenous and oral ampicillin and erythromycin at 24–32 weeks' gestation found a significant reduction in respiratory distress as well as a reduction in perinatal morbidity and maternal intra-uterine infection with an improvement in latency.[91] Three of twelve trials also found a significant benefit of antibiotics with respect to neonatal sepsis, and these are confirmed by meta-analyses[89,90] One trial suggested a reduction in intra-ventricular haemorrhaging with use of antibiotics.[81]

These findings need to be considered cautiously since prolonged antibiotic use might lead to resistant bacterial strains and a subsequent increase in the rate of neonatal and maternal morbidity. One study found a significantly increased risk of necrotising enterocolitis with maternal antibiotic therapy.[87]

Table 11.4 Prophylactic antibiotics following PPROM

Author	Year	Antibiotics	Results and comments
Dunlop et al[77]	1974	± Cephalexin (p.o.)	± Ritrodrine Reduced rate of stillbirth, RDS, NEC and IVH Improved survival
Amon et al[78]	1988	Ampicillin (i.v. then p.o.)	Increased pregnancy prolongation
Morales et al[79]	1989	Ampicillin (i.v.)	Reduced risk of chorioamnionitis
Debodinance et al[80]	1990	Mezlocillin (i.v.)	Reduced risk of chorioamnionitis
Johnston et al[81]	1990	Mezlocillin (i.v.) then ampicillin (p.o.)	Increased pregnancy prolongation Reduced risk of chorioamnionitis, endometritis + IVH
McGregor et al[82]	1991	Erythromycin (p.o.)	Increased pregnancy prolongation
Christmas et al[83]	1992	Ampicillin (i.v.) Gentamicin (i.v.) Clindamycin (i.v.) Ampicillin and clavulonate (p.o.)	Increased pregnancy prolongation
Kurki et al[84]	1992	Penicillin (i.v.)	Reduced risk of chorioamnionitis
Mercer et al[76]	1992	Erythromycin (p.o.)	Increased pregnancy prolongation Delay in clinical chorioamnionitis
McCaul et al[59]	1992	Ampicillin (i.v. then p.o.)	Reduction in maternal and neonatal sepsis Less RDS
Blanco et al[85]	1993	Cefizoxime (i.v.)	Increased pregnancy prolongation Increased neonatal survival Decrease in neonatal sepsis, RDS, IVH and NEC
Lockwood et al[86]	1993	Piperacillin (i.v.)	Increased pregnancy prolongation
Owen et al[87]	1993	Ampicillin (i.v.) then ampicillin or erythromycin (p.o.)	Decreased maternal sepsis Improved neonatal survival Increased risk of NEC
Ernest & Givner[88]	1994	Penicillin (i.v. then p.o.)	Decreased maternal sepsis
Lewis et al[92]	1995	Ampicillin ± sulbactam	Increased pregnancy prolongation
McGregor et al[47]	1996	Clindamycin (i.v.)	Reduction in bacterial vaginosis linked preterm birth + PPROM
Mercer et al[91]	1996	Ampicillin	Increased pregnancy prolongation Less RDS and maternal sepsis

In summary, antibiotic treatment for women with PPROM remote from term offers significant benefit with respect to pregnancy prolongation and reductions in clinically apparent intra-uterine infection and neonatal infectious morbidity. Further study is necessary to find the optimal treatment regimen since oral therapy does not appear to reduce significantly the incidence of infectious morbidity, though it does prolong pregnancy.[76,82] In addition, ampicillin-sulbactam treatment was found to be more effective than ampicillin alone, which suggests that an early, aggressive, broad-spectrum course of intravenous therapy is required.[92] The value of extended antibiotic treatment is unclear since this may lead to the development of resistant bacterial strains with an increase in infant and maternal morbidity. Intravenous antibiotics should be used initially, followed by a short course of oral therapy (5 days) using broad-spectrum agents together with agents which have activity against bacterial vaginosis related organisms.

SUMMARY

There is now overwhelming evidence that infection is a major cause of spontaneous early preterm labour. There is also increasing evidence that abnormal genital tract colonisation in the form of bacterial vaginosis in early pregnancy is a predictor of preterm labour. We are also developing a greater understanding of the microbiology of preterm labour.[95,96] From currently available evidence it would appear that, provided the choice of antibiotics is appropriate for the likely organisms or groups of organisms present, prophylactic antibiotics for those women at high risk of preterm labour (previous preterm birth, abnormal genital tract colonisation, PPROM) may be of help in prolonging pregnancy and reducing maternal and neonatal infectious morbidity for women in preterm labour. With the right choice of agent or combination of agents which will be active against bacterial vaginosis or bacterial vaginosis related organisms the current evidence suggests that for women in pre-term labour antibiotics maybe of help particularly if used in conjunction with tocolytics.

Caution should be exercised under these circumstances. There is no substitute for delivery of a baby in good condition and heroic efforts to delay delivery at gestational ages where survival rates are high may compromise both mother and fetus. Women in preterm labour of infectious aetiology are refractory to the use of tocolytics and are, therefore, at higher risk of the serious side effects with use of these drugs.

Preterm labour is either a physiological process occurring too early in pregnancy or more likely, due to a pathological trigger and infection is likely to be a trigger. Preterm labour approaching 37 weeks' gestation is more likely to be physiological in contrast to those labours just after 24 weeks which are certainly due to some pathology.

This being the case, the risk versus benefit of antibiotics for women in preterm labour is only likely to balance in favour of their use at very early gestations.

REFERENCES

1 Andrews W W, Goldenberg R L, Hauth J C. Preterm labor: emerging role of genital tract infections [Review]. Infect Agents Dis 1995; 4: 196–211

2 Meis P J, Ernest J M, Moore M L. Causes of low birth weight births in public and private patients. Am J Obstet Gynecol 1987; 156: 1165–1168

3 Colton T, Kayne H L, Zhang Y, Heeren T. A meta-analysis of home uterine activity monitoring. Am J Obstet Gynecol 1995; 173: 1499–1505

4 Anonymous. A multicenter randomized controlled trial of home uterine monitoring: active versus sham device. The Collaborative Home Uterine Monitoring Study (CHUMS) Group. Am J Obstet Gynecol 1995; 173: 1120–1127

5 Lamont R F, Elder M G. Serum levels of Ritodrine used for the management of preterm labour. J Obstet Gynaecol 1986; 7: 20–22

6 Besinger R E, Iannucci T A. Tocolytic therapy. In: Elder M G, Lamont R F, Romero R. (eds) Preterm labor. New York; Churchill Livingstone, 1997; 243–297

7 Niebyl J R, Lundstrom V, Green K. Premature labor and indomethacin. Am J Obstet Gynecol 1980; 136: 1014–1019

8 Ohlsson A. Treatments of preterm premature rupture of the membranes: a meta-analysis. Am J Obstet Gynecol 1989; 160: 890–906

9 Lettieri L, Vintzileos A M, Rodis J F, Albini S M, Salafia C M. Does `idiopathic' preterm labor resulting in preterm birth exist? Am J Obstet Gynecol 1993; 168: 1480–1485

10 Goepfert A R, Goldenberg R L. Prediction of prematurity [Review]. Curr Opin Obstet Gynecol 1996; 8: 417–427

11 Owen P, Patel N. Prevention of preterm birth [Review]. Baillière's Clin Obstet Gynaecol 1995; 9: 465–479

12 Gibbs R S, Romero R, Hillier S L, Eschenbach D A, Sweet R L. A review of premature birth and subclinical infection. Am J Obstet Gynecol 1992; 166: 1515–1528

13 Lamont R F, Fisk N M. The role of infection in the pathogenesis of preterm labour. Prog Obstet Gynaecol 1993; 10: 135–158

14 Mazor M, Chaim W, Horowitz S, Romero R, Glezerman, M. The biomolecular mechanisms of preterm labor in women with intra-uterine infection [Review]. Isr Med Sci 1994; 30: 317–322

15 Dombroski R A, Woodward D S, Harper J K et al. A rabbit model for bacterial-induced abortion by treatment of mice with antisera. Am J Obstet Gynecol 1990; 163: 1938–1947

16 Gravett M G, Haluska G J, Cook M J, Novy M J. Fetal and maternal endocrine response to experimental intra-uterine infection in rhesus monkeys. Am J Obstet Gynecol 1996: 174: 1725–1731

17 Romero R, Mazor M. Infection and preterm labor. Clin Obstet Gynecol 1988; 31: 553–583

18 Romero R, Sirtori M, Oyarzun E et al. Infection and labor: V. Prevalence, microbiology, and clinical significance of intraamniotic infection in women with preterm labor and intact membranes. Am J Obstet Gynecol 1989; 161: 817–824

19 Romero R, Fayek S, Avila C et al. The prevalence and microbiology of intraamniotic infection in twin gestation with preterm labor. Am J Obstet Gynecol 1990; 163: 757–761

20 Hillier S L, Nugent R P, Eschenbach D A et al. Association between bacterial vaginosis and preterm delivery of a low-birth-weight infant. The Vaginal Infections and Prematurity Study Group. N Engl J Med 1995; 333: 1737–1742

21 Lamont R F. Bacterial vaginosis. In: Studd J W W, Jardine-Brown C. (eds) The Yearbook of the Royal College of Obstetricians & Gynaecologists. London: Parthenon, 1995; 30: 149–160

22 Lamont R F, Taylor-Robinson D, Newman M, Wigglesworth J S, Elder M G. Spontaneous early preterm labour associated with abnormal genital bacterial colonisation. Br J Obstet Gynaecol 1986; 93: 804–810

23 Lamont R F, Taylor-Robinson D, Wigglesworth J S, Furr P M, Evans R T, Elder M G. The role of mycoplasmas, ureaplasmas and chlamydiae in the genital tract of women presenting in spontaneous early preterm labor. J Med Microbiol 1987; 24: 253–257

24 McDonald H M, O'Loughlin J A, Jolley P, Vigneswaran R, McDonald P J. Vaginal infection and preterm labor. Br J Obstet Gynecol 1991; 98: 427–435

25 Gravett M G, Nelson H P, DeRouen T, Critchlow C, Eschenbach D A, Holmes K K. Independent associations of bacterial vaginosis and *Chlamydia trachomatis* infection with adverse pregnancy outcome. JAMA 1986; 256: 1899–1903

26 Kurki T, Sivonen A, Renkonen O V, Savia E, Ylikorkala O. Bacterial vaginosis in early pregnancy and pregnancy outcome. Obstet Gynecol 1992; 80: 173–177

27 Meis P J, Goldenberg R L, Mercer B et al. The preterm prediction study: significance of vaginal infections. National Institute of Child Health and Human Development Maternal-Fetal Medicine Units Network. Am J Obstet Gynecol 1995; 173: 1231–1235

28 Holst E, Goffeng A R, Andersch B. Bacterial vaginosis and vaginal microorganisms in idiopathic premature labor and association with pregnancy outcome. J Clin Microbiol 1994; 32: 176–186

29 Hay P E, Lamont R F, Taylor-Robinson D. Bacterial vaginosis and preterm delivery. BMJ 1994; 308: 787–788

30 McDonald H M, O'Loughlin J A, Vigneswaran R, Jolley P T, McDonald P J. Bacterial vaginosis in pregnancy and efficacy of short course oral metronidazole treatment: a randomized controlled trial. Obstet Gynecol 1994; 84: 343–348

31 Morales W J, Schorr S, Albritton J. Effect of metronidazole in patients with preterm birth in preceding pregnancy and bacterial vaginosis: a placebo-controlled, double-blind study. Am J Obstet Gynecol 1994; 171: 345–349

32 McGregor J A, French J I, Parker R et al. Prevention of premature birth by screening and treatment for common genital tract infections: results of a prospective controlled evaluation. Am J Obstet Gynecol 1995; 173: 157–167

33 McGregor J A, French J I, Jones W et al. Bacterial vaginosis is associated with prematurity and vaginal fluid mucinase and sialidase: results of a controlled trial of topical clindamycin cream. Am J Obstet Gynecol 1994; 170: 1048–1059

34 Joesoef M R, Hillier S L, Wiknjosastro G et al. Intravaginal clindamycin treatment for bacterial vaginosis: effects on preterm delivery and low birth weight. Am J Obstet Gynecol 1995; 173: 1527–1531

35 Hauth J C, Goldenberg R L, Andrews W W, DuBard M B, Copper R L. Reduced incidence of preterm delivery with metronidazole and erythromycin in women with bacterial vaginosis. N Engl J Med 1995; 333: 1732–1736

36 Kass E H. Pyelonephritis and bacteraemia: a major problem in preventive medicine. Ann Intern Med 1962; 56: 46–53

37 Kincaid-Smith P, Bullen M. Bacteriuria in pregnancy. Lancet 1965; 1: 395–399

38 Little P J. The incidence of urinary infection in 5000 pregnant women. Lancet 1966; 2: 925–928

39 Robertson J G, Livingstone J R, Isdale M H. The management and complication of asymptomatic bacteriuria in pregnancy: report of a study on 8,275 patients. J Obstet Gynaecol Br Commonw 1968; 75: 59–65

40 Schieve L A, Handler A, Hershow R et al. Urinary tract infection during pregnancy: its association with maternal morbidity and perinatal outcome. Am J Public Health 1994; 84: 405–410

41 Romero R, Oyarzun E, Mazor M et al. Meta-analysis of the relationship between asymptomatic bacteriuria and preterm delivery/low birth weight. Obstet Gynecol 1989; 73: 576–582

42 Regan J A, Chao S, James L S. Premature rupture of membranes, preterm delivery, and group B streptococcal colonization in mothers. Am J Obstet Gynecol 1981; 141: 184–186

43 Alger L S, Lovchik J C, Hebel J R et al. The association of *Chlamydia trachomatis, Neisseria gonorrhoeae*, and group B streptococci with preterm rupture of the membranes and pregnancy outcome. Am J Obstet Gynecol 1988; 159: 397–404

44 Matorras R, Garcia-Perea, Madero R, Usandizaga J A. Maternal colonization by group B streptococci and puerperal infection; analysis of intrapartum chemoprophylaxis. Eur J Obstet Gynecol Reprod Biol 1990; 38: 203–207

45 Katz V L. Management of group B streptococcal disease in pregnancy. Clin Obstet Gynecol 1993; 36: 832–842

46 Klebanoff M A, Regan J A, Rao A V et al. Outcome of the Vaginal Infections and Prematurity Study: results of a clinical trial of erythromycin among pregnant women colonized with group B streptococcus. Am J Obstet Gynecol 1995; 172: 1540–1545

47 McGregor J A, French J I, Witkin S. Infection and prematurity: evidence-based approaches [Review]. Curr Opin Obstet Gynecol 1996; 8: 428–432

48 McGregor J A, French J I, Reller L B et al. Adjunctive erythromycin treatment for idiopathic preterm labor: results of a randomized, double-blinded, placebo-controlled trial. Am J Obstet Gynecol 1986; 154: 98–103

49 McGregor J A, French J I, Seo K. Adjunctive clindamycin therapy for preterm labor: results of a double-blind, placebo-controlled trial. Am J Obstet Gynecol 1991; 165: 867–875

50 Morales W J, Angel J D, O'Brien F W et al. A randomized study of antibiotic therapy in idiopathic preterm labor. Obstet Gynecol 1988; 72: 829–833

51 Winkler M, Baumann L, Ruchhaberle K E, Schiller E M. Erythromycin therapy for subclinical intra-uterine infections in threatened preterm delivery. A preliminary report. J Perinat Med 1988; 16: 253–256

52 Mazor M, Chaim W, Horowitz S, Leiberman J R, Glezerman M. Successful treatment of preterm labor by eradication of *Ureaplasma urealyticum* with erythromycin. Arch Gynecol Obstet 1993; 253: 215–218

53 Nadisauskiene R, Bergstrom S, Kilda A. Ampicillin in the treatment of preterm labor: a randomized, placebo-controlled study. Gynecol Obstet Invest 1996; 41: 89–92

54 Nadisauskiene R, Bergstom S. Impact of intrapartum intravenous ampicillin on pregnancy outcome in women with preterm labor: a randomized, placebo-controlled study. Gynecol Obstet Invest 1996; 41: 85–88

55 Newton E R, Dins Moor M J, Gibbs R S. A randomized, blinded, placebo-controlled trial of antibiotics in idiopathic preterm labor. Obstet Gynecol 1989; 74: 562–566

56 Newton E R, Shields L, Redgway III L E et al. Combination antibiotics and indomethacin in idiopathic preterm labor: a randomized double-blind clinical trial. Am J Obstet Gynecol 1991; 165: 1753–1759

57 Cox S M, Bohman V R, Sherman M L, Leveno K J. Randomized investigation of antimicrobials for the prevention of preterm birth. Am J Obstet Gynecol 1996; 174: 206–210

58 Romero R, Sibai B M, Caritis S et al. Antibiotic treatment of preterm labor with intact membranes: a multicenter, randomized, double blinded, placebo-controlled trial. Am J Obstet Gynecol 1993; 169: 764–774

59 McCaul J F, Perry K G, Moore J L et al. Adjunctive antibiotic treatment of women with preterm rupture of membranes or preterm labor. Int J Gynecol Obstet 1992; 38: 19- 24

60 Kaltreider D F, Kohl S. Epidemiology of preterm delivery. Clin Obstet Gynecol 1980; 23: 17–31

61 Romero R, Mazor M, Wu W K et al. Infection in the pathogenesis of preterm labour. Semin Perinatol 1988; 12: 262–279

62 Santhanam U, Avila C, Romero R et al. Cytokines in normal and abnormal parturition: elevated amniotic fluid interleukin-6 levels in women with premature rupture of membranes associated with intra-uterine infection. Cytokine 1991; 3: 155–163

63 Romero R, Yoon B H, Mazor M et al. A comparative study of the diagnostic performance of amniotic fluid glucose, white blood cell count, interleukin-6, and Gram stain in the detection of microbial invasion in patients with preterm premature rupture of membranes. Am J Obstet Gynecol 1993; 169: 839–851

64 Cotton D B, Hill L M, Strassner H T et al. The use of amniocentesis in preterm gestation with ruptured membranes. Obstet Gynecol 1984; 63: 38–48

65 Vintzileos A L, Campbell W A, Nochimson D J et al. Qualitative amniotic fluid volume versus amniocentesis in predicting infection in preterm premature rupture of the membranes. Obstet Gynecol 1986; 67: 579–583

66 Garite T J, Freeman R K. Chorioamnionitis in the preterm gestation. Obstet Gynecol 1982; 59: 539–545

67 Zlatnik F, Gellhaus T M, Benda J A et al. Histologic chorioamnionitis, microbial infection and prematurity. Obstet Gynecol 1990; 76: 355–359

68 Hillier S L, Martias J, Krohn M, Kiviat N, Holmes K K, Eschenbach D A. A case control study of chorioamniotic infection and histologic chorioamnionitis in prematurity. N Engl J Med 1988; 319: 972–977

69 Pankuch G A, Appelbaum P C, Lorenz R P et al. Placental microbiology and histology and the pathogenesis of chorioamniotis. Obstet Gynecol 1984; 64: 802–806

70 Nelson D M, Stempel L E, Zuspan F P. Association of prolonged premature rupture of membranes and abruptio placentae. J Reprod Med 1986; 31: 249–253

71 Vintzileos A M, Campbell W A, Nochimson D J et al. Preterm premature rupture of membranes: a risk factor for the development of abruptio placentae. Am J Obstet Gynecol 1987; 156: 1235–1238

72 Rotschild A, Ling E W, Putterman M L. Neonatal outcome after prolonged preterm rupture of the membranes. Am J Obstet Gynecol 1990; 162: 46–52

73 Nimrod C, Varela G, Hings F. The effect of very prolonged membrane rupture of fetal development. Am J Obstet Gynecol 1984; 148: 540–543

74 McGregor J A, Schoonmaker J N, Lunt B D, Lawellin D W. Antibiotic inhibition of bacterial-induced fetal membrane weakening. Obstet Gynecol 1990; 76: 124–128

75 Kirschbaum T. Antibiotics in the treatment of preterm labor [Review]. Am J Obstet Gynecol 1993; 168: 1239–1246

76 Mercer B, Moretti M, Rogers R, Sibai B. Antibiotic prophylaxis in preterm premature rupture of the membranes: a prospective randomized double-blind trial of 220 patients. Am J Obstet Gynecol 1992; 166: 794–802

77 Dunlop P D M, Crowley P A, Lamont R F, Hawkins D F. Preterm ruptured membranes, no contractions. J Obstet Gynaecol 1986; 7: 92–96

78 Amon E, Lewis S V, Sibai B M et al. Ampicillin prophylaxis in preterm premature rupture of the membranes: a prospective randomized study. Am J Obstet Gynecol 1988; 159: 539–543

79 Morales W J, Angel J L, O'Brien W F, Knuppel R A. Use of ampicillin and corticosteroids in premature rupture of the membranes: a randomized study. Obstet Gynecol 1989; 73: 721–726

80 Debodinance P, Parmentier D, Devulder G et al. IV. Peut-on reduire le risque infectieux neonatal dans les ruptures prematurees des membranes. F Gynecol Obstet Biol Reprod 1990; 19: 533–536

81 Johnston M M, Sanchez-Ramos L, Vaughn A J et al. Antibiotic therapy in preterm premature rupture of the membranes: a randomized prospective double-blind trial. Am J Obstet Gynecol 1990; 163: 743–747

82 McGregor J A, French J I, Seo K. Antimicrobial therapy in preterm premature rupture of membranes: results of a prospective, double-blind, placebo-controlled trial of erythromycin. Am J Obstet Gynecol 1991; 165: 632–640

83 Christmas J T, Cox S M, Andrews W et al. Expectant management of preterm ruptured membranes: effects of antimicrobial therapy. Obstet Gynecol 1992; 80: 759–762

84 Kurki T, Hallman M, Zilliacus R et al. Premature rupture of the membranes: effect of penicillin prophylaxis and long-term outcome of the children. Am J Perinatol 1992; 9: 11–16

85 Blanco J, Iams J, Artal R et al. Multicenter double-blind prospective random trial of ceftizoxime vs placebo in women with preterm premature ruptured membranes (PPROM). Am J Obstet Gynecol 1993; 168: 378 (Abstract)

86 Lockwood C J, Costigan K, Ghidini A et al. Double-blind placebo-controlled trial of piperacillin prophylaxis in preterm membrane rupture. Am J Obstet Gynecol 1993; 169: 970–976

87 Owen J, Groome L J, Hauth J C. Randomized trial of prophylactic antibiotic therapy after preterm amnion rupture. Am J Obstet Gynecol 1993; 169: 976–981

88 Ernest J M, Givner L B. A prospective randomized placebo-control trial of penicillin in preterm premature rupture of membranes. Am J Obstet Gynecol 1994; 170: 516–521

89 Mercer B, Arheart K. Antimicrobial therapy in expectant management of preterm premature rupture of the membranes. Lancet 1995; 346: 1271–1279

90 Egarter C, Leitich H, Karas I I et al. Antibiotic treatment in premature rupture of membranes and neonatal morbidity: a meta-analysis. Am J Obstet Gynecol 1996; 174: 589–597

91 Mercer B, Miodovnik M, Thurnau G et al. the NICHD-MFMU Network: a multi-center randomized mass trial of antibiotic versus placebo therapy after preterm premature rupture of the membranes [Abstract]. Am J Obstet Gynecol 1996; 174: 304

92 Lewis D F, Fontenot M T, Brooks G G et al. Latency period after preterm premature rupture of the membranes: a comparison of ampicillin with and without sulbactam. Obstet Gynecol 1995; 86: 392–395

93 Norman K, Pattison R E, de Souza J, de Jong P, Moller G, Kirsten G. Ampicillin and metronidazole treatment in preterm labour: a multicentre, randomised controlled trial. Br J Obstet Gynaecol 1994; 101: 404–408

94 Lamont R F. New approaches in the management of preterm labour of infective aetiology. Br J Obstet Gynaecol 1998; 105: 134–137

95 Rosenstein I J, Morgan D J, Sheehan M, Lamont R F, Taylor-Robinson D. Bacterial vaginosis in pregnancy. Distribution of bacterial species in different Gram stain categories of the vaginal flora. J Med Microbiol 1996; 45: 120–126

96 Chin B M, Lamont R F. The microbiology of preterm labour and delivery. Cont Rev Obstet Gynaecol 1997; 9: 285–296

97 Svare J, Langhoff-Roos J, Andersen L et al. Ampicillin-metronidazole treatment in idiopathic preterm labour: a randomised controlled multicentre trial. Br J Obstet Gynaecol 1997; 104: 892–897

98 McDonald H M, O'Loughlin H A, Vigneswaran R. Impact of metronidazole therapy on preterm birth in women with bacterial vaginosis flora (Gardnerella vaginalis): a randomised, placebo controlled trial. Br J Obstet Gynaecol 1997; 104: 1391–1397

99 American Academy of Pediatrics. Revised guidelines for prevention of early onset Group B Streptococcal (GBS) infection. Pediatrics 1997; 99: 489–496

Gurleen Sharland

Diagnosis and management of fetal cardiac abnormalities

Detailed descriptions of the cross-sectional appearance of the normal human fetal heart were published by several authors in 1980.[1,2] More recently, the normal cardiac structures have been identified in the fetus in the first trimester, allowing earlier detection of a cardiac abnormality.[3] A high degree of diagnostic accuracy in the detection of fetal congenital heart disease can now be expected by units experienced in performing the technique.[4-7] A systematic approach to the examination of the fetal heart will enable the confirmation of normality easily and, in cases with congenital heart malformations, will ensure an accurate diagnosis. This is best achieved by checking the connections of the heart. Additional cardiac anomalies can be sought once the major connections have been checked. There are 6 cardiac connections to consider, 3 on each side of the heart. These are the venous-atrial connection, the atrio-ventricular connection and the ventriculo-arterial connection. On the right side of the heart, the inferior and superior vena cavae drain to the right atrium, which then connects through the tricuspid valve to the right ventricle, which in turn gives rise to the pulmonary artery. On the left side of the heart, the left atrium receives the pulmonary veins. The left atrium then connects via the mitral valve to the left ventricle which gives rise to the aorta. The method of imaging these connections must be learnt in order to detect major forms of congenital heart disease.

THE NORMAL FETAL HEART

The four chamber view

Pulmonary venous connection and atrioventricular connections
The most easily obtained view of the fetal heart is the four-chamber view, which is achieved in a horizontal section of the fetal thorax just above the

Dr Gurleen Sharland, Senior Lecturer in Fetal and Paediatric Cardiology, Honorary Consultant, Fetal Cardiology, Guy's Hospital, 15th Floor Guy's Tower, St Thomas Street, London SE1 9RT, UK

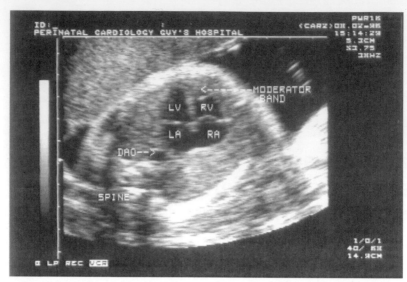

Fig. 12.1 The fetal heart is seen in a four chamber projection with the apex nearest to the ultrasound beam. One complete rib is visualised in the section. DAO = descending aorta, LA = left atrium, LV = left ventricle, RA = right atrium, RV = right ventricle. Note the moderator band which is a normal feature of the right ventricle.

diaphragm. Examination of this view will demonstrate the pulmonary veins and atria, the atrioventricular connections and the two ventricles. Thus, three of the six connections are seen in this one view alone, and clues to the normality of the great arteries can be identified. The appearance of the four-chamber view will vary according to the orientation of the fetus to the ultrasound beam. Figure 12.1 illustrates the image obtained when the apex of the heart is closest to the transducer, whereas in Figure 12.2 the ultrasound beam is perpendicular to the

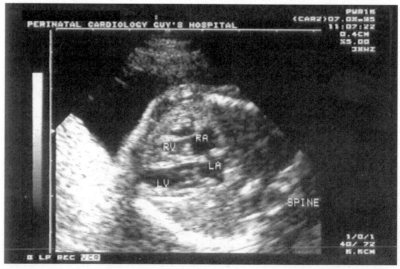

Fig. 12.2 The fetal heart is seen in a four chamber projection with the ultrasound beam perpendicular to the interventricular septum. In this projection the ventricular walls and the septum appear thicker than in Figure 12.1. LA = left atrium, LV = left ventricle, RA = right atrium, RV = right ventricle.

interventricular septum. In this latter projection, the ventricular walls and septum will appear thicker as illustrated in the image.

Important features of a four chamber view that should always be noted are:

1　The heart occupies about a third of the thorax and the apex points out of the left anterior thorax.

2　There are two atria of approximately equal size.

3　There are two ventricles of approximately equal size and thickness. Both show equal contraction in the moving image.

4　The atrial and ventricular septa meet the two atrioventricular valves (mitral and tricuspid) at the crux of the heart forming an offset cross. This offset cross appearance is because the septal leaflet of the tricuspid valve inserts slightly lower in the ventricular septum than the mitral valve.

5　The two atrioventricular valve (mitral and tricuspid) are seen to open equally in the moving image.

6　The interatrial defect, the foramen ovale is patent in fetal life. It is usually guarded by the foramen ovale flap valve, which can usually be seen flickering in the left atrium.

7　The interventricular septum should appear intact.

8　The pulmonary venous connections to the back of the left atrium should be identified (Fig. 12.3).

It should be noted that after 28 weeks' gestation the right ventricle may look slightly dilated compared with the left in the normal fetus.

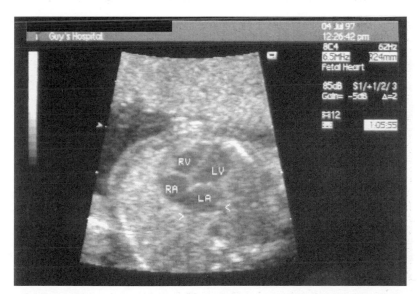

Fig. 12.3 The fetal heart is seen in a four chamber projection. At least two of the four pulmonary veins (shown by the two arrows) can be seen to be draining into the pack of the left atrium. LA = left atrium, LV = left ventricle, RA = right atrium, RV = right ventricle.

Views of the two great arteries

Ventriculo-arterial connections

The great arteries (aorta and pulmonary artery) can be imaged in both horizontal and longitudinal projections.[8] Angulating the transducer cranially from the four-chamber and towards the right shoulder demonstrates the aorta arising in the centre of the chest from the left ventricle and sweeping out into the right thorax (Fig. 12.4). The horizontal section cranial to this plane will

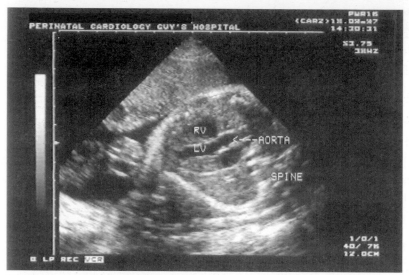

Fig. 12.4 Angulating cranially and towards the right shoulder demonstrates a long axis view of the left ventricle. The aorta arises from the left ventricle and is directed towards the right. LV = left ventricle, RV = right ventricle.

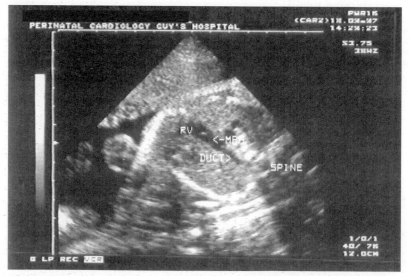

Fig. 12.5 The horizontal section cranial to the plane in Figure 12.4 demontrates the pulmonary artery. This artery arises anteriorly, close to the chest wall and is directed straight back towards the spine. The ductal connection to the descending aorta is also demonstrated. MPA = main pulmonary artery, RV = right ventricle.

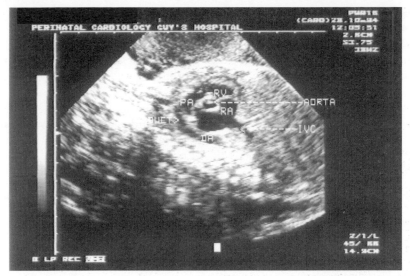

Fig. 12.6 The ductal arch, comprising of the pulmonary artery, duct and descending aorta is illustrated in this view, which also shows the right heart connections. DA = descending aorta, IVC = inferior vena cava, PA = pulmonary artery, RA = right atrium, RV = right ventricle.

demonstrate the pulmonary artery (Fig. 12.5). This artery arises anteriorly, close to the chest wall and is directed straight back towards the spine. Angulating the transducer towards the left shoulder in a longitudinal view demonstrates the right heart connections and the ductal arch (Fig. 12.6). This arch is formed by the pulmonary artery, arterial duct and its connection to the descending aorta. Thus, this arch arises anteriorly and is a wide sweeping arch. The aortic arch can also be imaged in a longitudinal section of the fetus, but by angulating the transducer towards the right shoulder in this instance (Fig. 12.7). The aorta normally arises

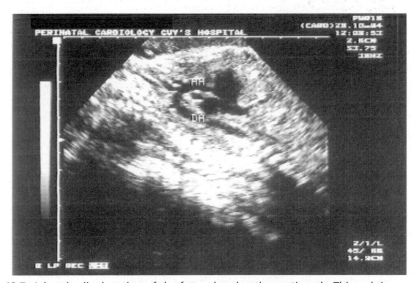

Fig. 12.7 A longitudinal section of the fetus showing the aortic arch. This arch is a tight hooked arch and two of the three head and neck vessels can clearly be seen arising from it. AA = ascending aorta, DA = descending aorta.

in the centre of the thorax and forms a tight hook shape with the head and neck vessels arising from the crest of the arch.

The following are important features of the great arteries and allow major anomalies of the great arteries to be excluded:

1   Two arterial valves should always be seen.

2   The aorta arises from the centre of the chest and is wholly committed to the left ventricle. It gives rise to the aortic arch, which can be identified by head and neck vessels.

3   The pulmonary artery arises from the right ventricle and is a branching vessel giving rise to the branch pulmonary arteries and the arterial duct.

4   The great arteries are similar in size, but the pulmonary artery at the valve ring may be slightly bigger than the aorta.

5   The pulmonary valve is anterior and cranial to the aortic valve.

6   The great arteries cross over at their origin.

7   The arch of the aorta is of similar size to the pulmonary artery and duct and is complete.

CARDIAC ABNORMALITIES

Segmental examination of the connections of the heart will allow detection of abnormalities at the venous-atrial, atrio-ventricular and ventriculo-arterial junctions. Additional anomalies can then also be sought. Some of the more common abnormalities are discussed below.

Atrioventricular septal defect

There is a defect in the lower part of the atrial septum and the inlet part of the ventricular septum, at the crux of the heart. The size of both the atrial and the ventricular component can be variable. A common atrioventricular valve bridges the defect and there is loss of the normal differential insertion of the two atrioventricular valves. An example is shown in Figure 12.8A,B. Atrioventricular septal defects are one of the commonest forms of heart disease seen in prenatal life.[9] This type of defect is commonly associated with chromosomal anomalies, in particular with trisomy 21, although it can occur with other chromosome anomalies.[10] It is also frequently found associated with atrial isomerism, although it can occur with normal situs in patients with normal chromosomes.

Tricuspid atresia

There is no connection between the right atrium and right ventricle and no opening valve can be seen between these two chambers. The four chamber view in the fetus will be abnormal as a patent tricuspid valve is not seen and the right ventricular chamber is small or may even be indiscernible (Fig. 12.9).

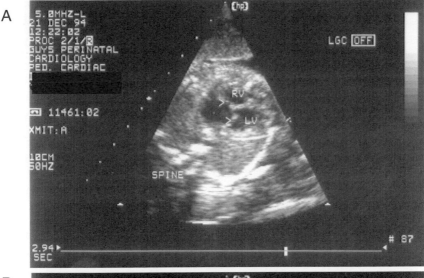

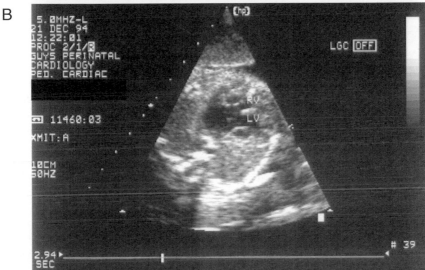

Fig. 12.8 (A) An example of an atrioventricular septal defect with the common valve shown in systole. The valve is indicated by the two arrowheads. Note the loss of differential insertion at the crux of the heart. **(B)** In diastole both atria communicate with both ventricles. LV = left ventricle, RV = right ventricle.

There is no demonstrable flow across the anterior atrioventricular valve on colour flow mapping. Typically, there is a ventricular septal defect, which can be of variable size and this will influence the size of the right ventricular cavity. Tricuspid atresia is rarely associated with extracardiac anomalies.

Mitral atresia

The mitral valve is not patent in this condition and the four chamber view will be abnormal as an opening mitral valve is not seen and the left ventricle is small. (Fig. 12.10). There is no demonstrable flow across the posterior

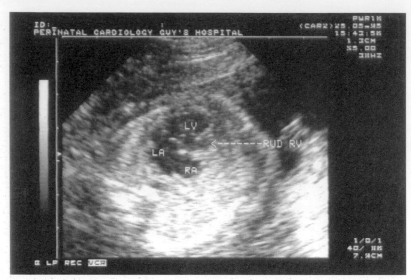

Fig. 12.9 An example of tricuspid atresia where a patent tricuspid valve is not seen and the right ventricular chamber is very small. There is an associated ventricular septal defect. LA = left atrium, LV = left ventricle, RA = right atrium, Rud RV = rudimentary right ventricle.

atrioventricular valve on colour flow mapping. Mitral atresia can occur in three settings. It most commonly occurs in association with aortic atresia in the hypoplastic left heart syndrome (Fig. 12.11). Alternatively, mitral atresia can occur with a ventricular septal defect with either a normally connected but patent aorta, or with double outlet right ventricle (Fig. 12.12).

In fetal life, mitral atresia has a significant association with chromosomal anomalies (18%), usually trisomy 18, but 13, 21 and translocation/deletion syndrome are also possible.[10]

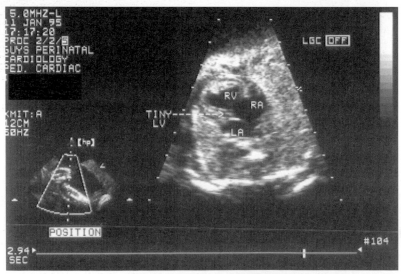

Fig. 12.10 An example of mitral atresia with an indiscernible left ventricle. LA = left atrium, LV = left ventricle, RA = right atrium, RV = right ventricle.

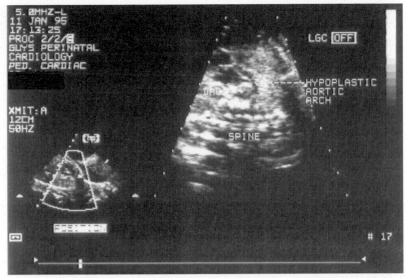

Fig. 12.11 A view of a very hypoplastic ascending aorta and aortic arch in hypoplastic left heart syndrome. DAO = descending aorta.

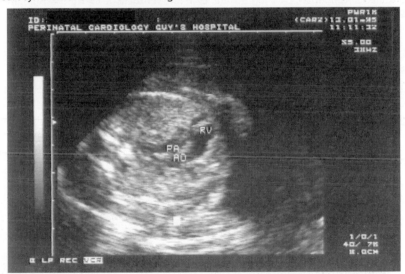

Fig. 12.12 A view of the great arteries in mitral atresia with double outlet right ventricle. Both the great arteries arise from the right ventricle with the aorta being anterior to the pulmonary artery. AO = aorta, PA = pulmonary artery, RV = right ventricle.

Tricuspid dysplasia and Ebstein's anomaly

Tricuspid valve abnormalities are often detected in the fetus because of cardiomegaly.[11] The four chamber view will be abnormal due to the cardiomegaly, which is a result of right atrial and ventricular enlargement. In tricuspid valve dysplasia the tricuspid valve appears thickened and nodular (Fig. 12.13). In Ebstein's anomaly, the attachment of the septal leaflet of the tricuspid valve is displaced into the right ventricle. There is a variable degree of tricuspid regurgitation. Secondary lung hypoplasia as a result of long-standing

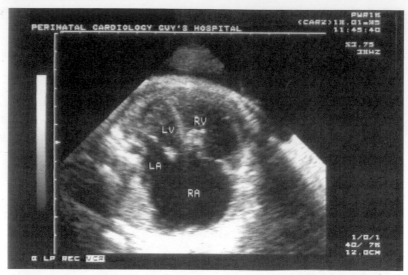

Fig. 12.13 An example of tricuspid valve dysplasia. There is marked cardiomegaly, with the right atrium in particular being enlarged. The tricuspid valve appears thickened and nodular. LA = left atrium, LV = left ventricle, RA = right atrium, RV = right ventricle.

compression from severe cardiomegaly can be a life threatening associated feature. Obstruction to the right ventricular outflow tract is common in the form of pulmonary stenosis or atresia.

Tricuspid dysplasia can be difficult to distinguish from Ebstein's malformation, as the two overlap each other in terms of anatomical findings.[12] The differentiation is not important in fetal life as the prognosis is similar when diagnosed *in utero*. Tricuspid dysplasia is uncommonly associated with extracardiac lesions but chromosomal anomalies can occur.

Ebstein's malformation is rarely associated with extracardiac anomalies.

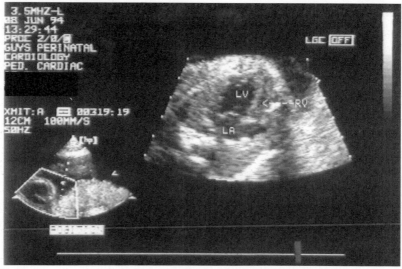

Fig. 12.14 An example of pulmonary atresia with an intact interventricular septum where the right ventricle is hypertrophied. LA = left atrium, LV = left ventricle, RV = right ventricle.

Critical pulmonary stenosis and pulmonary atresia with intact ventricular septum

Obstruction at the level of the pulmonary valve can be partial (stenosis) or complete (atresia). Usually the right ventricle is hypertrophied and contracts poorly (Fig. 12.14). The tricuspid valve movement is restricted and there may be a jet of tricuspid regurgitation at high velocity. If the pulmonary valve can be visualised, it will be noted that it is either restricted in its movement or does not open. In pulmonary atresia there will be no forward flow detectable into the pulmonary artery, but reverse flow from the arterial duct is frequently seen, as the branch pulmonary arteries fill retrogradely from the duct. In pulmonary stenosis, an antegrade jet of flow at a high velocity may be detected, but in many of the severe cases there will also be retrograde flow from the arterial duct. The pulmonary artery may be smaller than normal for the gestational age and is often smaller than the aorta.[13]

Critical aortic stenosis

There is obstruction to flow through the aortic valve which is usually severe or critical if detected in the fetus.[14] In severe cases, the left ventricle may be dilated and poorly contracting with evidence of increased echogenicity of the ventricular walls and papillary muscles of the mitral valve (Fig. 12.15). The mitral valve will be restricted in opening and there may be mitral regurgitation at high velocity. The aortic valve may appear thickened and the aortic Doppler may be increased depending on the degree of left ventricular compromise.

Coarctation of aorta

The aortic arch can be partially obstructed as in coarctation of the aorta, or it may be completely interrupted. Coarctation can occur as an isolated defect or as a component of a complex malformation. In its isolated form in fetal life, the

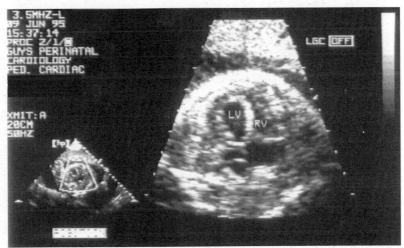

Fig. 12.15 An example of critical aortic stenosis. The left ventricle is dilated with increased echogenicity of the ventricular walls. This correlates with endocardial fibroelastosis. LV = left ventricle, RV = right ventricle.

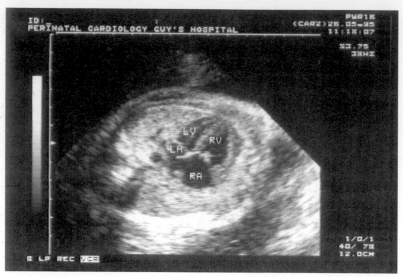

Fig. 12.16 The four chamber view in an example of coarctation of the aorta. The right sided structures appear dilated compared with the left. LA = left atrium, LV = left ventricle, RA = right atrium, RV = right ventricle.

narrowing is preductal and there is usually associated hypoplasia of the isthmus and transverse arch.[15] One of the difficulties with this diagnosis *in utero* is that the coarctation shelf lesion is not seen and the diagnosis is suspected on other soft signs.[16] The first clue to the diagnosis is asymmetry of the four chamber view, with the right ventricle dilated relative to the left (Fig. 12.16). The pulmonary artery will appear dilated compared with the aorta. The aortic arch is narrowed in the horizontal views, especially in comparison with the pulmonary artery and arterial duct.[17]

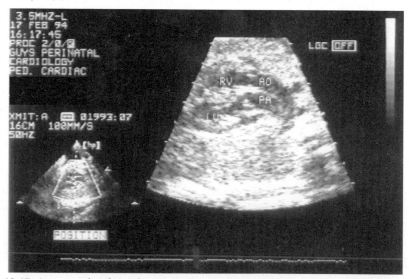

Fig. 12.17 An example of simple transposition with the aorta arising anteriorly from the right ventricle and the pulmonary artery arising from the left ventricle. The two arteries arise in parallel orientation. AO = aorta, LV = left ventricle, PA = pulmonary artery, RV = right ventricle.

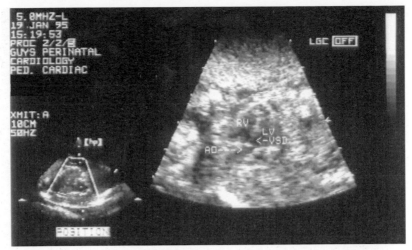

Fig. 12.18 An example of an aorta overriding a ventricular septal defect, where the aorta arises astride the crest of the ventricular septum. AO = aorta, LV = left ventricle, RV = right ventricle, VSD = ventricular septal defect.

Transposition of the great arteries

The aorta (artery forming the arch with head and neck vessels) arises from the right ventricle and the pulmonary artery (the branching great artery) from the left ventricle. The relative positions of the two arteries is abnormal as the aorta arises anterior and in parallel orientation to the pulmonary artery. The normal 'cross-over' of the great arteries is, therefore, not found and the two great arteries arise in parallel orientation (Fig. 12.17). The aortic arch will form a wide sweeping arch instead of the normal tight hooked arch. In simple transposition the interventricular septum is intact. However, transposition can occur with a ventricular septal defect, or with more complex heart disease.

Tetralogy of Fallot

This condition is made up of four components, anterior deviation of the aorta, a ventricular septal defect, infundibular pulmonary stenosis and right ventricular hypertrophy. The four chamber view of the fetal heart is usually normal. On long-axis views of the left ventricle the ventricular septal defect and aortic override are seen as illustrated in Figure 12.18. The other features of tetralogy, subpulmonary stenosis and right ventricular hypertrophy may not always be evident in the fetus. The pulmonary artery is usually smaller than the aorta (Fig. 12.19). Tetralogy of Fallot is commonly associated with extracardiac malformations. These include omphalocoele and diaphragmatic hernia in addition to trisomy 21, 13, 18 and additions/deletions.[18]

Pulmonary atresia with a ventricular septal defect

The four chamber view of the fetal heart may be normal. There is ventricular septal defect in the outlet septum and the aorta overrides the crest of the ventricular septum. In most cases no main pulmonary artery can be identified,

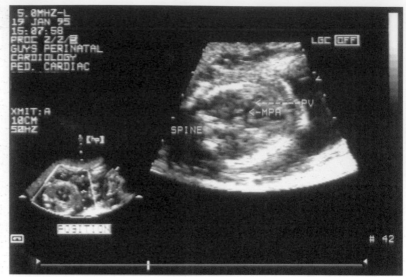

Fig. 12.19 A small pulmonary artery which was detected in association with aortic override (Fig. 12.18) in an example of tetralogy of Fallot. PV = pulmonary valve, MPA = main pulmonary artery.

although branch pulmonary arteries can sometimes be found. It may be difficult to distinguish tetralogy from a case with pulmonary atresia if the main pulmonary artery is very small. It may also be difficult to distinguish this condition from a common arterial trunk. This condition can be associated with chromosomal defects and has been associated with the Di George syndrome.

Common arterial trunk

A single great artery arises from the heart, overriding a ventricular septal defect and gives rise to both the aortic arch and the branch pulmonary arteries.

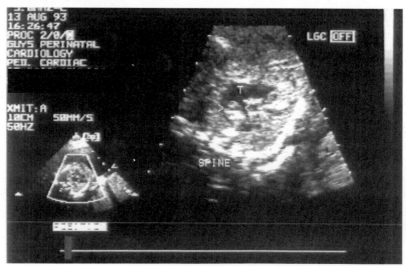

Fig. 12.20 In this example of a common arterial trunk, the branch pulmonary arteries (arrowheads) can be identified arising from the common trunk (T).

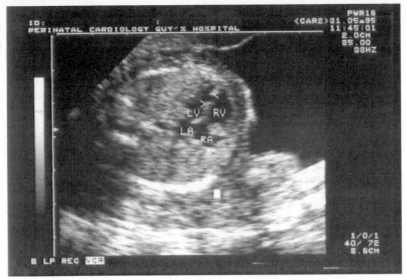

Fig. 12.21 An example of a mid-trabecular ventricular septal defect (shown by arrowheads). LA = left atrium, LV = left ventricle, RA = right atrium, RV = right ventricle.

The four chamber view may be normal. The truncal valve is often thickened and dysplastic. There may be turbulence at the truncal valve and an increase in truncal velocity. There may also be truncal valve regurgitation. The branch pulmonary arteries can be identified arising from the common trunk (Fig. 12.20).[19] This condition can be associated with chromosomal anomalies and the Di George syndrome.

Ventricular septal defect

A defect in the ventricular septum can occur in any part of the ventricular septum. A ventricular septal defect can occur in isolation or may be a component of many complex forms of congenital heart disease. A defect in the outlet or perimembranous ventricular septum will be detected in the subaortic position in the long axis view of the left ventricle. A defect in the inlet septum will be seen in the four chamber views of the fetal heart and will cause loss of differential insertion of the atrioventricular valves. A trabecular defect can be found in any part of the muscular septum and is usually evident in a four chamber view (Fig. 12.21). Ventricular septal defects are commonly associated extracardiac structural anomalies and karyotypic anomalies.[9,10]

MANAGEMENT AND OUTCOME

It has now become accepted that a different spectrum of disease is seen in prenatal life from that observed in those who survive to infancy.[9,20] There is a higher incidence of associated extracardiac lesions, including non-immune fetal hydrops,[21] compared with postnatal life and, in addition, a significant number of affected pregnancies may result in a spontaneous intra-uterine loss.[22,23] These factors will influence the outcome for prenatally diagnosed congenital heart disease and must be taken into account at the time of counselling. Since there is a high association with other anomalies it is prudent to recommend or organise further investigations to exclude any associated lesions. The finding of an associated anomaly may influence the parents' decision about how to proceed. Additionally, some forms of cardiac lesions are progressive in nature, so that obstructive lesions can change in severity and there may be a reduced rate of growth observed in the chambers or arteries as a result of reduced blood flow.[14,16,17,24,25] Although progression is usually to a more severe form of lesion, rarely it can be to a less severe form.[26]

Following the diagnosis of a cardiac malformation, the clinician should be able to provide the parents with detailed information about the problem. This includes an accurate description of the anomaly, along with information regarding the need for surgical intervention and the type of surgery available for the condition, the number of procedures likely to be required, the mortality and morbidity associated with this, and the overall long-term outlook for the child. The parents need to understand all these facts before they can make any decisions about how to proceed. Thus, it is vital to make an accurate a diagnosis as soon as possible and to involve a paediatric cardiologist in the discussion with the parents. The prognosis is very variable and will depend on the nature of the lesion. It is normal for parents to be extremely distressed at the time of disclosure of an abnormality and further information is likely to be required after the initial explanations. A single consultation with the parents often does not resolve parental anxiety or provide them with adequate understanding of the problem. The majority of parents require continuing support and are likely to need more than one consultation in order to absorb and understand the implications of the ultrasound findings. Information leaflets and contact with other parents who have had a child affected with a similar problem are invaluable. In order to help deal with the needs of the parents, in our own unit we now have the services of a full time nurse counsellor, who is present during the consultations with the parents and provides continuing support for them.

The major decision the parents face, when a severe cardiac defect is diagnosed in early pregnancy, is whether they wish to continue with the pregnancy or whether they wish to interrupt it. Termination of pregnancy is an option available before 24 weeks of gestation, but, as stressed above, the parents should have accurate and adequate information before making their final choice. Should a termination take place, it is vital to try and obtain permission for autopsy in order to confirm the diagnosis and to look for any associated malformations. Ideally this should be performed by a pathologist who is familiar with the examination of congenital heart anomalies. This information is vital when counselling parents for recurrence risks in future pregnancies. In continuing pregnancies, appropriate arrangements should be made to restudy the fetal heart in later pregnancy, as some lesions may progress, and some will be at risk of developing non-immune fetal hydrops. The parents can meet the paediatricians, paediatric cardiologists, and paediatric cardiac surgeon likely to be looking after their baby. In some conditions, it may be beneficial for the neonate to transfer antenatal care to allow delivery in a unit with paediatric cardiology facilities available on site.

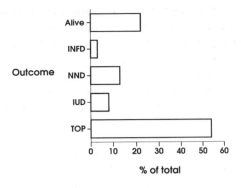

Fig. 12.22 The outcome of 1737 consecutive cases of congenital heart disease diagnosed prenatally at Guy's Hospital between 1980–1996. INFD = death in infancy, IUD = spontaneous intra-uterine death, NND = neonatal death, TOP = termination of pregnancy.

Once the fetus is mature, delivery can be timed to occur when appropriate personnel are available. Vaginal delivery should be possible in most cases as most babies with severe congenital heart defects are unlikely to have problems until after delivery. The advantage of prenatal diagnosis is that it allows immediate cardiac assessment of the neonate and avoids late diagnosis after an infant has become cyanotic or acidotic.

The outcome of 1737 consecutive structural cardiac abnormalities diagnosed at Guy's Hospital between 1980 and 1996 is shown in Figure 12.22. During this time, 54% of parents opted to stop the pregnancy following prenatal diagnosis. However, the termination rate in our unit has fallen significantly over the past few years (Fig. 12.23). There are several reasons accounting for the changes that have occurred in our fetal cardiology practice over the last few years. Increasing experience of ultrasonographers in obstetric units has improved the detection rate of some of the correctable forms of congenital heart disease, such as transposition of the great arteries. Although the detection rate for the great artery abnormalities remains poor overall, there has been a slow but steady improvement. The introduction of nuchal fold screening is another factor, as many chromosomal anomalies are detected before referral for fetal echocardiography, resulting in interruption of

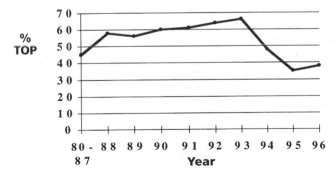

Fig. 12.23 The percentage of parents electing termination of pregnancy each year following the prenatal detection of congenital heart disease at Guy's Hospital.

pregnancy in some instances before the fetal heart is evaluated, even though there may be a cardiac defect present.[27] Advances in surgical techniques have improved some treatment options, such as the arterial switch procedure for transposition of the great arteries, or new treatment options have been developed for some conditions, such as the Norwood procedure for the management of the hypoplastic left heart syndrome. Additionally, there has been an improvement in the survival rate seen in the last few years in the offspring of pregnancies that have continued. This to some degree probably reflects the improvement in detection rates of correctable lesions and also the changes in surgical practice. The survival rate of the continuing pregnancies seen between 1980–1993 in our unit was 41%.[9,18] Of the pregnancies that continued in between 1994–1996, just over 60% are surviving. Although these children are still young and some could still have clinical problems, there does seem to be a notable improvement in the numbers surviving.

KEY POINTS FOR CLINICAL PRACTICE

- A systematic approach to examination of the fetal heart will enhance the detection of structural cardiac abnormalities and will enable an accurate diagnosis of congenital heart disease to be made

- Once an abnormality has been detected appropriate counselling must be provided and adequate support given to the parents

- Associated extracardiac abnormalities should be sought for

- Plans for the remainder of pregnancy, delivery, and postnatal management should be made using a team approach

- In cases resulting in termination of pregnancy, permission for autopsy should be sought to confirm the ultrasound diagnosis

---

REFERENCES

1 Allan L D, Tynan M J, Campbell S, Wilkinson J, Anderson R H. Echocardiographic and anatomical correlates in the fetus. Br Heart J 1980; 44: 444–451
2 Kleinman C S, Hobbins J C, Jaffe C C , Lynch D C, Talner N S. Echocardiographic studies of the human fetus: prenatal diagnosis of congenital heart disease and cardiac dysrhythmias. Pediatrics 1980; 65: 1059–1067
3 Allan L D, Santos R, Pexieder T. Anatomical and echocardiographic correlates of normal cardiac morphology in the late first trimester fetus. Heart 1997; 77: 68–72
4 Allan L D, Chita S K, Sharland G K, Fagg N L K, Anderson R H, Crawford D C. The accuracy of fetal echocardiography in the diagnosis of congenital heart disease. Int J Cardiol 1989; 25: 279–288
5 Huhta J C, Strasburger J F, Carpenter R J, Reiter A. Fetal echocardiography: accuracy and limitations in the diagnosis of cardiac disease [Abstract]. J Am Coll Cardiol 1985; 5: 387
6 Allan L D, Chita S K, Al-Ghazali W, Crawford D C, Tynan M J. Doppler echocardiographic evaluation of the normal human fetal heart. Br Heart J 1987; 57: 528–533
7 Sharland G K, Chita S K, Allan L D. The use of colour Doppler in fetal echocardiography. Int J Cardiol 1990; 28: 229–236
8 Allan L D. Manual of fetal echocardiography. Lancaster: MTP, 1986

9 Allan L D, Sharland G K, Milburn A et al. Prospective diagnosis of 1,006 consecutive cases of congenital heart disease in the fetus. J Am Coll Cardiol 1994; 23: 1452–1458

10 Allan L D, Sharland G K, Chita S K, Lockhart S, Maxwell D J. Chromosomal anomalies in fetal congenital heart disease. Ultrasound Obstet Gynecol 1991; 1: 8–11

11 Sharland G K, Chita S K, Allan L D. Tricuspid valve dysplasia or displacement in intrauterine life. J Am Cardiol 1991: 17; 944–949

12 Lang D, Oberhoffer R, Cook A et al. The pathological spectrum of malformations of the tricuspid valve in prenatal and neonatal life. J Am Coll Cardiol 1991: 17; 1161–1167

13 Hornberger L K, Benacerraf B R, Bromley B S, Spevak P J, Sanders S P. Prenatal detection of severe right ventricular outflow tract obstruction: pulmonary stenosis and pulmonary atresia. J Ultrasound Med 1994; 13: 743–750

14 Sharland G K, Chita S K, Fagg N et al. Left ventricular dysfunction in the fetus: relation to aortic valve anomalies and endocardial fibroelastosis. Br Heart J 1991; 66: 219–224

15 Hornberger L K, Sahn D J, Kleinman C S, Copel J, Silverman N H. Antenatal diagnosis of coarctation of the aorta: a multicenter experience. J Am Coll Cardiol 1994; 23: 417–423

16 Sharland G K, Chan K, Allan L D. Coarctation of the aorta: difficulties in prenatal diagnosis. Br Heart J 1994; 71: 70–75

17 Sharland G K. Left heart disease in the fetus. MD thesis, University of London, 1993

18 Allan L D, Sharland G K. The prognosis in fetal tetralogy of Fallot. Pediatr Cardiol 1992; 13: 1–4

19 de Araujo L M, Schmidt K G, Silverman N H, Finkbeiner W E. Prenatal detection of truncus arteriosus by ultrasound. Pediatr Cardiol 1987; 8: 261–263

20 Allan L D, Crawford D C, Anderson R H, Tynan M J. Spectrum of congenital heart disease detected echocardiographically in prenatal life. Br Heart J 1984; 54: 523–526

21 Knilans T K. Cardiac abnormalities associated with hydrops fetalis. Semin Perinatol 1995; 19: 483–492

22 Copel J A, Pilu G, Kleinman C S. Congenital heart disease and extracardiac anomalies: associations and indications for fetal echocardiography. Am J Obstet Gynecol 1986; 154: 1121–1132

23 Sharland G K, Lockhart S M, Chita S K, Allan L D. Factors influencing the outcome of congenital heart disease detected prenatally. Arch Dis Child 1990; 64. 284–287

24 Hornberger L K, Sanders S P, Rein Azaria J J T, Spevak P J, Parness I A, Colan S D. Left heart obstructive lesions and left ventricular growth in the midtrimester fetus: a longitudinal study. Circulation 1995; 92: 1531–1538

25 Hornberger L K, Sanders S P, Sahn D J, Rice M J, Spevak P J, Benacerraf B R. In utero pulmonary artery and aortic growth and potential for progression of pulmonary outflow tract obstruction in tetralogy of Fallot. J Am Coll Cardiol 1995; 25: 739–745

26 Sharland G K, Qureshi S A. Closure of the ventricular component of an atrioventricular septal defect during fetal life. Cardiol Young 1995; 5: 272–274

27 Hyett J, Moscoso G, Nicolaides K. Abnormalities of the heart and great vessels in first trimester chromosomally abnormal fetuses. Am J Med Gen 1997; 69: 207–216

James J. Walker

Current thoughts on the pathophysiology of pre-eclampsia/eclampsia

Pre-eclampsia/eclampsia has been recognised as a clinical entity since the times of Hippocrates.[1] In 1916, Zweifel first termed 'toxaemia' the disease of theories.[2] Many of the causal theories attributed to pre-eclampsia/eclampsia describe pathological features of the clinical presentation which are the result rather than the cause of the disease process.[3] It has been called many things and has been thought to be a neurological, renal, hepatic, hypertensive and more recently a placental disorder. The truth is that it is probably all these things in different people and is certainly more than just hypertension in pregnancy.[4] This chapter attempts to clarify the current thoughts on the aetiology of this perplexing condition and what help these give to the clinical management.

PRE-ECLAMPSIA AS A MODULAR CONDITION

The presentation and progression of this condition is so varied that it is sometimes difficult to imagine it is one disease (Table 13.1). The reason for this variation is that it is the result of both pathological change and maternal response. In different women, the rate of progression and the organ systems affected can be different (Fig. 13.1). There needs to be an initial placental trigger but it is the maternal response that probably modifies the disease presentation and progression. Since research into pre-eclampsia usually studies only one component of the disease, the results from different groups are often contradictory and they may be measuring changes of maternal adaptation rather than of pathology. They may be beneficial or harmful to the mother. By trying to understand the variations of disease presentation and progression, management of the affected women can become clearer and the

Prof. James J. Walker MD FRCP(G) FRCP(E) FRCOG, Department of Obstetrics and Gynaecology, St James's University Hospital, Beckett Street, Leeds LS9 7TF, UK

Table 1.1 Evidence in support of the multiple modular approach to pre-eclampsia

Poor placentation
    Deficient trophoblast invasion
    Failure of adaptation of maternal vessels
    Increased incidence of placental insufficiency

Hyperplacentosis
    Increased incidence in twin pregnancy
    Increased incidence in diabetic pregnancy
    Increased incidence in rhesus incompatibility
    Association with molar pregnancy

Fetal/placental response
    Need for placenta to be present to develop the disease
    Need for placenta to be present for continuation of disease
    Increase release of placental villus emboli
    Abnormalities of villus formation

Systemic reaction
    Activation of circulating neutrophils
    VCAM-1 is elevated in the serum
    Abnormalities of lymphocyte function
    Increased cytokine activity
    Increased lipid peroxide production

Maternal response
    Decreased cellular protection from free radical activity
    Generalised membrane instability
    Diminished vascular endothelial function
    Increased vascular resistance/vasoconstriction
    Hypertension
    Renal impairment
    Convulsion
    Liver impairment
    Platelet consumption
    Haemolysis

outcomes more predictable. The one thing, that is agreed by all, is that a placenta is required for the development and maintenance of pre-eclampsia and delivery, with removal of the placenta, remains the ultimate cure.[4]

THE PLACENTA AS THE TRIGGER TO PRE-ECLAMPSIA

Pre-eclampsia only occurs in the presence of the placenta. It is usually, but not always, associated with placental insufficiency and intra-uterine growth restriction (IUGR). Hypertension in pregnancy does not cause growth retardation but co-exists with the placental lesions resulting in the restriction of growth.

Both normal and abnormal implantation is likely to be influenced by maternal/fetal immunological interaction. Implantation of the developing embryo is influenced by immunologically active cells in the decidua, particularly large granular macrophages and lymphocytes.[5] These cells appear to be important to the mother's ability to recognise the invading trophoblast and respond appropriately to it. This is an unique immunological event. Since implantation can occur in the absence of decidua, it would appear that its main

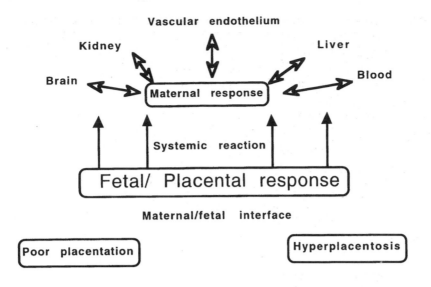

Fig. 13.1 A diagram of the components of the pathophysiology of pre-eclampsia that make up the multisystem disorder.

role is to protect the mother from the excessive placental invasion. An abnormal or excessive maternal immunological response may lead to a deficient implantation and poor placentation.

It used to be thought that there was a barrier between the fetal and maternal tissue, but it is now known that there is direct contact between the maternal cells, both decidual and blood, and the placental trophoblastic cells. These cells do not express the usual polymorphic class I and II MHC antigens that are responsible for the normal immune response.[5] Some of the cells express a unique HLA-G encoded class I MHC molecule and are believed to play a role in the maternal/fetal immune response. There is also evidence of immuno-suppression by the placental hormones. All these changes allow the trophoblastic cells to invade deep into the maternal tissues, particularly the spiral arterioles.

The trophoblastic cells proliferate markedly and differentiate into villous trophoblast which form the placenta and non-villous trophoblast which invade the decidua and the maternal spiral arterioles. It is the invasion of the decidua around and within the lumen of the maternal vessels that convert them into the classic funnel-shaped vessels which supply the intervillous space.[6] The degree of the invasion varies in different pregnancies and it is the failure of these changes that precede the placental insufficiency of later pregnancy.

The ability of the placenta to exchange nutrients and gases between the fetus and the mother is largely dependent on blood flow, both from the mother and the fetus. By 24 weeks, the invasion is complete and the maximum potential blood flow to the placenta decided. In pre-eclampsia, deficient implantation results in a reduction of maternal placental blood flow. The fetus will grow normally until it outgrows this maximum placental function at which time intra-uterine growth restriction occurs. This will occur at different gestations and to a different degree depending on the scale of the abnormality.

Secondary damage can occur causing atherosclerosis and thrombosis in the placental bed which can precipitate a sudden deterioration. This reduced blood flow can be demonstrated by uterine artery Doppler velocity wave form abnormalities in patients who are destined to develop pre-eclampsia and IUGR as early as 24 weeks.[7]

These placental blood flow abnormalities give rise to interference with fetal oxygenation and growth. It is now thought that utero–placental ischaemia is responsible for pre-eclampsia.[4] It is believed that placental ischaemia results in the release of a substance 'Factor X'. Therefore, the maternal systemic changes seen in pre-eclampsia may be in response to factors released secondarily to placental ischaemia.[4] It would not be surprising if the placenta responded in some way to the increasing fetal demands and the presence of ischaemia. This could be physiological in nature in an attempt to overcome the deficiencies or pathological in nature because of ischaemic damage.

The story is not that simple, however, as the placental lesion is not specific to pre-eclampsia. Similar findings are found in intra-uterine growth restriction (IUGR).[8] Other factors are required to turn placental insufficiency in to the systemic pathology of pre-eclampsia. Whether this is an excessive release of this Factor X, or an abnormal response to it, is more difficult to assess. It is the maternal reaction to any placental factor that produces the signs and symptoms of pre-eclampsia.

THE MATERNAL DEBRIS THEORY

The substance responsible for the systemic reaction may be fragments of placental villi. The development of villi in women with placental insufficiency are abnormal in form, with excessive elongation and lack of the normal terminal budding.[9] This could make them more likely to fragment. Villus membranes have been shown to affect the function of the vascular endothelium.[10] However, this affect is achieved by villus material from normal placentas and there is no increase of the effect from membranes from placentas from pre-eclamptic women. This would suggest that the problem relates to either an increase in substance release from the ischaemic placenta or an abnormal reaction in the mothers who develop pre-eclampsia or a combination of both. This could be mediated through an activation of the maternal systemic immune system.

MATERNAL IMMUNOLOGY

Various workers have demonstrated increased activation and functional abnormalities of maternal neutrophils (Table 13.2).[11,12] Immunocytochemical studies have localised neutrophil elastase in term placenta, decidua and myometrium in women with PET.[13] The cell-adhesion molecule, VCAM-1 is elevated in the peripheral serum. Neutrophil activity is partly mediated through this adhesion molecule which encourages adhesion to the vascular endothelium.[14] These immunological reactions could be part of the mechanism of maternal/fetal interaction which results in the abnormalities of

Table 13.2 Evidence for and against an immunological basis to pre-eclampsia

For
More common in primigravida
More common in twin pregnancies
Incidence increased by change of partner
A higher incidence of HLA homozygosity
Against
No increase in ABO, HLA or Y-linked compatibility
The incidence is similar in monozygotic and dizygotic twin pregnancies
Similar placental findings are found in intra-uterine growth retardation

implantation and invasion or could be the maternal systemic response to the placental reaction.

Any increase in the systemic neutrophil activity may be partly responsible for the maternal endothelial cell dysfunction.[15] This may be by direct cellular effects or through release of cytokines and free radicals which affect cellular function. Increased cytokines in pre-eclampsia have been shown to affect the production of prostacyclin and thromboxane in human mononuclear-cells,[16] and may have similar effects on vascular endothelial function. In various studies, TNFα has been shown to be increased in PET and this has been related to a specific polymorphism of the promoter region of the gene.[17] This study suggests that a susceptibility to the disease may relate to a particular genotype which results in an overreaction of inflammatory stimuli.

Therefore, the mother would appear to mount a local reaction within the placental bed. There is also evidence of a general systemic immunological reaction and this may explain the multisystem nature of the condition. An increase in the release of villus debris may be a result of the local immunological reaction or secondarily to placenta ischaemia. This would have further systemic effects.

However, anyone who looks after women with pre-eclampsia will be impressed by the variation of presentation and severity. No two women appear to present or respond in the same way. There appears to be little correlation between blood pressure level, proteinuria, platelet count, clinical symptoms and risk of convulsion. Although the risk of IUGR is increased, it is not certain. These changes would appear to be dependant on differing maternal responses.

MATERNAL RESPONSE

The fundamental abnormality in women presenting with pre-eclampsia is cellular dysfunction (Fig. 13.1). Although this has been primarily quoted as a vascular endothelial disorder, other tissue sites are also involved such as the liver, renal and brain as well as the circulating blood cells. The areas affected in any given women are different and may be related to changes in the immunological response, free radical activity or the ability of the different cell types to protect themselves against free radical attack.[18]

The most common physical presentation of pre-eclampsia is hypertension. This has led to the believe that this is the fundamental pathological change.

This is now known to be not true, but a vascular endothelial cell dysfunction is certainly part of the disease process, though not permanent endothelial damage.[19] A fully functioning vascular endothelium is important for the normal physiological changes of pregnancy. Various studies have demonstrated that serum from a pre-eclamptic woman initially increases prostacyclin or nitric oxide production from normal vascular endothelium in vitro.[20,21] This suggests that the endothelium of pre-eclamptic women may react differently from normal. Therefore, maternal response has a role in the disease process.

However, the vascular endothelial cell may not be unique in this response. Other cell types may be equally, or more severely, dysfunctional. Abnormalities in various cells types could explain the immunological activity, red cell fragility, platelet activation, hepatocyte dysfunction, glomerular endotheloisis and neuronal sensitivity. Therefore, almost all the clinical manifestations of pre-eclampsia can be explained by cellular dysfunction secondary to a response to circulating factors in the maternal blood. The degree of which the cell is affected will depend on the cell's ability to protect itself.

Cellular protection

Normally, cells have multiple levels of protection from extracellular attack. This is particularly true of the cell membrane which is so central to cell survival and function. The red cell in women with pre-eclampsia is deficient in intracellular free radical scavengers opening them to increased damage and membrane instability.[18,22] Levels of anti-oxidant activity correlate with plasma levels of prostacyclin and thromboxane in women with pregnancy-induced hypertension.[23] These changes, particularly those found with superoxide dismutase (SOD), have also been found in neutrophils. However, normal superoxide-dismutase gene activity has been found in pregnancy-induced hypertension. Therefore, the decreased SOD activity would appear to be a secondary phenomenon.[24] Using nuclear magnetic resonance (NMR), measurement of the oxidation across cell membranes can be made. This shows increasing oxidation with disease severity, although the correlations are not absolute, suggesting the degree of oxidation or the protection from it differs between affected women.[25] Changes in the membrane stability can lead to an influx of calcium into the cell producing increased activity of the cell and changes in membrane rigidity. Alterations in the membrane of the red cell can alter blood rheology and the tendency to lyse and can explain many of the clinical findings in this condition. Recent work has shown that red cell membranes in PET are more fragile to saline dilution and more likely to lyse.[25] This could explain the haemolysis seen in this condition. Although these changes have been studied in the red cell, there is no reason to think that similar abnormalities are not found in other body cells, particularly those in contact with blood such as the vascular endothelium.

HEREDITARY FACTORS

Many studies have suggested that pre-eclampsia is a familial disease. Since there appears to be a wide patient variation in presentation and progression of the disease, it seems likely that there may be genetic factors that modulate the process, the so called 'modulator genes'. Recent studies in Iceland has confirmed this family linkage and the results are consistent with a single gene dominance with 48% inheritance.[26] This work has led to investigations of gene linkage within the family groups.

Angiotensinogen: a candidate gene involved in pre-eclampsia?

In a study of several generations of women, Arngrimsson et al[27] found further evidence for the role of AGT or a neighbouring gene in the predisposition to pre-eclampsia. This was true for women with both proteinuric and non-proteinuric pre-eclampsia. When proteinuric pre-eclampsia was studied, an increased significance level was observed. However, in the five families where the index pregnancy had eclampsia, no significant linkage was observed. This suggests that the genetic factor may be related to the hypertension of pre-eclampsia and the risk of convulsion is related to another, maybe genetic, cause.

TNFα gene in pre-eclampsia

As already mentioned, TNFα can affect cells in many ways, including altering the balance between oxidant and anti-oxidant status, changing the pattern of prostaglandin production and affecting expression of several cell surface components. In a small study, TNFα mRNA expression was significantly elevated in pre-eclamptic patients compared with the control groups.[17] The high expression of TNFα may be associated with the TNF1 allele, whose frequency was found to be markedly increased in pre-eclamptic patients. These suggest that TNFα may have a major role in mediating endothelial disturbances, and that some women are predisposed to excessive TNFα production to any given stimuli. This would make liable to a more severe form of the disease making this one of the possible 'modifier genes'.

Factor V Leiden abnormality

A common mutation in the factor V gene, the Leiden mutation, is the most frequent genetic cause of resistance to activated protein C. In one study, 14 of 158 women with severe pre-eclampsia (8.9%) were heterozygous for the Leiden mutation compared with 17 of 403 normotensive gravid controls (4.2%).[28] This difference was statistically significant. These data suggest that carriers of the factor V Leiden mutation are at increased risk for severe pre-eclampsia. It is interesting to note that these women are also at increased risk for deep venous thrombosis, a known association with pre-eclampsia.

The eNOS gene in pre-eclampsia

Pregnancy-induced hypertension been called a manifestation of endothelial-cell dysfunction. One of the substances affected may be nitric oxide, although the studies are not conclusive. Nitric oxide is produced by nitric oxide synthase (NOS) of which there are various types. One is eNOS, or endothelial

NOS. The role of the *eNOS* gene in the development of a familial pregnancy-induced hypertension was evaluated by analysis of linkage among affected sister pairs. There was a statistically increased allele sharing among affected sisters. These results support the localisation of a familial pregnancy-induced hypertension susceptibility locus in the region of chromosome 7q36 encoding the *eNOS* gene.[29]

Other studies have failed to show linkage with the superoxide dismutase (SOD) and renin genes. However, it is obvious that many genes may be involved, all producing a different effect on the disease process and modifying its presentation. Large multicentre studies are required to discover the relative role of genetics, and these loci in particular, in the pathophysiology of pre-eclampsia.

HOW DO THESE FINDINGS CORRELATE WITH THE PATHOPHYSIOLOGY SEEN?

The classic presenting symptoms in pre-eclampsia are hypertension, oedema and proteinuria.

Hypertension

Since vascular dysfunction is an accepted primary lesion in pre-eclampsia, it is not surprising that hypertension occurs. Although sensitivity to vaso-active substances has been reported over many decades, the exact mechanisms of the rise in blood pressure are not clear. There is no doubt that there is an upset in prostaglandin biochemistry, most likely to be related to changes in production of prostacyclin,[30] but similar changes have been implicated in nitric oxide and endothelin production. There are probably nitric oxide-dependent and nitric oxide-independent mechanisms of vasodilatation.

Nitric oxide synthesis can be determined by measuring urinary levels of nitrites and nitrates, oxidation products of NO. Measurement of nitrites and nitrates in the blood or urine of normal pregnant and hypertensive pregnant women revealed no difference between the groups.[31,32] These studies did not support a major role for nitric oxide in the development of pre-eclampsia.

Therefore, the picture is not clear. Vasodilatatory substances may or may not be deficient in pre-eclampsia. This suggests that these abnormalities are not the fundamental problem but may play a part in the response mechanisms which can ameliorate the disease process if they functional normally. The dysfunction of the vascular endothelial cell found in pre-eclampsia may be the reason for the failure of adequate response.

For whatever reason, women with pre-eclampsia have a varying degree of hypertension which is the primary risk factor for the mother.

Oedema

Oedema is normal in pregnancy and the oedema found in pre-eclampsia may just be an exaggeration if what is normally seen. There is no doubt that there is an increase capillary leak which is probably due to a combination of increased postcapillary resistance, increased capillary leak and decreased blood osmotic pressure.[33] These changes make tissue oedema more likely. This results in the potentially life threatening pulmonary oedema which can occur, especially postpartum, when there is an increased cardiac return. It is important to realise that these women can have heart failure with normal levels of central venous pressure and are particularly prone to fluid overload. Around 30% of women will have increased intrathoracic water prior to delivery. This has led to the development of protocols that tend to 'run them dry'.[34]

Proteinuria

Protein is always present in urine in small amounts and this increases in normal pregnancy. The presence of measurable protein can be due to an increase in the 'normal' renal leakage or a specific increase from renal damage. The amount of protein found in the urine will depend on the amount passing across the glomerulus and the amount reabsorbed by the tubules.

The classic lesion of pre-eclampsia is glomerular endotheliosis. This is not a sign of damage but a pathophysiological change that will recover within days of delivery. It is always associated with proteinuria which consists mostly of albumin which implies leaks across the glomerular membrane. Therefore, in the majority of women, the presence of proteinuria confirms the presence of endotheliosis and the diagnosis of pre-eclampsia but is not necessarily a marker of disease severity. Although proteinuria is associated with an increase in the morbidity for both mother and baby, there is no evidence that the level of proteinuria correlates with degree of risk. In more severe disease, the proteinuria is less specific, being associated with tubular proteins that are markers of tubular damage which may relate to, at least in the short term, renal impairment, but this is uncommon and renal failure is a relatively rare complication in pre-eclampsia in the absence of sepsis or coagulation abnormalities. When it occurs, it is almost always acute tubular necrosis which should recover with correct management. This tubular damage will also interfere with uric acid reabsorbtion from the tubule.

Uric acid

Uric acid is formed from xanthine by the action of xanthine oxidase, and is the chief end product of purine metabolism. In non-pregnant subjects, daily excretion varies between 500–800 mg of urate, and plasma uric acid levels vary between 0.24 and 0.36 mmol/l. Urate clearance varies between 6 and 12 ml/min. Renal handling of urate and subsequent urinary excretion is estimated to cover two-thirds of the daily elimination of uric acid. The bulk of plasma urate is freely filterable. Most (98%) is initially re-absorbed and the largest part of excreted urate (80–85%) derives from secondary tubular secretion. Tubular secretion of urate is dependent on renal tubular blood flow. In addition, a variety of factors influence the renal excretion of uric acid, these include volume status, the renin-angiotensin system, catecholamines, urinary solute excretion, plasma ketoacids, plasma glucose, and plasma cortisol.

Production of uric acid during pregnancy has been described as unaltered, but pregnant women excrete considerably more uric acid than when they are not pregnant. During pregnancy, urate clearance increases to between 12 and 20 ml/min and plasma levels decrease to 0.18–0.26 mmol/l. This increase in uric acid excretion is probably mainly caused by the physiologic hypervolemia of pregnancy and increased renal blood flow. Sodium restriction or use of diuretics are known to cause an increase in serum uric acid levels. In the third trimester, plasma uric acid levels may increase to concentrations equivalent to nonpregnant values. The hyperuricemia of pregnancy-induced hypertension is partly due to the failure of tubular secretion but placental ischaemia may contribute to the elevation of uric acid in PET secondary to ischaemia. The levels of uric acid also correlate with levels of oxidative stress.[25] Therefore, pre-eclamptic hyperuricemia is probably caused by a combination of increased production, intrarenal (peritubular) vasoconstriction and hypovolemia. In pre-eclampsia, a rise in uric acid can be seen to be a marker of the systemic disease process and increased risk rather than simply a sign of renal involvement.

Platelet activity

The platelet count does not change significantly during pregnancy, although there may be a slight fall during the last 8 weeks of pregnancy. Burrows and Kelton[35] reported a mean platelet count of $225 \times 10^9/l$ with 95% confidence intervals being $109-341 \times 10^9/l$. These levels are below accepted non-pregnant normals. About 5% had mild to moderate thrombocytopenia with apparently normal outcomes.

Platelet life-span is significantly shorter in pregnancy-induced hypertensive disorders, in particular when complicated by fetal growth retardation and there is a good correlation between platelet life-span and the presence of hyperuricemia, suggesting that they are makers of a similar disease process.

Many studies in women with pregnancy induced hypertension and pre-eclampsia have reported changes in platelet numbers, platelet survival and mean platelet volume (MPV) which have been interpreted as evidence of increased platelet consumption. Changes in platelet size may antedate the clinical findings.[36] This is thought to be secondary to intravascular platelet aggregation and increased adhesion to damaged vascular endothelium.

Hepatic lesions

The most characteristic feature of the hepatic lesion in eclampsia is its variability in extent and severity. The classic hepatic lesion associated with severe pre-eclampsia is periportal or focal parenchymal necrosis and periportal lake haemorrhages. Fibrin–fibrinogen deposition in the hepatic sinusoids has been noted to occur as an early feature of pre-eclampsia. In severe pre-eclampsia, large deposits of fibrin-like material may obstruct blood flow in sinusoids and cause hepatic capsular distension. Hepatic capsular distension may cause upper epigastric pain, 'stomach upset', a feeling of upper abdominal pressure or banding. Haemorrhage can occur beneath the liver capsule and may be so extensive as to cause rupture of the capsule with massive haemorrhage into the peritoneal cavity. This remains one of the rare but severe causes of maternal mortality. It would appear that hepatic lesions are patient specific rather than related directly to disease severity. The common

DIC	
Aetiology	Thromboplastins, thrombin, fibrin
Pathology	Intravascular fibrin
Pregnancy association	Abruptio placentae
Fibrinogen levels	Low
Platelet count	Mild to moderately decreased
Red cells	Slight to moderate fragmentation
Micro-angiopathy	
Aetiology	Endothelial cell damage, platelet activation, deficient production of vasodilator autocoids
Pathology	Intravascular platelet aggregation and deposition
Pregnancy association	Pre-eclampsia/HELLP syndrome
Fibrinogen levels	Normal or high
Platelet count	Moderate to markedly decreased
Red cells	Moderate to marked fragmentation

coagulation abnormalities that are seen in pre-eclampsia are due to hepatic dysfunction and not disseminated intravascular coagulation (DIC) which is rare and not a fundamental part of pre-eclampsia in the absence of placental abruption. Table 13.3 shows the major differences between DIC and microangiopathy.

This grouping of coagulation abnormalities accompanied by microangiopathy, with extensive endothelial cell damage and subsequent platelet activation has been described as HELLP syndrome, haemolysis, elevated liver enzymes and low platelets.[37] This is not a separate disease state but a subsyndrome of pre-eclampsia associated with a more adverse outcome.

Neurological

Although eclampsia remains the primary presentation in many parts of the world, it is now relatively rare in the UK with an incidence of around 1/2000 pregnancies.[38] The reason for this dramatic fall in this specific complication is difficult to work out. There is no doubt that earlier intervention and delivery has played a role, but since the cause of the convulsion is unclear, it is difficult to attribute responsibility. There may be different genetic and environmental factors at play. The fall in incidence is not related to antihypertensive drugs or the use of magnesium sulphate. Cerebral oedema and neuronal irritation are the possible direct stimuli to convulsion maybe explaining why postpartum eclampsia has not fallen as quickly as the antenatal presentation. It is postpartum that the women is most prone to tissue oedema. A controlled stable delivery with strict fluid balance and blood pressure control may lead to further drops in the incidence of this still dangerous presentation of pre-eclampsia.

SUMMARY

The pathophysiology of pre-eclampsia can be separate into three parts.

1 Abnormalities of placentation, evidence of which can be found early in pregnancy before the clinical manifestations of the disease are apparent. Pre-eclampsia is also associated with excessive placentation, as in twin and molar pregnancies. The stimulus would be produced either from the ischaemic, small, poorly implanted placenta of classic pre-eclampsia or from a large placenta found in a multiple pregnancy. This suggests that the placenta may be the source of a 'Factor X' that can cause the systemic manifestations of the condition. This factor could be some form of placental debris or an inflammatory reaction leading to activated neutrophils and production of reactive oxygen species and lipid peroxides.

2 Abnormalities of platelet/vessel wall interaction, leading to increased vascular sensitivity and platelet consumption. The vascular activity also appears to antedate the clinical signs of pre-eclampsia. These changes may be mediated through a dysfunction of the vascular endothelial cell which is part of a generalised cellular dysfunction. The degree of dysfunction and which structures are affected varies between women.

3 Maternal response to these changes which will modify the way that the disease is manifest, the severity of the signs and symptoms and the outcome for mother and child. Investigations should be aimed at looking for evidence of the systemic involvement and the maternal reaction. This will help to understand the disease progression and target treatment at the most likely beneficial areas.

KEY POINTS FOR CLINICAL PRACTICE

- There may be a strong family history
- Hypertension may not be the primary presenting symptom
- The placenta is the initial trigger to disease development
- The presentation of pre-eclampsia is very varied and any body system can be affected
- Maternal response is the main controller of disease severity
- Upper abdominal pain is a concerning feature suggestive of HELLP syndrome
- Eclampsia is not an inevitable progression from pre-eclampsia
- Pulmonary oedema can occur with a normal CVP due to capillary leak

REFERENCES

1 Chesley L C. Evolution of concepts of eclampsia. In: Bonnar J, MacGillivary I, Symonds E M. (eds) Pregnancy hypertension. Lancaster: MTP Press, 1980; 1–4

2   Zweifel P. Eklampsie. In: Doderlein A.(ed) Handbuch der Gerburtshilfe, II. Wiesbaden: Bergman, 1916; 672–676

3   Chesley L C. False starts in the study of pre-eclampsia-eclampsia. Obstet Gynecol Annu 1976; 5: 177–187

4   Roberts J M, Redman C W G. Pre-eclampsia – more than pregnancy-induced hypertension. Lancet 1993; 341: 1447–1451

5   Sargent I L. Maternal and fetal immune responses during pregnancy. Exp Clin Immunoglobulins 1993; 10: 85–102

6   Wells M, Bulmer J N. The human placental bed: histology, immunocytochemistry and pathology. Histopathology 1988; 13: 483–498

7   Bower S, Bewley S, Campbell S. Improved prediction of pre-eclampsia by 2-stage screening of uterine arteries using the early diastolic notch and color Doppler imaging. Obstet Gynecol 1993; 82: 78–83

8   Sheppard B L, Bonnar J. An ultrastructural study of utero-placental spiral arteries in hypertensive and normotensive pregnancy and fetal growth retardation. Br J Obstet Gynaecol 1981; 88: 695–705

9   Kingdom J C, Macara L M, Whittle M J. Fetoplacental circulation in health and disease. Arch Dis Child 1994; 70: 161–163

10 Cockell A P, Learmont J G, Smarason A K, Redman C W G, Sargent I L, Poston L. Human placental syncytiotrophoblast microvillous membranes impair maternal vascular endothelial function. Br J Obstet Gynaecol 1997; 104: 235–240

11 Chen G, Wilson R, Cumming G, Walker J J, McKillop J H. Production of prostacyclin and thromboxane-a(2) in mononuclear-cells from pre-eclamptic women. Am J Obstet Gynecol 1993; 169: 1106–1111

12 Greer I A, Dawes J, Johnston T A, Calder A A. Neutrophil activation is confined to the maternal circulation in pregnancy-induced hypertension. Obstet Gynecol 1991; 78: 28–32

13 Butterworth B H, Greer I A, Liston W A, Haddad N G, Johnston T A. Immunocytochemical localization of neutrophil elastase in term placenta decidua and myometrium in pregnancy-induced hypertension. Br J Obstet Gynaecol 1991; 98, 929-933

14 Lyall F, Greer I A, Boswell F, Macara L M, Walker J J, Kingdom J C P. The cell-adhesion molecule, vcam-1, is selectively elevated in serum in pre-eclampsia – does this indicate the mechanism of leukocyte activation? Br J Obstet Gynaecol 1994; 101: 485–487

15 Roberts J M. Pre-eclampsia – not simply pregnancy-induced hypertension. Hosp Pract 1995; 30: 25

16 Chen G, Wilson R, McKillop J H, Walker J J. The role of cytokines in the production of prostacyclin and thromboxane in human mononuclear-cells. Immunol Invest 1994; 23: 269-279

17 Chen G, Wilson R, Wang S H, Zheng H Z, Walker J J, McKillop J H. Tumor-necrosis-factor-alpha (tnf-alpha) gene polymorphism and expression in pre-eclampsia. Clin Exp Immunol 1996; 104: 154–159

18 Wisdom S J, Wilson R, McKillop J H, Walker J J. Antioxidant systems in normal pregnancy and in pregnancy-induced hypertension. Am J Obstet Gynecol 1991; 165: 1701–1704

19 Roberts J M, Hubel C A, Taylor R N. Endothelial dysfunction yes, cytotoxicity no. Am J Obstet Gynecol 1995; 173: 978–979

20 Degroot C J M, Davidge S T, Friedman S A, Mclaughlin M K, Roberts J M, Taylor R N. Plasma from pre-eclamptic women increases human endothelial-cell prostacyclin production without changes in cellular enzyme-activity or mass. Am J Obstet Gynecol 1995; 172: 976–985

21 Baker P N, Davidge S T, Roberts J M. Plasma from women with pre-eclampsia increases endothelial-cell nitric-oxide production. Hypertension 1995; 26: 244–248

22 Chen G, Wilson R, Cumming G, Walker J J, Smith W E, McKillop J H. Intracellular and extracellular antioxidant buffering levels in erythrocytes from pregnancy-induced hypertension. J Hum Hypertens 1994; 8: 37–42

23 Chen G, Wilson R, Cumming G, Walker J J, Smith W E, McKillop J H. Prostacyclin, thromboxane and antioxidant levels in pregnancy-induced hypertension. Eur J Obstet Gynecol Reprod Biol 1993; 50: 243–250

24 Chen G, Wilson R, Boyd P et al. Normal superoxide-dismutase (*sod*) gene in pregnancy-induced hypertension - is the decreased *sod* activity a secondary phenomenon? Free Radic Res 1994; 21: 59–66

25 Spickett C M, Reglinski J, Smith W E, Wilson R, Walker J J, McKillop J. Erythrocyte glutathione balance and membrane stability during pre-eclampsia. Free Radic Biol Med 1997; In press

26 Arngrimsson R, Bjornsson S, Geirsson R T, Bjornsson H, Walker J J, Snaedal G. Genetic and familial predisposition to eclampsia and pre-eclampsia in a defined population. Br J Obstet Gynaecol 1990; 97: 762–769

27 Arngrimsson R, Purandare S, Connor M et al. Angiotensinogen – a candidate gene involved in pre-eclampsia. Nat Genet 1993; 4: 114–115

28 Dizontownson D S, Nelson L M, Easton K, Ward K. The factor-V Leiden mutation may predispose women to severe pre-eclampsia. Am J Obstet Gynecol 1996; 175: 902–905

29 Arngrimsson R, Hayward C, Nadaud S et al. Evidence for a familial pregnancy-induced hypertension locus in the *eNOS*-gene region. Am J Hum Genet 1997; 61: 354–362

30 Greer I A, Walker J J, Cameron A D, McLaren M, Calder A A, Forbes C D. Prostacyclin in normal and hypertensive pregnancy. Am J Obstet Gynecol 1985; 153: 710–712

31 Curtis N E, Gude N M, King R G, Marriott P J, Rook T J, Brennecke S P. Nitric-oxide metabolites in normal human-pregnancy and pre-eclampsia. Hypertens Pregn 1995; 14: 339–349

32 Brown M A, Tibben E, Zammit V C, Cario G M, Carlton M A. Nitric-oxide excretion in normal and hypertensive pregnancies. Hypertens Pregn 1995; 14: 319–326

33 Brown M A, Zammit V C, Lowe S A. Capillary permeability and extracellular fluid volumes in pregnancy-induced hypertension. Clin Sci 1989; 77: 599–604

34 Walker J J. Care of the patient with severe pregnancy induced hypertension. Eur J Obstet Gynecol Reprod Biol 1996; 65: 127–135

35 Burrows R F, Kelton J G. Perinatal thrombocytopenia. Clin Perinatol 1995; 22: 779

36 Walker J J, Cameron A D, Bjornsson S, Singer C R, Fraser C. Can platelet volume predict progressive hypertensive disease in pregnancy? Am J Obstet Gynecol 1989; 161: 676–679

37 Weinstein L. Syndrome of hemolysis, elevated liver enzymes, and low platelet count: a severe consequence of hypertension in pregnancy. Am J Obstet Gynecol 1982; 142: 159–167

38 Leitch C R, Cameron A D, Walker J J. The changing pattern of eclampsia over a 60 year period. Br J Obstet Gynaecol 1997; 104: 917–922

Michael Maresh

Diabetes in pregnancy

Diabetes occurs in about four per thousand pregnancies in the UK and, as such, is the most common pre-existing medical disorder in pregnancy. The majority of these women are type I insulin dependent diabetic women with only a small proportion in the UK having type II non-insulin dependent diabetes. Whilst maternal mortality is rare, with only 3 maternal deaths being reported between 1991 and 1993,[1] perinatal mortality and morbidity is high. From the data that is available for type II diabetes, it would appear that mortality and morbidity are similarly raised to that in type I diabetes.

Although no recent national data are available, surveys from two English regions suggest that perinatal mortality is probably increased about 5-fold[2,3] and congenital malformations up to 10-fold.[2] This shows that the St Vincent declaration target of adverse pregnancy outcomes being of a similar level to that of non-diabetic women[4] is not being achieved. Internationally, reports from individual tertiary centres suggest that perinatal mortality can be reduced to levels similar to that found in non-diabetic women[5] and congenital malformations reduced significantly, albeit still raised above normal.[6]

The UK situation may be partly explained by the fact that despite repeated recommendations that all pregnant women with diabetes should be looked after by one obstetrician only in each hospital and in a joint clinic with a single physician, this is still not occurring as more than one obstetrician is involved in 49% of units and only 57% having a joint clinic.[7] With regard to congenital malformations, if these are to be further reduced, issues regarding pre-pregnancy care need to be addressed.

The subject of glucose tolerance in pregnancy and gestational diabetes is confused by variable definitions and a lack of well controlled research resulting in frequent debates in the literature[8,9] as to its relevance. Minor degrees of glucose intolerance are not associated with an adverse pregnancy outcome, whilst more marked abnormalities are almost certainly putting the fetus at

Dr Michael Maresh, Consultant Obstetrician and Gynaecologist, Saint Mary's Hospital for Women and Children, Central Manchester Healthcare NHS Trust, Hathersage Road, Manchester M13 0JH, UK

similarly increased risks in late pregnancy as those found with women with established diabetes. Accordingly, before discussing the management of diabetes, issues surrounding gestational diabetes mellitus and impaired glucose tolerance will be discussed.

GESTATIONAL DIABETES MELLITUS AND IMPAIRED GLUCOSE TOLERANCE

Definitions

Glucose concentration in blood is a continuous variable and, as such, any cut-off for normality is arbitrary. Currently, abnormalities are diagnosed using the 75 g oral glucose tolerance test (GTT). The thresholds recommended by the World Health Organization (WHO) to define impaired glucose tolerance (IGT)[10] are: (i) fasting glucose ≤ 7.8 mmol/l; and (ii) 2 h glucose ≥ 8 mmol/l and ≤ 11.0 mmol/l. Diabetes mellitus (DM) is defined if: (i) fasting glucose > 7.8 mmol/l; and/or (ii) 2 h glucose > 11.0 mmol/l. It can thus be seen that there is a continuum between normality, IGT and DM.

The WHO criteria were based on non-pregnant populations and there are well recognised changes in pregnancy, particularly in the third trimester. These are a slower cellular response to a glucose load – 'insulin resistance' – despite the increased insulin secretion which occurs as pregnancy progresses. This results in a higher post prandial glucose concentration and also a marginal decrease in fasting glucose concentrations.[11] Population studies in the third trimester suggest that about 10% of apparently normal women have IGT using the WHO definition.[12] This promotes doubt about the relevance of the diagnostic criteria in pregnancy. A multicentre European study confirmed these findings[13] and recommended higher cut offs based primarily on 95th percentiles after a 75 g oral GTT: (i) 1 h glucose ≥ 10.5 mmol/l; and 2 h glucose ≥ 9 mmol/l and ≤ 11.0 mmol/l.

The fasting values obtained in the European study were not totally consistent between centres and a consensus would be that the normal fasting concentration should be < 6 mmol/l. These values have also been recommended by Hadden[14] and by the Report of the Pregnancy and Neonatal Care Group of the St Vincent's Task Force.[7] It is recommended that the term gestational impaired glucose tolerance (GIGT) should be used and that future studies investigating the relevance of the condition should use these rather than WHO criteria. The prevalence of GIGT will depend on the characteristics of the population as abnormalities of glucose tolerance are more common in older and more obese women and also women from the Indian subcontinent. Typically, about 2% may have GIGT using the recommended definition above and about 0.5% have GDM.

Risks

Maternal risks
As GIGT is associated with maternal obesity and obese mothers are more likely to have overweight babies, the risk of caesarean section is likely to be higher.

Rarely, impaired glucose tolerance in pregnancy may deteriorate rapidly to diabetes and, occasionally, ketoacidosis develops. Warning the patient of typical symptoms and testing the urine for glucose and ketones should prevent significant risks to the mother. In addition it has been estimated that about 1 in 10 000 women are pregnant during the insidious development of insulin dependant diabetes.[15] The deterioration of glucose tolerance in pregnancy may cause rapid worsening of diabetes in these cases with the development of ketoacidosis. Routine urine testing for glucose and ketones in any woman unexpectedly ill in pregnancy should minimise risks.

The major risk to the mother is that of the increased risk in later life of developing diabetes mellitus. Extrapolating from long term follow up studies,[16,17] the risk of having diabetes mellitus was found to be 36% at 24 years with an additional 25% having IGT. Many other shorter length studies support this.[18]

Fetal risks

Pregnancies in women with type II non-insulin dependent diabetes almost certainly have the same risks to the fetus as those with type I insulin dependent diabetes (see below). Of women diagnosed during pregnancy to have gestational diabetes mellitus, approximately 1 in 4 will have a diabetic glucose tolerance test after pregnancy (i.e. type II diabetes mellitus) and will, therefore, almost certainly have had undiagnosed diabetes prior to pregnancy and thus have put their fetus at these increased risks.

With regard to IGT, the one randomised controlled trial of treating or not treating was not large enough to show a significant difference in perinatal mortality (3.6% treated, 8.5% untreated).[19] Previous non randomised studies had suggested an increased risk.[20] While there is a need for randomised studies addressing both mortality and morbidity, one can conclude that today the increased risk of a fetus dying *in utero* from maternal IGT is likely to be minimal as long as the IGT does not develop into diabetes mellitus.

Neonatal risks

Birthweight is increased in babies born to mothers with impaired glucose tolerance in pregnancy. However, if the mothers are treated, the major reason for this increase in birthweight is not the severity of the glucose tolerance, but the increased maternal obesity.[21] Increased size at birth puts the neonate at risk of traumatic delivery. Minor morbidity from maternal IGT almost certainly occurs such as neonatal hypoglycaemia and polycythaemia. While this may require admission to a special care nursery, there is no evidence of significant prolonged neonatal morbidity.[21]

Long term risks to the child and adult

As there is an association between IGT in pregnancy and the subsequent development of maternal type II diabetes, which has a strong genetic tendency, one would expect an increased incidence of DM developing in the offspring of mothers who had IGT in pregnancy. Some studies in selected populations have suggested such an association.[22] Long-term studies (which have no knowledge of glucose tolerance in the index pregnancy) have suggested it is the lighter babies who are most at risk.[23]

Screening for IGT and DM in pregnancy

The purpose of the screening test is to subject a minimum number of women to the diagnostic test – the oral GTT – (high specificity) and yet to detect as many as possible cases (high sensitivity). Ideally, screening should be performed at the initial visit in order to detect the rare, previously undiagnosed cases of subclinical DM. This is particularly justifiable in some groups, e.g. IGT or DM in a previous pregnancy or in high risk women such as older Indian women with multiple potential diabetic features. As glucose tolerance worsens with pregnancy, the screening test should be repeated again even if an earlier test has been negative. As a compromise, 28 weeks is usually considered an appropriate gestation for screening as most cases should be diagnosable by then and there may be an opportunity still to influence outcome. A number of screening tests are available, but the evaluation of some of these tests antedated the use of WHO criteria and, therefore, the sensitivity and specificity of the tests are only approximate. These are now discussed.

Potential diabetic features

These are features in women's history which predisposes them to an increased risk of developing IGT or DM in pregnancy. They include: (i) diabetes in a first degree relative (e.g. mother, sister); (ii) maternal obesity (> 120% ideal body weight); (iii) previous large baby (> 4 kg); (iv) previous unexplained stillbirth; and (v) previous abnormal glucose tolerance. To these can be added factors developing in pregnancy such as glycosuria (see below) and hydramnios. The prevalence of potential diabetic features varies enormously from population to population. The sensitivity of this as a screening method is about 50% and the specificity about 66%.[24,25]

Glycosuria

Testing for glycosuria at each antenatal visit remains a cheap, simple and established method of screening. Random glycosuria in the third trimester is present in about 15% of women with a 2 h GTT value > 8.6 mmol/l and in about 40% of women with a 2 h GTT value > 11 mmol/l.[22] While sensitivity is thus low, the specificity is high with about 90% of the pregnant population not having random glycosuria.[26]

Random blood glucose estimation

This is widely used, but only has a sensitivity of about 40%, although has a high specificity of about 90%.[27,28] The sensitivity is based on the concept of

Table 14.1 Proposed screening methods appropriate for women who are not at high risk of having IGT or GDM.[7]

1	The urine should be tested for glycosuria at every antenatal visit
2	Timed laboratory blood glucose measurements should be made at the booking visit and at 28 weeks' gestation and when glycosuria of 1+ or more is detected
3	A 75 g 2 h oral GTT should be performed if the timed blood glucose concentrations are => 6 mmol/l in the fasting state or 2 h after food or alternatively if the blood glucose concentration is => 7 mmol/l within 2 h of food

noting the time of sampling and relating it to the last meal. The suggested thresholds for performing a GTT were values of 6.4 mmol/l if sampled < 2 h after a meal and 5.8 mmol/l if > 2 h.[29]

Glycosylated haemoglobin
There have been many studies investigating the use of this as a screening test, but they have shown it to be of low sensitivity.

Glucose load
The only screening test for IGT with both high sensitivity (79%) and specificity (83%) is the 50 g glucose load given without dietary preparation with measurement of the blood glucose concentration 1 h later.[24] However, despite attempts to introduce this to the UK over the last 15 years only 6% of maternity units are currently using it.[7]

Fasting glucose and potential diabetic features
Combining a fasting blood glucose measurement with potential diabetic features have been found to have a sensitivity in the order of 90%, although a specificity of about 50%.[27,30] Whether testing in the fasting state in large numbers of women can be routinely achieved remains in doubt.

Conclusion on screening methods
In view of the practicalities of trying to ensure as many women as possible are screened with a method which can be easily implemented in a system of antenatal care now given predominantly in the community the scheme summarised in Table 14.1, which would be appropriate for women who are not at high risk of having IGT or GDM, has been proposed.[7] The sensitivity and specificity of such a system has not been evaluated, but it would almost certainly be an improvement on the current screening programmes in the UK. The criteria for abnormalities in the glucose tolerance test are as recommended above.

PRE-PREGNANCY CARE

There are multiple reasons why pregnancies should be planned in women with pre-existing diabetes and these are summarised in Table 14.2. These should include general measures such as checking rubella status, advice on smoking and use of folate supplementation. Good diabetic control at the time of conception is associated with a reduced risk of congenital malformations[31,32] and there is no evidence that hypoglycaemia has adverse effects. As the malformations particularly associated with diabetes (neural tube, cardiac and the caudal regression syndrome) occur between the 5th–9th weeks of pregnancy, assessing the women at 6 weeks of pregnancy to try to optimise control is too late. Non-insulin dependent diabetic women should be changed from oral hypoglycaemic agents and those on insulin have their control carefully assessed. If they previously have not adjusted their insulin dosage themselves before, this may be an ideal opportunity to learn this, particularly if their control is unsatisfactory. In addition, they need to be taught how to cope with hypoglycaemia (e.g. use of glucagon). It is also an opportunity to

Table 14.2 Pre-pregnancy assessment.

> Diabetes control/appropriate medication
> Understanding of pregnancy management
> Weight/diet
> Blood pressure/appropriate medication
> Retinopathy
> Nephropathy
> Autonomic neuropathy
> Ischaemic heart disease
> Smoking
> Rubella status
> Folic acid supplementation

discuss their current insulin regimen. For instance, it may be worth considering a multiple dose regimen of three short acting insulin injections pre-prandially and one long acting dose.

Complications associated with diabetes need to be assessed. Any significant retinopathy should be treated as this may deteriorate during pregnancy. Renal impairment needs to be assessed and, if moderately impaired, the woman needs to be warned that premature delivery is almost certainly going to occur and occasionally at a non-viable stage. However, she can be told that renal function deterioration should not be accelerated by a pregnancy. Older women with long standing diabetes should be considered to be at increased risk of ischaemic heart disease. Those with autonomic neuropathy need to be warned about the possibility of severe vomiting which can occur throughout pregnancy with a gastric autonomic neuropathy. If hypertension is present, it should be controlled with drugs which are suitable during pregnancy. Angiotensin converting enzyme (ACE) inhibitors, which are widely used in women with diabetes, are contra-indicated because of possible teratogenesis and effects on fetal renal function which may cause oligohydramnios. Atenolol has been associated with a reduction in birthweight.

There is also the opportunity to review the diet (see below) and try to ensure that the woman is of appropriate weight. This is particularly a problem with type II diabetic women where, if overweight, enormous doses of insulin may be necessary in pregnancy.

There is no one ideal strategy to ensure that as many as possible pregnancies are planned after all the above has been undertaken. All health professionals who are involved with women with diabetes during their reproductive years need to ensure that adequate contraception is being used. Those in primary care have a major role. The obstetrician has a role in the education of other health professionals. Physicians looking after diabetic women, particularly those involved with adolescents, have a major role. This is demonstrated by Steel who has achieved up to 60% of pregnant women having had pre-pregnancy assessment.[32] Specific pre-pregnancy clinics have only a minor role as the people who most need such a service tend not to attend. However, they do allow the woman to meet the team who will look after her during pregnancy which should encourage her to attend early in pregnancy. Diabetes specialist nurses and midwives all have their role in trying to ensure women are prepared prior to pregnancy. The use of computerised diabetic registers can also be used to ensure women in the relevant age group are particularly targeted.

Finally, it is important pre-pregnancy to point out to the woman the amount of effort which may be required from her in pregnancy to achieve optimum control. This may well impact on work, family and social life and needs to be understood. One advantage of women coming to meet the team in a joint pregnancy diabetic clinic prior to pregnancy is that there is an opportunity to discuss such issues with pregnant women who are attending the clinic that day.

ANTENATAL DIABETES MANAGEMENT

Early pregnancy may be characterised by great difficulty with diabetic control due to the pregnancy effects on insulin effectiveness and by hyperemesis. Urinary testing for ketonuria is mandatory if blood glucose concentrations are high. This needs to be backed up by emergency medical advice being available. At their first visit, women must be given written information on how to obtain such advice. Hospitalisation may be required if hyperemesis cannot be readily managed with anti-emetics.

The aim of diabetic control is that the woman should be normoglycaemic as this is likely to result in a normal pregnancy outcome. This means that one should be aiming for pre-prandial glucose values of less than 6 mmol/l. Whilst this may be achievable much of the time in a recently diagnosed diabetic woman with some residual endogenous insulin production, this may not be so easy in those with long-standing diabetes. Women must not be criticised if their control is not good, but constructively helped and not made to feel to blame. There is general agreement that home blood glucose monitoring should be done daily, 3 times pre-prandially and once at bedtime. Night time testing may be of value sometimes as pre-breakfast hyperglycaemia may be as a result of nocturnal hypoglycaemia. Post-prandial testing appears to be of less value and is not routinely performed. Measurement of glycosylated haemoglobin (monthly) or glycosylated plasma proteins (fortnightly) are an additional useful indicator of diabetes control. Again, the objective is that the results are in the laboratory's normal range for the non-diabetic person.

The most widely used insulin regimen in the UK is that of giving a once daily injection of a long/intermediate acting insulin with short acting insulin being given pre-prandially.[7] With this type of regimen, women feel much happier about making minor adjustments to their insulin dosage on the basis of their home glucose monitoring. Regimes of twice daily injections of short and intermediate insulin mixtures should not be routinely changed in pregnancy if satisfactory control is being achieved. Subcutaneous insulin infusion systems are extremely rarely used. Women with impaired glucose tolerance or gestational diabetes should be started on insulin if their pre-prandial glucose concentrations are persistently ≥ 6 mmol/l.

Hypoglycaemia is worrying for the woman, but almost certainly will occur from time to time with the tight diabetic control required for pregnancy. Women should be reassured that hypoglycaemia will not affect the fetus. However, they and their partner and other close associates need to be warned of this and be able to recognise the symptoms. The woman needs to have a glucagon kit and her partner instructed on how to use it.

The dietary advice give for diabetes in general applies equally to pregnancy.[33] Complex carbohydrate should provide about 50% of the total calories which should be well distributed throughout the day. A high fibre diet is beneficial with 30–50 g fibre advised daily. With regard to the energy requirement, 30–35 kcal/kg pre-pregnant ideal body weight is recommended. Such guidelines need to be individualised to take account of cultural and life-style circumstances. The services of a dietician is necessary for satisfactory pregnancy care. Women with type II diabetes are frequently overweight and their weight gain may need to be severely limited by careful dietary modification. Dietary advice is the initial treatment in all women with impaired glucose tolerance and gestational diabetes mellitus. Dietary restriction not only reduces post prandial hyperglycaemia, but also fasting glucose concentrations, presumably through reduced insulin resistance. However, if pre-prandial concentrations are initially ≥ 8 mmol/l dietary restrictions will almost certainly not be sufficient.

Antenatal medical complications

Medical complications (Table 14.3), such as worsening hypertension, retino-pathy and neuropathy, need to be detected early. Antihypertensive medication may need to be commenced or modified. Typical agents used are methyldopa or nifedipine. β-Blockers are also used although labetalol tends to be preferred to atenolol. ACE inhibitors are not used because of their possible effects on fetal renal function. A blood pressure no higher than 140–150/90–95 is usually aimed for, as this is thought to minimise the risk of renal damage which is a major source of morbidity in the long term in diabetes.

Microalbuminuria is frequent in diabetes and proteinuria should be routinely checked for at every visit. If present, 24 hourly estimations on a monthly basis may be helpful. Serum albumin should also be checked along with renal function blood tests. Usually protein leakage increases without significant deterioration in serum creatinine concentrations. If the serum creatinine concentration is rising persistently, then consideration must be given to termination of the pregnancy. If the nephrotic syndrome develops and yet renal function and blood pressure are stable, diuretics may be helpful to prolong pregnancy a little more. Differentiation from pre-eclampsia (which is claimed to be more common in diabetes) may be difficult, but pre-eclampsia is usually

Table 14.3 Medical complications in diabetic pregnancy.

Diabetic ketoacidosis
Hypoglycaemia
Nephrotic syndrome
Visual deterioration/retinopathy
Severe hypertension
Vomiting (gastric neuropathy)
Ischaemic heart disease

associated with fetal growth restriction, thrombocytopenia and hyperuricaemia. Once again, the experience from looking after many such patients through centralisation of care is likely to be beneficial.

Impaired vision is a major handicap in the long-term and retinopathy may deteriorate during pregnancy, particularly in association with improved diabetic control. Regular retinal assessment by an experienced physician or ophthalmologist is essential with laser therapy as indicated. The centralisation of care to one pregnancy team again facilitates an integrated approach.

Other medical complications such as autonomic neuropathy which can affect the stomach and cause persistent vomiting are rare, but can cause major management problems. Even less common is ischaemic heart disease which does need to be considered in the older diabetic woman.

ANTENATAL OBSTETRIC MANAGEMENT

Screening for fetal abnormalities

Women with established diabetes probably have a slightly higher risk of miscarriage[2] and, therefore, should be given the chance of having an early viability ultrasound scan. As the incidence of malformations is increased, particularly if diabetes control is suboptimal, detailed fetal anomaly scanning should be offered at around 20 weeks' gestation. In particular, this should look for abnormalities of the neural tube, heart, kidneys and sacral region (sacral agenesis, short femurs). Cardiac abnormalities are sometimes not detected on routine anomaly scanning and if control is poor, referral to a tertiary centre for a fetal cardiac scan should be considered. Transposition of the great vessels is the most common major cardiac abnormality found in association with diabetes (Table 14.4).

Table 14.4 Feto-maternal complications in diabetic pregnancy

Miscarriage
Congenital anomalies
Fetal growth restriction
Excessive fetal growth
Hydramnios
Premature delivery
Antenatal asphyxia
Pre-eclampsia

Chromosomal abnormalities are not increased in association with diabetes, but because women with diabetes appreciate the potential severity of their own condition, the possibility of having a baby with a chromosomal abnormality needs discussion. Serum screening tests such as AFP and HCG need careful interpretation in diabetic pregnancy because of differences in the normal ranges in women with diabetes. As a result of the above, karyotyping by amniocentesis tends to be more widely used than in the general population.

Fetal growth assessment

Assessment of fetal growth is important as both excessive fetal growth and growth restriction are well recognised complications of diabetic pregnancy. The relationship between diabetes and growth is complex and involves factors such as: (i) the blood supply, which may be impaired in diabetes due to vascular disease; (ii) arterial blood pressure which may be elevated or artificially lowered through treatment; and (iii) diabetes control which undoubtedly is relevant, although the data are confusing with, for example, birthweight not correlating well with the third trimester blood glucose control. Almost certainly, the original Pedersen hypothesis[34] is correct with maternal hyperglycaemia causing fetal hyperglycaemia and subsequent fetal hyper-insulinaemia with resulting fetal overgrowth. However, it may be that once fetal growth acceleration has commenced, it is impossible to reverse this, although it may be that further growth acceleration can be prevented through tight diabetic control.

As fetal growth restriction is associated with an increased risk of antenatal asphyxia or death and possible long-term handicap and as fetal macrosomia is associated with the same type of problems, as well as intrapartum trauma and other short term neonatal problems (see below), assessment of fetal growth is essential. While clinical assessment, including fundal height measurements is important, this should be supplemented by ultrasound. Measurement of fetal abdominal circumference should be performed on a 2–4 weekly basis from about 24 weeks' gestation in women with established diabetes and in those with impaired glucose tolerance or gestational diabetes from 28–30 weeks. Fetal bony measurements are not affected by maternal diabetes so comparison with ultrasound head measurements will usually demonstrate if growth acceleration is present. If deviations from normal growth centiles are observed, then measurements should be repeated after 2 weeks and antenatal fetal monitoring (see below) commenced. Consideration with regard to delivery may also be required (see below).

Antenatal fetal monitoring

It is well recognised that maternal diabetes is associated with an increased risk of antenatal stillbirth which is of the order of a 5-fold increase.[2] An understanding of the probable aetiologies allows a more logical approach to management, although it must be stated initially that no one test applied to all women in a non-individualised way will be successful. This again explains why published results from individual referral centres[5] are better than reviews based on regional results.[2] A number of factors are likely to be associated with antenatal asphyxia and death: (i) maternal vascular disease may cause impaired uterine spiral artery blood supply; (ii) placental release of oxygen impaired through poor diabetic control causing a higher percentage of glycosylated haemoglobin and reduction in oxygen release;[35] (iii) growth accelerated fetuses will have increased oxygen demands which may not be capable of being fully met; and (iv) mild maternal hyperglycaemia (e.g. 8–10 mmol/l) causes fetal hyperglycaemia and fetal acidaemia.[36]

The various tests available have their limitations. Doppler umbilical artery blood flow profile monitoring is not a useful screening test,[37,38] but should be used as in normal pregnancy if there is concern about fetal growth restriction as an abnormal test is likely to be predictive of subsequent problems. Biophysical profile testing has to be carefully interpreted as one component, the amniotic fluid volume, may be independently affected by diabetic control and another, fetal breathing, by the blood glucose concentration at the time of testing.

Antenatal cardiotocography, as it is a screening test for fetal acidaemia, should be a useful test. Serial cardiotocographic traces may demonstrate the relationship between suspicious or abnormal traces and blood glucose control. However, in order to be useful in predicting fetal demise, it would need to be done frequently (ideally every day) and in addition if hyperglycaemia, e.g. ≥ 8 mmol/l is persistent.

In view of the above, one can make some broad generalisations. In the presence of normal fetal growth and amniotic fluid volume on ultrasound and if maternal normoglycaemia exists, then no specific monitoring should be needed other than with normal pregnancy such as maternal fetal movement counting. If fetal growth restriction is detected with abnormal umbilical artery Doppler profiles, typically in association with maternal hypertension and nephropathy, then admission or daily assessment with cardiotocography, supplemented as indicated by biophysical assessment would be required. If excessive fetal growth is present, but growth continues, and normoglycaemia is present, then outpatient assessment on a weekly basis is usually sufficient until about 35 weeks. If control is suboptimal or there is a suggestion on ultrasound that growth, previously accelerating, it now slowing then daily assessment is advisable. Timing of delivery will depend on many factors and is discussed further below. It cannot be emphasised enough that the stillbirth rate in diabetic pregnancy is about 1 in 40[2] and that under these circumstances guidelines can only be general with such complex cases and the role of the experienced team is paramount to reduce this risk. Women with impaired glucose tolerance are not at increased risk of antenatal stillbirth and should not require intensive monitoring unless there are other indications. Those with gestational diabetes may be at increased risk and similar considerations are required as for women with established diabetes.

LABOUR AND DELIVERY

Timing of delivery

As may be appreciated from the above, timing of delivery has to be individualised depending on the presence and severity of the various fetal and maternal complications.

If elective pre-term delivery is contemplated, usually as a result of maternal problems, then steroid therapy to enhance fetal lung maturation needs to be considered. Since this antagonises insulin activity it has to be done in hospital with frequent blood glucose determinations (e.g. 2 hourly). Usually intravenous insulin, with a sliding scale regimen, is required. Doses of up to 10–14 units of insulin per hour are often required. If hyperglycaemia of this degree is present, fetal cardiotocography is required. In view of this disruption to diabetic control with its attendant fetal risks, steroid therapy is not usually given on a weekly prophylactic basis, but is reserved for when pre-term delivery appears imminent.

Surfactant production may be impaired with maternal diabetes and occasionally amniocentesis for assessment may be indicated. If borderline, then this may be a reason to give steroid therapy if not already given. The combination of diabetes, excessive amniotic fluid, caesarean delivery and slight prematurity does put the neonate at high risk of pulmonary problems such as transient tachypnoea of the newborn.

Since between 25–40% of neonates are typically found to be macrosomic,[39] a common decision which is required is to consider induction when vaginal delivery still remains a feasible alternative. Estimation of fetal weight with ultrasound has the same limitations as in non-diabetic pregnancy. When the fetal abdominal circumference exceeds 36 cm, neonatal macrosomia becomes probable.[40] Accordingly, induction of labour for suspected mild macrosomia is often practised at 37–38 weeks' gestation.

In uncomplicated well controlled diabetes with normal fetal growth, pregnancy should be allowed to continue until 39–40 weeks whilst awaiting spontaneous labour. Most women seem to request induction by term. This would be a reasonable approach as, even in these cases, there is still a slight risk of antenatal stillbirth. In addition, there will have been an enormous investment of effort from the woman and her family and possible detrimental effects on her health, so that a pregnancy loss at this stage would be unacceptable.

Mode of delivery

Caesarean section rates are extremely high in diabetic pregnancy. In the 1980 UK survey, the rate for women with established diabetes was 58%[41] and in a regional survey in 1994 the rate was 62%.[3] Even in reports from specialised centres, the caesarean rate is higher than a normal population, but this is not surprising as there is a higher proportion of complicated pregnancies.

Attempting vaginal delivery with suspected mild fetal macrosomia clearly has a risk of some degree of dystocia and, therefore, for women who are being looked after in small units, where immediate experienced help may not always be at hand, there should be serious consideration for an elective caesarean section. Similarly, in units not used to managing intravenous insulin and sliding scale regimens (see below), major diabetic control problems with possible fetal effects can occur and caesarean may, therefore, be safer.

There is, therefore, no correct caesarean section rate. All women should be at least first considered for vaginal delivery rather than the converse which tends to occur. One of the differences about being looked after in a central referral unit, rather than the nearest maternity unit, is that vaginal delivery is probably more likely to occur and where there is a choice of hospitals to attend, women should be made aware of local policy.

Management of labour

Insulin regimens

Prior to induction or elective caesarean, consideration needs to be given as to whether or not the previous day's long acting insulin should be reduced. If induction of labour with prostaglandins and a relatively unfavourable cervix is being performed then often women can be managed by having snacks and short acting doses of insulin until labour is established. Women admitted in labour, particularly if multiparous, may well not need any additional insulin. Labour itself is associated with a reduced insulin requirement. The key to diabetes management is hourly assessment of blood glucose concentrations using a bedside meter. With this it should be possible to have women not immobilised with intravenous infusions and pumps until necessary. Such regimens are highly efficient and are usually required once the women is in active labour. Typically 10 g of dextrose are given hourly using a 10% dextrose infusion and insulin is given separately using an infusion pump. Usually rates of between 0.5–2.0 units insulin/h are required. All units should have their own written guidelines on the delivery unit for this with a sliding scale of insulin dosage dependent on the maternal glucose concentration. Normoglycaemia (i.e. < 7 mmol/l) should be aimed for, as this will reduce the risk of neonatal hypoglycaemia. Women with impaired glucose tolerance and gestational diabetes mellitus rarely become hyperglycaemic in labour so insulin is not usually required.

Fetal monitoring
Continuous fetal heart rate monitoring should be used and, if suspicious or abnormal, the maternal blood glucose concentration should be initially rechecked as hyperglycaemia can cause fetal acidaemia.[36] If hyperglycaemia exists, this should be rapidly corrected, but if there is an abnormal trace with normoglycaemia fetal blood sampling should be performed as with normal practice.

Progress in labour
Normal progress in labour should occur but, if there is concern about primary dysfunctional labour, oxytocin can be considered. This should not be given in a glucose solution to facilitate diabetic control. A secondary arrest phenomenon, particularly in a multiparous woman, should usually be managed by caesarean section rather than oxytocin in case of unsuspected disproportion.

As long as labour is progressing at an acceptable rate, then there is no need to set arbitrary time limits. The combination of a sliding scale, intravenous insulin regimen and adequate analgesia, such as an epidural, should allow many primiparous women to have a safe and comfortable labour with resultant vaginal delivery. A caesarean for a first delivery will result in a very high chance of a subsequent caesarean.

If there is a suspicion of macrosomia then the most experienced obstetrician available in the hospital should be present in the second stage.

Caesarean section
Caesarean delivery should be conducted in a routine fashion. Clearly a slightly larger incision may be required for a macrosomic baby and this, combined with the possibility of marked maternal obesity, means that the procedure should not be left to the inexperienced. Prophylactic antibiotics should be given for both elective and emergency procedures. Women with diabetes are more likely than the general population to have risk factors for thromboembolism so that

measures should be taken to minimise this risk. Diabetic control should be managed using the locally agreed sliding scale insulin regimen for the peri-operative period.

POST DELIVERY CARE

Maternal care

Diabetes management

Once the placenta has delivered, the hormones responsible for the antagonism to insulin rapidly disappear from the maternal circulation so the insulin requirement reverts to that of prior to pregnancy. For type I insulin dependent diabetic women, the simplest insulin adjustment is to advise them to return to their pre-pregnancy regimen. Monitoring blood glucose should continue at this time as before, but women need not in this interim period be quite so concerned about normoglycaemia as they will want to avoid any hypoglycaemic attacks whilst caring for a baby.

Women with type II (non-insulin dependant diabetes) will usually have been on oral hypoglycaemic drugs or just dietary advice alone prior to pregnancy. Their insulin should be stopped post delivery and blood glucose concentrations checked to see as to whether they need to return to therapy. The same should apply to women with gestational diabetes. Some of these women may have had undiagnosed type II diabetes anyway. Women with only impaired glucose tolerance need not have regular blood glucose checks. All women with gestational diabetes and impaired glucose tolerance should have a glucose test performed 6–12 weeks post delivery. Even if this is normal, women should be warned of the risks of developing abnormal glucose tolerance in future. Extrapolating from long-term follow up studies,[16,17] the risk of having diabetes mellitus was 36% at 24 years follow-up with an additional 25% of women having impaired glucose tolerance. Obesity increases this risk and women should be recommended to avoid obesity through care with their diet and regular exercise. An annual check of fasting or post-prandial glucose concentration should permit early diagnosis of any deterioration of glucose tolerance.

Breast feeding

Breast feeding should be encouraged in all women with diabetes. This will be made harder by a higher chance of feeding problems through prematurity and also the possible need for supplementation if there is neonatal hypoglycaemia. Accordingly, particular support will be often required by midwives. An additional 40–50 g carbohydrate is advised during lactation.[42] Normally women with type I diabetes increase their input of carbohydrate rather than reducing their insulin requirement.

Contraception

In view of what has been mentioned with regard to pre-pregnancy care, avoiding any unplanned pregnancies is important post delivery and adequate contraception must be used. This can be discussed again at the 6 week post natal check which is best performed by the hospital team rather than by those in the community. Intra-uterine contraceptive devices are suitable in diabetic women and the same contra-indications apply as with the general population. Combined oral contraceptive pills have only a slight effect on glucose tolerance. Data to support a specific choice of preparation are lacking. Norethisterone or low-dose norgestrel preparations combined with 30–35 µg ethinyloestradiol appear suitable. Long-term usage is probably inadvisable, but many women wish to limit permanently their family size by sterilisation. Non-permanent methods such as condoms and diaphragms are effective contraceptives with no direct risks to health and, therefore, can be encouraged in those not ready for permanent contraception.

Neonatal management

Infants born to mothers with type I or type II diabetes do not need routine admission to the special care neonatal unit. However, they should be assessed by an experienced paediatrician at or shortly after delivery. Careful cardiac assessment is required because of the possibility of cardiac anomalies not diagnosed on antenatal ultrasound scanning and cardiac septal hypertrophy which is often found in diabetes. Neonatal complications are listed in Table 14.5. Many of these complications could have resulted from fetal hyperinsulinaemia, the central concept in the Pedersen hyperglycaemia–hyperinsulinaemia hypothesis.[34] Simple neonatal assessment by checking respiratory rate and routine blood tests should be all that is required for monitoring neonatal progress. Hypoglycaemia is quite common, particularly if the mother's diabetic control in pregnancy has not been ideal. Neonatal glucose concentration should be assessed 1–2 h after birth and then 4–6 hourly for the first 24–48 h. Values less than 2 mmol/l are common and should be initially managed by oral feeds. However, if < 1 mmol/l, then intravenous glucose is normally given.

Table 14.5 Neonatal complications.

Traumatic delivery, e.g. Erb's palsy
Developmental anomalies, e.g. cardiac
Cardiac septal hypertrophy
Transient tachypnoea of the newborn
Pulmonary surfactant deficiency
Hypoglycaemia
Polycythaemia
Hypocalcaemia
Hypomagnesaemia
Jaundice

REFERENCES

1 Department of Health. Report on Confidential Enquiries into Maternal Deaths in the United Kingdom 1991–1993. London: HMSO, 1996
2 Casson I F, Clarke C A, Howard C V et al. Outcomes of pregnancy in insulin dependent diabetic women: results of a five year population cohort study. BMJ 1997; 315: 275–280

3 Hawthorne G, Robson S, Ryall E A et al. Prospective population based survey of outcome of pregnancy in diabetic women: results of the Northern Diabetic Pregnancy Audit, 1994. BMJ 1997; 315: 279–281

4 Workshop report. Diabetes care and research in Europe: the Saint Vincent declaration. Diabet Med 1990; 7: 360

5 Kitzmiller J L, Gavin L A, Gin G D et al. Pre-conception care of diabetes mellitus; predictive value of maternal glycemic profile. Am J Obstet Gynecol 1987; 156: 1089–1095

6 Damm P, Molsted-Pedersen L. Significant decrease in congenital malformations in newborn infants of an unselected population of diabetic women. Am J Obstet Gynecol 1989; 161: 1163–1167

7 Jardine Brown C, Dawson A, Dodds R et al. Report of the Pregnancy and Neonatal Care Group. Diabet Med 1996; 13: S43–S53

8 Jarrett R J. Should we screen for gestational diabetes? BMJ 1997; 315: 736–737

9 Soares J de A C, Dornhorst A, Beard R W. The case for screening for gestational diabetes. BMJ 1997; 315: 737–739

10 World Health Organization. Expert Committee: Diabetes Mellitus Technical Report Series. Geneva: WHO, 1980; 646

11 Lind T, Billewicz W Z, Brown G. A serial study of changes occurring in the oral glucose tolerance test during pregnancy. J Obstet Gynaecol Br Commonw 1973; 80: 1033–1039

12 Gillmer M D G, Bickerton N J. Advances in the management of diabetes in pregnancy: success through simplicity. In: Bonnar J. (ed) Recent Advances in Obstetrics and Gynaecology. Edinburgh: Churchill Livingstone, 1994; 51–78

13 Lind T. A prospective multicentre study to determine the influence of pregnancy upon the 75 g oral glucose tolerance test. In: Sutherland H W, Stowers J M, Pearson D W M. (eds). Carbohydrate metabolism in pregnancy and the newborn IV. Berlin: Springer, 1989: 209–226

14 Hadden D R. Medical management of diabetes in pregnancy. Ballière's Clin Obstet Gynaecol 1991; 5: 369–394

15 Buschard K, Buck I, Molsted-Pedersen L et al. Increased incidence of true type I diabetes acquired during pregnancy. BMJ 1987; 294: 275–279

16 O'Sullivan J B. Subsequent morbidity among gestational diabetic women. In: Sutherland H W, Stowers J M. (eds) Carbohydrate metabolism in pregnancy and the newborn. Edinburgh: Churchill Livingstone 1984: 174–180

17 O'Sullivan J B. The Boston gestational diabetes studies: review and perspectives. In: Sutherland H W, Stowers J M, Pearson D W M. (ed) Carbohydrate metabolism in pregnancy and the newborn. London: Springer, 1989; 287–294

18 Dornhorst A, Bailey P C, Anyaoku V et al. Abnormalities of glucose tolerance following gestational diabetes. Q J Med 1990; 284: 1219–1228

19 O'Sullivan J B. Prospective study of gestational diabetes and its treatment. In: Stowers J M, Sutherland H W. (eds) Carbohydrate metabolism in pregnancy and the newborn. Edinburgh: Churchill Livingstone 1975: 195–204

20 O'Sullivan J B, Charles D, Mahan C M et al. Gestational diabetes and perinatal mortality rate. Am J Obstet Gynecol 1973; 116: 901–904

21 Maresh M J A, Beard R W, Bray C S et al. Factors predisposing to and outcomes of gestational diabetes. Obstet Gynecol 1989; 74: 342–346

22 Pettitt D J, Knowler W C, Baird H R et al. Gestational diabetes: infant and maternal complications of pregnancy in relation to third trimester glucose tolerance in the Pima Indians. Diabetes Care 1980; 3: 458–464

23 Hales C N, Barker D J P, Clark P M S et al. Fetal and infant growth and impaired glucose tolerance at age 64. BMJ 1991; 303: 1019–1022

24 O'Sullivan J B, Mahan C M, Charles D et al. Screening criteria for high risk gestational diabetic patients. Am J Obstet Gynecol 1973; 116: 895–900

25 Beard R W, Gillmer M D G, Oakley N W et al. Screening for gestational diabetes. Diabetes Care 1980; 3: 468–471

26 Sutherland H W, Stowers J M, McKenzie C. Simplifying the clinical problem of glycosuria in pregnancy. Lancet 1970; i: 1069–1071

27 Jowett N I, Samanta A K, Burden A C. Screening for diabetes in pregnancy: is a random blood glucose enough? Diabet Med 1987; 4: 160–163

28 Nasrat A A, Johnstone F D, Hasan S A M. Is random plasma glucose an efficient screening test for abnormal glucose tolerance in pregnancy? Br J Obstet Gynaecol 1988; 95: 855–860

29 Lind T, Anderson J. Does random blood glucose sampling outdate testing for glycosuria in the detection of diabetes during pregnancy. BMJ 1984; 289: 1569–1571

30 Mortensen H B, Molsted-Pedersen L, Kuhl C et al. A screening procedure for diabetes in pregnancy. Diabetes Metab 1985; ii: 249–253

31 Mills J L, Knopp R H, Simpson J L et al. Lack of relation of increased malformation rates in infants of diabetic mothers to glycemic control during organogenesis. N Engl J Med 1988; 318: 671–676

32 Steel J M, Johnstone F D, Hepburn D A, Smith A F. Can prepregnancy care of diabetic women reduce the risk of abnormal babies? BMJ 1990; 301: 1070–1074

33 British Diabetic Association. Dietary recommendations for people with diabetes. An update for 1990s. Diabet Med 1992; 2: 189–202

34 Pedersen J. The pregnant diabetic and her newborn – problems and management. Copenhagen: Munksgaard, 1977

35 Madsen H. Fetal oxygenation in diabetic pregnancy. Dan Med Bull 1986; 33: 64–74

36 Salvesen D R, Brudenell J M, Proudler A J, Crook D, Nicolaides K H. Fetal pancreatic β-cell function in pregnancies complicated by maternal diabetes mellitus: relationship to fetal acidemia and macrosomia. Am J Obstet Gynecol 1993; 168: 1363–1369

37 Salvesen D R, Higueras M T, Mansur C A, Freeman J, Brudenell J M, Nicolaides K H. Placental and fetal Doppler velocimetry in pregnancies complicated by maternal diabetes mellitus. Am J Obstet Gynecol 1993; 168: 645–652

38 Johnstone F D, Steel J M, Haddad N G, Hoskins P R, Greer I A, Chambers S. Doppler umbilical artery flow velocity waveforms in diabetic pregnancy. Br J Obstet Gynaecol 1992; 99: 135–140

39 Fraser R B. Diabetic control in pregnancy and intrauterine growth of the fetus. Br J Obstet Gynaecol 1995; 102: 275–277

40 Pedersen J F, Molsted-Pedersen L. Sonographic estimation of fetal weight in diabetic pregnancy. Br J Obstet Gynaecol 1992; 99: 475–478

41 Beard R W, Lowy C. The British Survey of Diabetic Pregnancies. Commentary. Br J Obstet Gynaecol 1982; 89: 783–786

42 Ferris A M, Neubauer S H B, Bendel R B, Green G W, Ingardia C J, Reece E A. Perinatal lactation protocol and outcome in mothers with and without insulin dependent diabetes mellitus. Am J Clin Nutr 1993; 57: 43–48

20.

21.

22.

23.

24.

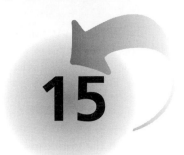

Jennifer M. Best   K. Shanti Raju   John Cason

Human papillomavirus infections and their importance in obstetrics

Human papillomavirus (HPVs) infections of the female genital tract are associated with genital warts and cervical carcinoma. Until recently, little attention has been paid to genital HPV infections during pregnancy since such infections were believed to be sexually transmitted. However, recent studies have demonstrated that these viruses, like many other micro-organisms, may be efficiently transmitted from mother-to-child at birth. The long-term implications of these findings are at present unknown. This chapter describes the evidence for the perinatal transmission of genital HPVs – particularly for those HPVs associated with cervical carcinoma – and discusses the obstetric implications of these observations.

PAPILLOMAVIRUSES

The papillomaviruses genus comprises of many similar DNA viruses which form part of the as *Papovaviridae*. Distinct papillomaviruses have been shown to infect many animal species including humans. Individual papillomaviruses demonstrate strict species-specificity and to date, more than 80 human papillomavirus (HPV) genotypes as well as many sub-types and variants have been described.[1,2] Papillomaviruses have a distinct target cell specificity: all are epitheliotropic in their natural host and may be divided into those which infect mucosal/genital sites (mucosatropic) and those which target cutaneous

Dr Jennifer M. Best, Reader in Virology, The Richard Dimbleby Laboratory of Cancer Virology, Department of Virology, The Rayne Institute, St Thomas' Hospital Campus, Lambeth Palace Road, London SE1 7EH, UK

Ms K. Shanti Raju, Senior Lecturer in Obstetrics and Gynaecology, Department of Obstetrics and Gynaecology, St Thomas' Hospital Campus, Lambeth Palace Road, London SE1 7EH, UK

Dr John Cason, Senior Lecturer in Virology, The Richard Dimbleby Laboratory of Cancer Virology, Department of Virology, The Rayne Institute, St Thomas' Hospital Campus, Lambeth Palace Road, London SE1 7EH, UK

surfaces. HPV infections are characteristically confined to the epithelium, penetrating down to the basal cells, but there is no evidence to suggest that they enter the bloodstream.

Papillomavirus particles consist of non-enveloped, icosahedral protein capsids 55 nm in diameter which contain a single copy of circular, double-stranded DNA of about 8000 base pairs in length. HPV genomes encode for six early proteins (involved with viral replication) and two late proteins which form the viral capsids.[3] HPV virions are stable to heat and desiccation[4] and have been detected in fomites, clothing and even the smoke from the laser ablation of lesions.[5]

Papillomaviruses are difficult to propagate in conventional cell cultures in vitro and there is no convenient animal model. Thus native viral antigens are unavailable for serological studies. However, HPV proteins expressed as synthetic peptides or as proteins produced in prokaryotes or eukaryotes have been used as antigens in serological and cell-mediated immunity assays. As a consequence, whilst HPVs can be detected by electron microscopy individual types cannot be identified using serological methods. Recent developments, in particular the production of HPV virus-like particles (VLP), may eventually permit the development of convincing immuno-assays. However, at present, these tests tend to be insensitive and their specificity is not well established.

Identification and typing of individual HPVs currently relies upon the detection of viral DNA. Techniques used include the 'gold-standard' method of Southern blot hybridization with HPV type-specific probes, as well as dot-blots, filter *in situ* hybridization and the (DNA/RNA) Hybrid Capture™ technique.[6,7] However, amplification techniques, particularly the polymerase chain reaction (PCR), are now preferred by most workers due to their high sensitivity.

GENITAL PAPILLOMAVIRUS INFECTIONS

Genital infection with mucosal HPVs may result in clinical, sub-clinical or latent manifestations. HPV types 2, 6 or 11 may cause benign exophytic epithelial proliferations (*condylomata acuminata: CA* [genital warts]). This is a distressing condition which causes discomfort and inconvenience. The incidence of CA is increasing in many Western countries, where it is now considered to be the most common sexually-transmitted disease. One estimate of the occurrence of CA in England suggested an incidence of about 85 000 cases in 1993.[8] HPV-2, 6 and 11 infections may also produce subclinical flat warts and latent infections. Indeed, the latter may be very common as studies using HPV-6 VLPs have indicated a seroprevalence of 19% amongst women with no history of CA.[9] Similarly, a recent PCR-based study of HPV-6/11 DNA indicated a 54% prevalence rate in swabs from women with normal vaginal histology.[10]

In contrast to HPV-6 and HPV-11, other genital HPVs such as types 16 or 18 may cause inapparent flat warts that can only be visualised after the application of acetic acid. Such flat warts may progress to cervical intra-epithelial neoplasia (CIN) and sometimes to cervical cancer. Cervical carcinoma is the second most common cause of female cancer deaths in the world.[11] In England and Wales, despite an established cervical screening programme, about 1800 cervical cancer deaths still occur each year.

Thus, the mucosatropic HPV types 2, 6 and 11 are now considered to belong to a 'low-cancer risk' group, whilst HPV types 16, 18, 31, 33, 35, 45, 51, 52 and 56, are commonly described as 'high-cancer risk'. The basis of this classification is that DNA of high, but not low, risk HPVs is: (i) consistently detected in most high-grade CIN lesions and in about 95% of all cases of cervical cancers world-wide;[12–14] (ii) integrated into the host genomic DNA in cervical cancers;[15] (iii) present in the majority of cell-lines derived from cervical cancers (*e.g.* CaSki, SiHa, HeLa and XH-1);[16] and (iv) able to transform rodent and human keratinocytes.[17] Three early proteins have transforming activity. E6 protein promotes the ubiquitin-dependent degradation of p53, a tumour suppressor protein which acts to down-regulate the progression of a cells into the replicative cycle, or to induce apoptosis of cells which have sustained irreparable DNA damage. Similarly, E7 protein of the high-risk HPVs binds to pRb, another tumour suppressor protein which also down-regulates progression of cells to mitosis.[18] The E5 protein is a mitogen with weak transforming activity which acts via co-operation with the epidermal-derived growth factor receptor.

TRANSMISSION OF MUCOSAL HUMAN PAPILLOMAVIRUSES

Low-risk HPVs

Low-risk HPVs are sexually transmitted, but may also be detected in children as a result of mother-to-child transmission and sexual abuse (below). Infected children may occasionally develop juvenile laryngeal papillomatosis (JLP), which can persist as the life-threatening condition of recurrent respiratory papillomatosis.

The presence of genital warts as evidence of sexual abuse is somewhat controversial. One study concluded that most cases of CA in girls are acquired sexually.[19] This view was supported by observations such as vaginal wash samples from 5 of 15 (33%) sexually abused girls were positive for HPV DNA compared to none of 17 controls, when tested by Southern blotting.[20] However, in another study of four cases of childhood CA, only one had other evidence of sexual abuse.[21] Similarly, a report of an 11-year-old girl with CA (whose father had penile CA) failed after investigation, to find evidence for sexual abuse.[22] A larger study of 500 children with CA concluded that sexual abuse was not an adequate explanation for all lesions.[23] In the latter paper, children with no history of sexual abuse developed genital warts between the ages of 1–6 years. In contrast, children with a history of sexual abuse tended to develop CA about a year later in life. Thus, whilst a few authors may still regard CA in children as sufficient grounds to pursue sexual abuse cases,[24] most workers acknowledge that infant infection with low-risk HPVs may result from vertical transmission. Indeed, this route of infection is believed to explain the occurrence of JLP.[25–27] Whilst JLP is rare, the fact that up to 30% of pregnant women, with no history of CA, may have antibodies to HPV-6[9] suggests vertically-acquired latent HPV-6 infections may be common. Similarly, another group using HPV-11 L1 VLPs have demonstrated IgG and IgM antibodies, respectively, in 16% and 19% of pregnant women and, in 5% and 0% of their new-born infants.[28]

In cases of vertical transmission of low-risk HPVs, it is presumed that virus is acquired by the infant during passage through the birth canal, but this is based largely on anecdotal evidence and case reports. One report documents a mother with CA at the time of delivery who gave birth to an infant who developed CA 2 years later. This genital wart contained the same two low-risk HPV genotypes as the mother's lesions.[29] Severe anogenital warts in a 17 month-old girl with AIDS-related complex were also believed to have been acquired from the mother.[30] Current evidence suggests that CA may develop more than 21 months after perinatal HPV infection.[23,29,31] In the case of JLP, one study indicates that perinatally-acquired virus may have a latent period of up to 12 years.[29] Thus, for low-risk HPVs, virus may be transmitted from mother-to-child to cause persistent subclinical infections which may develop into lesions many years later.

Low-risk HPVs may also be acquired *in utero* by ascending infection. Tang et al[32] described an infant born with a large anogenital wart, which may have resulted from an ascending infection due to premature rupture of membranes. Similarly, it was suggested that prenatal, rather than horizontal, transmission of HPV had occurred when another child – delivered by caesarean section from a women with anogenital warts – developed CA 2.5 years later when the mother was free from lesions.[33]

Whilst some viruses (e.g. human immunodeficiency virus: HIV) may be transmitted via breast milk,[34,35] it seems unlikely that HPVs are present in milk, since these viruses do not have a viraemic phase and are not associated with breast lesions. Certain retroviruses can be transmitted vertically via the gametes and there is one report of HPV DNA sequences in purified human sperm cells.[36] However, this again seems an unlikely mode of transmission for HPVs given their high specificity for keratinocytes.

Other routes of infection, such as hetero-inoculation, for example from bathing with an infected mother, have also been suggested as possible means of transmission of low-risk HPVs to infants.[37] HPV DNA may also be transmitted via HPV contaminated fomites[38] or clothing.[39] HPV-2 associated CA may also occur as a result of autoinoculation.[40]

High-risk HPVs

Until recently, high-risk HPVs were believed to cause only genital infections and be transmitted by sexual contact; this view was reinforced by the fact that high-risk HPVs are associated with cervical carcinoma which exhibits the epidemiological characteristics of a sexually-transmitted disease.[11] Sexual-transmission of high-risk HPVs was believed to be dependent upon a reservoir of infected males with subclinical/latent penile HPV infections.[41–43]

The evidence that high-risk HPVs are exclusively sexually-transmitted is now being critically reappraised, since high-risk HPVs have been detected in populations such as virgins, infants and, children (below) and it is now recognised that they may also infect the buccal mucosa and are associated with

Table 15.1 Evidence supporting the non-sexual transmission of high-risk HPVs

Non-sexual transmission of high-risk HPVs Variety of sites susceptible to high-risk HPV infection   (cervix, vagina, periungal, prostate, buccal cavity and larynx) High-risk HPV DNA common in asymptomatic women Often poor concordance between high-risk HPV infections of partners High-risk HPV DNA in samples from virgins Antibodies to high-risk HPVs in sera from prepubertal children High-risk HPV DNA is common in buccal cavities of prepubertal children
Perinatal transmission of high-risk HPVs Increased detection of high-risk HPV DNA in pregnancy High-risk HPV DNA in buccal and genital swabs of new-borns Maternal viral load predicts infection of infant Concordant high-risk HPV sequence variants in mother and child Persistence of high-risk HPVs for at least 2 years in children infected at birth High-risk HPV mRNA in 2-year-olds infected at birth

See text for specific references.

oral carcinomas.[44] Indeed, it would be surprising if high-risk papillomaviruses were not transmitted from mother-to-child, since many other micro-organisms are transmitted in this way (e.g. herpes simplex virus, hepatitis B virus and HIV, *Treponema pallidum*, *Chlamydia trachomatis* and *Neisseria gonorrhoeae*).[45] There is also strong evidence that low-risk HPVs (see above)[25–27] and JC polyomavirus[46] are transmitted from parent-to-child. Recent studies have now shown that perinatal transmission of high-risk HPVs may be common (Table 15.1), however the subject remains controversial as some workers find it hard to accept that sexual activity may not be the main route of transmission.

Sexual transmission of high-risk HPVs
The prevalence of high-risk HPV infections was believed to be low among women with normal cervical smears, but this was based upon results obtained using insensitive methods to detect viral DNA. Introduction of PCR tests which permit the detection of small quantities of viral DNA, has revealed that HPV-16 DNA is common amongst young women with no evidence of CIN.[47–49] This fact has led some to conclude that sexual activity is not correlated with risk of HPV-16 infection.[50]

Authors of some studies investigating sexual transmission of high-risk HPVs have reported a low concordance of HPV genital infections between heterosexual partners. Hippelainen et al[51] showed that of 270 couples investigated for genital HPV DNA by filter *in situ* hybridisation, both partners of 66 couples were positive whereas, only 15 (23%) of these had identical HPV types. Whilst women with low-risk HPV infections had male partners with identical HPV-types in 50% and 37% of cases, respectively, the rate of concordance was much lower amongst those with HPV-16 or HPV-18 infections (24% and 16%). Another study of heterosexual partners using dot-blot assays found a concordance between partners with HPV-16 infections of

57% and of just 29% for HPV-18.[52] Unfortunately, interpretation of such studies is often confounded by the inclusion of short-term and non-monogamous partnerships.

In a viral DNA sequencing study, Ho and colleagues[53] investigated HPV-16 genomic variants in 8 HPV-16 DNA positive heterosexual couples: whilst 4 couples had identical HPV-16 genomic variants, 4 had mismatched variants. The authors subsequently formed the opinion that sexual transmission of HPV-16 does occur, but with low frequency.

High-risk HPV infections amongst sexually-inexperienced populations
Whilst some workers were unable to detect HPV DNA in swabs from virginal women,[54] or in cervical-vaginal specimens from young girls who had not been abused,[20] others have found HPV DNA in vulval swabs from 9 of 61 (14.8%) women who claimed no history of sexual intercourse.[55] Jochmus-Kudielka et al[56] also investigated vulval swabs from 24 asymptomatic virgins by PCR using HPV-16 primers and, in 5 cases (21%), HPV-16 DNA was detected. Similarly, 3 of 15 (20%) women who claimed to have never experienced vaginal intercourse with a man were positive at the vulva, but not at the cervix.[57] One group was, however, able to detect HPV DNA at the cervices of 4 of 13 (31%) virgins.[49]

The caveat which is attached to these observations is that the true virginal state of the women in some studies may be questionable. One investigation dealt with women in China, interviewed at compulsory pre-marital screening for sexually-transmitted diseases: a less than ideal setting to elicit truthful sexual histories.[55] Whilst acquisition of high-risk HPVs may occur in virgins vulval, rather than cervical, HPV infections are most common. Nevertheless, investigations of young[58] and adult[59] females indicate that external genital HPV infections are usually indicative of internal (cervico-vaginal) infection.

High-risk HPV infections in infants and children

Few groups have investigated the occurrence of high-risk HPV infections amongst children; this, no doubt, is due to the infrequency of high-risk HPV-associated lesions among children. There are occasional reports of children with CA which contain HPV-16,[60,61] or HPV-16 and HPV-18[24,37,62] and a report of a 12 year-old child with a laryngeal carcinoma that contained HPV-18 and HPV-33.[63] In a recent study, minor hyperplastic growths of the oral mucosa were found in 21 of 98 (21%) children and one child had a papilloma containing HPV-16 DNA.[64]

Evidence that high-risk HPV infections occur among children came initially from the observation that foreskins from 3 of 70 (4.3%) unselected healthy new-borns were HPV DNA positive, two (2.8%) of which contained HPV-16 DNA detected in dot-blot assays.[65] Further indications that childhood HPV-16 infections occur were provided by seroprevalence studies. Anti-HPV-16 E4 antibodies have been demonstrated in 30–40% of sera from children and adolescents up to 20 years of age.[56] In another study of 1707 sera from individuals aged 1–95 years, anti-HPV-16 E4 antibodies were common (20%) in sera from children and teenagers, but not from adults (1%), which led the authors to conclude that HPV-16 infections may occur frequently in early life.[66]

Other groups have confirmed these findings and demonstrated antibodies to HPV-16 capsid proteins in 25–44% of children when peptides or recombinant DNA derived proteins were used as antigens.[67–69] In addition, 80 of 200 (40%) sera from children aged between 1 month and 10 years had IgM antibodies which bound in immuno-assays to an HPV-16 L2 protein which had been expressed in insect cells via a recombinant baculovirus.[70,71] Whilst detection of antibodies in childrens' sera which react with assembled HPV-16 VLPs may be uncommon,[72] a study which compared the prevalence of antibodies to HPV-16 VLPs and an HPV-16 E2 peptide in sera from 155 children, antibodies to the former were rare (4.5%), but to the latter, common (44.5%).[69] One explanation of these data may be that antibodies to the capsid proteins may only persist for a short time, whereas antibodies to early proteins, which are produced throughout infection, may occur at higher titre.

PCR studies have confirmed such serological findings. Jenison et al[67] reported the detection of HPV-16 DNA in buccal cells from 19% of children under 6 years of age. Oral scrapings from 33 of 95 (35%) of children aged between 1 and 11 years were HPV DNA positive, 16 (17%) of which were HPV-16/18 or HPV-6/11.[64] Similarly, in an ongoing study of HPV-16 infections of the buccal cavities of 300 schoolchildren aged 3–11 years in London, UK, we have found a prevalence of about 40% using a sensitive PCR (Rice et al, unpublished data).

Perinatal transmission of high-risk HPVs

Detection of high-risk HPVs during pregnancy
The prevalence of genital HPV infections appears to increase during pregnancy though data regarding the occurrence of different HPV genotypes are controversial.[73] Some reports suggest that pregnancy has no discernible effect on the frequency of detection of HPV infections.[74] Others have noted that HPV-16 infections may be common during pregnancy when samples were analysed by Southern blotting.[75,76] Rando et al[76] reported that 52.5% of patients were HPV DNA positive in the third trimester of pregnancy, whilst only 17% were positive post-partum. Schneider et al[75] reported that 28% of pregnant women and 12% of non-pregnant controls were HPV positive, with HPV-16 being the dominant genotype detected amongst the former group. A PCR based study of cytologically normal women found that HPV positivity *per se* was slightly greater amongst pregnant rather than non pregnant women, but when just HPV types 16 and 18 were considered, significant differences were not found.[77] These differences may be due to the use of PCRs, which being more sensitive, can detect low levels of viral DNA amongst non-pregnant women that are missed when less sensitive detection methods are used. Use of a quantitative PCR would determine whether higher levels of HPV DNA are detected during pregnancy. Increases in detection of HPV infections during pregnancy could result from two factors which permit an increase in viral replication. These are namely: hormonal changes, which encourage HPV replication; and transient immunosuppression – both of which are associated with pregnancy.

Detection of high-risk HPV DNA in mothers and their infants
Transmission of HPVs from mother-to-infant at birth was first proposed by Sedlacek who showed that HPV DNA could be detected by Southern blotting

in nasopharyngeal aspirates from 11 of 23 (48%) infants born to HPV DNA positive mothers.[78] However, whilst HPV DNA in maternal cervical cells was genotyped, that in infant samples was not. Others have reported HPV DNA in oropharyngeal cells from 2 of 72 (2.8%) infants delivered to HPV positive mothers,[79] but these authors used the ViraPap/ViraType™ kit which is neither as sensitive, nor as specific, as the Southern blotting method used by Sedlacek and colleagues.

One report of 3 year-old children and their HIV infected mothers in Zaire revealed that whilst 10 of 81 (12.3%) children were positive for high-risk HPV DNA this did not correlate with the HPV status of the mothers.[80] This ambiguity may again be explained by the insensitivity of the Virapap/Viratype™ kit used or, alternatively, that transient HPV infections amongst mothers had regressed since delivery.

Convincing evidence of perinatal transmission of high-risk HPVs comes from PCR studies in which HPV-16 or HPV-18 DNA was demonstrated on swabs from the external genitalia and/or buccal cavities of 50% of 24 h-old infants delivered to HPV-16 or HPV-18 infected mothers.[81] Whilst at 24 h, HPV-16 DNA positive infants might just be smeared with infected maternal cells, high-risk HPV DNA persisted in at least half of the infants until they were 6 weeks of age and at 6 months of age, over half of the children remained positive. Thirteen of these HPV-16 DNA positive children were followed to 2 years of age and remained persistently infected[71,82] and four of these children had detectable HPV-16 mRNA indicating that replicative infections had been established (Biswas, Cason, Raju and Best, unpublished data).

Fredericks et al[83] also demonstrated high-risk HPV DNA by PCR analysis of samples from the genital tracts of mothers and buccal cavities of their infants when swabs were taken 6 weeks after parturition. HPV DNA was detected in cervical epithelial cells of 11 of 30 (37%) women and in buccal cells from 8 of 11 (73%) infants born to HPV positive women. Concordant HPV-18 infections occurred in 6 mothers and their infants. Whilst these data suggest HPV-18 may be transmitted at birth from mother-to-child, it remains possible that some children acquired infection from another source during the period between delivery and testing. Similar data have also been published by other laboratories.[64]

Not all studies have detected high rates of vertical transmission of HPVs. A PCR study using the MY09/11 primers by Smith et al[84] found that just 12% of mothers and 1% of their neonates were HPV DNA positive. Whilst the low transmission rate may be due to the fact that 65% of mothers who were HPV-positive during the third trimester were negative at the time of delivery, it seems more likely that these results are explained by the insensitivity of the assay used.[6]

Indeed, assay sensitivity is a fundamental issue when considering the detection of high-risk HPV DNA in samples from children, since the quantity of viral DNA present in such samples is usually low. As a result, infant viral DNA is impossible to detect using the insensitive Hybrid Capture™ technique, difficult to reveal in PCRs using HPV generic primers such as MY09/MY11 but may be detected by sensitive 'in-house' PCRs (Table 15.2).[6] Similarly, manipulation of the sample (e.g. phenol/chloroform extraction) is liable to result in sample loss and false negative results.

Table 15.2 Detection of HPV-16 DNA in maternal and infant samples by two methods

Sample	Method A	Method B
Maternal	20/61 (32.8%)	32/61 (52.5%)
Infant		
24 h	11/62 (17.7%)	27/62 (43.5%)
6 weeks	9/38 (23.7%)	23/38 (60.5%)
6 months	0/18 (0%)	9/18 (50%)

Data for cervical scrapes from 61 mothers and buccal and genital swabs from their 62 infants (at 24 h, 6 weeks and 6 months of age) are expressed as the number of individuals which were PCR positive (for infants at one or both sites) over the number tested and, in parentheses, the percentage positive. Samples were pelleted by centrifugation, treated with proteinase K, and then analysed by PCR. Method A involved screening samples in PCRs using the HPV-consensus MY09/11 primers and then typing using the HPV-type specific primers of van den Brule et al (see Pakarian et al[81]). Method B involved screening using an in house PCR/Southern blot and primers located in the E5 open reading frame of HPV-16.[7] Unpublished data, Kaye, Best and Cason.

Source and routes of infant infections with HPVs

Passage of the neonate through an infected birth canal probably explains both the source and route of high-risk HPV DNA in infants. Indeed, estimation of the viral load in the genital tracts of HPV-16 DNA positive pregnant women revealed that women who transmitted infection to their infants had significantly greater quantities of HPV-16 DNA than those who did not.[85] Furthermore, amongst 13 HPV-16 DNA positive children, we have also shown that mothers are usually the source of infant infections by using DNA sequencing to detect concordant HPV-16 variants in maternal and infant samples.[82] Other evidence for a maternal source of infant infections comes from a report of two mothers with dual HPV-16/HPV-18 infections who both produced infants who were similarly co-infected.[81]

It is also possible that ascending HPV infections occur, causing infection *in utero*. Whilst HPVs are generally considered not to have a viraemic phase, one highly contentious paper has reported HPV-16 and HPV-18 DNA in cord-bloods of neonates delivered of mothers with HPV DNA in their peripheral blood cells:[86] these findings remain to be confirmed. Nevertheless, ascending infections may occur via ruptured membranes. Indeed, transplacental HPV-16/18 infections have been reported, a situation previously described for low-risk HPVs.[32] HPV DNA has been detected in 75% (12 of 16) of amniotic fluids from cervix-HPV DNA positive pregnant women, implying that ascending infections may occur.[87] Further studies are required to confirm these findings. In addition, it seems probable that like the low-risk HPVs (above) other routes of high-risk HPV transmission to infants and children exist (e.g. horizontal spread, auto-inoculation and exposure to contaminated clothing).

Thus, there is now convincing evidence that both high- and low-risk HPVs may be transmitted from mother to infant. The following major issues remain to be resolved: (i) the rate of infection by this route; (ii) whether ascending infections amongst women with intact membranes are common; (iii) the prevalence of high-risk HPV infections amongst prepubertal girls; (iv) whether the cervix is infected with high-risk HPVs amongst prepubertal girls' and (v) whether childhood infections predispose to cervical disease in later life, or confer protection against re-infections.

The significance of vertical transmission in explaining the epidemiology of high-risk HPV-infections may have been under-estimated by others since: (i) between 5–40% of the young female population may have asymptomatic HPV-16 infections;[49,88,89] (ii) this may increase to about 52% during pregnancy;[75] and (iii) HPV-16/18 appear to be transmitted vertically in 50–73% of children born to infected mothers.[81,83] Thus, 26–38% of children may be infected with high-risk HPVs at birth.

The implications of infection with high-risk HPVs during infancy are currently unknown and warrant further study. For example, infection of children with high-risk HPVs could result in solid immunity and protection against re-infections. Alternatively, infection at birth – before the infant's immune system is mature – might lead to HPV-specific immunological tolerance, persistence of such infections and/or a reduced ability to clear high-risk HPV re-infections in later life.

MANAGEMENT

Since there is no effective anti-viral therapy for high-risk HPV infections, there is at present no rationale for testing pregnant women for HPVs, since such knowledge is likely only to create anxiety. Similarly, treatment of pregnant women with low-risk HPV infections for overt genital warts with non-specific agents such as podophylotoxin or podophylin would be contra-indicated as these drugs are mutagenic and largely ineffective with recurrences being common.

It could be argued that HPV testing of mothers was justified on the grounds that the option of caesarean section could be offered to those who proved to be viral DNA positive. However, the lesion associated with perinatal infection with low-risk HPVs – JLP – is a rare condition and, for the high-risk HPVs, there is as yet no evidence to demonstrate that infection of the infant results in predisposition to cervical carcinoma in later life. Indeed, our recent results indicate that, whilst high-risk HPVs may be frequently acquired perinatally, other infants may acquire infection via horizontal spread, indicating that elective caesarean delivery would confer no significant long-term protection.

THE FUTURE

Since it is clear that high-risk HPVs play an essential role in the aetiology of cervical carcinoma, many workers are investigating the possibility that it may be feasible to prevent or treat HPV infections, respectively, by prophylactic and/or therapeutic vaccination. Indeed, phase 1 clinical trials of a therapeutic vaccine using recombinant *vaccinia* viruses containing HPV-16 and HPV-18 E6 and E7 open reading frames have provided encouraging results in that the constructs appear to be immunogenic and safe.[90] Potential prophylactic vaccine candidates include virus-like particles expressed in eukaryotic cells.

Given the occurrence of childhood infections, it may be necessary to administer prophylactic vaccines against high-risk HPV infections in early childhood, in a manner analogous to the approach used to prevent perinatal hepatitis B infections (HBV). HBV vaccination at birth prevents infection of most infants born to HBV positive mothers, with the attendant risk of cirrhosis of the liver and hepatoma. A prophylactic HPV vaccine given soon after birth may also prevent persistent infant infections.

ACKNOWLEDGEMENTS

We wish to thank Professor J.E. Banatvala (Department of Virology, St Thomas' Hospital, London, UK) for constructive discussions during the preparation of this text, and are grateful for financial support from the Special Trustees of St Thomas' Hospital, The Richard Dimbleby Cancer Fund and the Wellcome Trust.

REFERENCES

1 De Villiers E M. Heterogeneity of the human papillomavirus group. J Virol 1989; 63: 4898–4903
2 Icenogle J P, Sathya P, Miller D L et al. Nucleotide and amino acid sequence variation in the L1 and E7 open reading frames of human papillomavirus types 6 and 16. Virology 1991; 184: 101–107
3 Pfister H, Fuchs P. Papillomaviruses: particles, genome organisation and proteins. In: Syrjanen K, Gissmann L, Koss L G. (eds) Papillomaviruses in human disease. Berlin: Springer, 1987; 6–15.
4 Smotkin D. Virology of human papillomaviruses. Clin Obstet Gynecol 1989; 32: 117–126
5 Kashima H K, Kessis T, Mounts P et al. PCR identification of human papillomavirus DNA in CO_2 laser plume from recurrent respiratory papillomatosis. Otolaryngol Head Neck Surg 1991; 104: 191–195
6 Cavuslu S, Mant C, Starkey W G et al. Analytic sensitivities of hybrid capture, consensus and type-specific PCRs for the detection of human papillomavirus type 16 DNA. J Med Virol 1996; 49: 319–324.
7 Cavuslu S, Starkey W G, Kaye J N et al. Detection of human papillomavirus type-16 (HPV-16) DNA utilising microtitre-plate based amplification reactions and a solid-phase enzyme-immunoassay detection system. J Virol Methods 1996; 58: 59–69
8 Lacey C J N, Fairley I. Medical therapy of genital human papilloma virus related disease. Int J STD AIDS 1995; 6: 399–407
9 Carter J J, Wipf G C, Hagensee M E et al. Use of human papillomavirus type 6 capsids to detect antibodies in people with genital warts. J Infect Dis 1995; 172: 8–11
10 Cui M H, Liu Y Q, Li H L, Li S R. Human papillomavirus in condyloma acuminata and other benign lesions of the female genital tract. Chin Med J 1996; 107: 703–708
11 Munoz N, Bosch F X. Epidemiology of cervical cancer. In: Munoz N, Bosch F X, Jensen O M. (eds) Human papillomavirus and cervical cancer. Lyon: International Agency for Research on Cancer, 1989; 9–40
12 Syrjanen K, Parkkinen S, Mantyjarvi R et al. Human papillomavirus type as an important determinant of the natural history of human papillomavirus infections of the uterine cervix. Eur J Epidemiol 1985; 1: 180–187
13 Labeit D, Back W, Weizsacker F V et al. Increased detection of HPV-16 virus in invasive, but not early cervical cancers. J Med Virol 1992; 36: 131–135
14 Bosch F, Manos M, Munoz N et al. Prevalence of human papillomavirus in cervical cancer: a worldwide perspective. J Natl Cancer Inst 1995; 8: 796–802
15 Gissmann L, Schwartz E. Persistence and expression of human papillomavirus DNA in genital cancer. In: Papillomaviruses, Ciba Foundation Symposium 120. Chichester: Wiley, 1986; 190–207

16 Yee C, Krishnan-Hewlett I, Baker C C et al. Presence and expression of human papillomavirus sequences in human cervical cell lines. Am J Pathol 1985; 119: 361–366

17 Jewers R J, Hildebrandt P, Ludlow J W et al. Regions of human papillomavirus type 16 oncoprotein required for the immortalization of human keratinocytes. J Virol 1992; 66: 1329–1335

18 Tidy J A, Wrede D. Tumor suppressor genes: new pathways in gynaecological cancer. Int J Gynaecol Cancer 1992; 2: 1–8

19 Herman-Giddens M E, Gutman L T, Berson N L, the Duke Child Protection Team. Association of coexisting vaginal infections and multiple abusers in female children with genital warts. Sex Transm Dis 1988; 54: 63–67

20 Gutman L T, St Claire K, Herman-Giddens M E et al. Evaluation of sexually abused and non-abused young girls for intravaginal human papillomavirus infection. Am J Dis Child 1992; 146: 694–699

21 Sait M A, Garg B R. Condylomata acuminata in children: report of 4 cases. Genitourin Med 1985; 61: 338–342

22 Giryes H, Grunwald M H, Hammer R, Halevy S. Evaluation of sexual abuse in an infant with condylomata acuminatum. Harefuah 1995; 129: 548–550

23 Ingram D L, Everett V D, Lyna P R et al. Epidemiology of adult sexually transmitted disease agents in children being evaluated for sexual abuse. Pediatr Infect Dis J 1992; 11: 945–950

24 Hanson R M, Glasson M, McCrossin I et al. Anogenital warts in childhood. Child Abuse Negl 1990; 13: 225–233

25 Quick C A, Watts S L, Krzyzek R A, Faras A J. Relationship between condylomata and laryngeal papollomata. Ann Otol Laryngol 1980; 89: 467–471

26 Shah K, Kashima H, Polk B F et al. Rarity of cesarean delivery in cases of juvenile onset respiratory papillomatosis. Obstet Gynecol 1986; 68: 795–799

27 Gissmann L, Wolnik L, Ikenberg H et al. Human papillomavirus types 6 and -11 DNA sequences in genital and laryngeal papillomas and in some cervical cancers. Proc Natl Acad Sci USA 1983; 80: 560–563

28 Heim K, Christensen N D, Hoepfl R et al Serum IgG, IgM, and IgA reactivity to human papillomavirus types 11 and 6 virus-like particles in different gynecologic patient groups. J Infect Dis 1995; 172: 395–402

29 Menton M, Neeser E, Walker S et al. Condylomata acuminata in pregnancy. Is there an indication for caesarean section? Gerburt-Frauenheilkd 1993; 53: 681–683

30 Laraque D. Severe anogenital warts in a child with human immunodeficiency virus infection. N Engl J Med 1989; 320: 1220–1221

31 De Jong A R, Weiss J C, Brent R L. Condylomata acuminata in children. Am J Dis Child 1982; 136: 704–706

32 Tang C K, Shermeta D W, Wood C. Congenital condylomata acuminatum. Am J Obstet Gynecol 1978; 131: 912–913

33 Obalek S, Jablonska S, Favre M et al. Condylomata acuminata in children: frequent association with human papillomaviruses responsible for cutaneous warts. J Am Acad Dermatol 1990; 23: 205–213

34 Van de Perre P V, Simonon A, Msellati P et al. Post natal transmission of human immunodeficiency virus type 1 from mother to infant. N Engl J Med 1991; 325: 593–598

35 Thiry L, Sprecher-Goldberger S, Jonckheer T et al. Isolation of AIDS virus from cell-free breast milk of three healthy virus carriers. Lancet 1985; ii: 891–892

36 Chan P J, Su B C, Kalugdan T et al. Human papillomavirus gene sequences in washed human sperm deoxyribonucleic acid. Fertil Steril 1994; 61: 982–985

37 Gibson P E, Gardner S D, Best S J. Human papillomavirus types in anogenital warts of children. J Med Virol 1990; 30: 142–145

38 Ferenczy A, Bergeron C, Richart R M. Human papillomavirus DNA in fomites on objects used for the management of patients with genital human papillomavirus infections. Obstet Gynecol 1989; 74: 950–954

39 Bergeron C, Ferenczy A, Richart R. Underwear: contamination by human papillomavirus infection. Epidemiol Rev 1990; 10: 122–163

40 Obalek S, Misiewicz J, Jablonska S et al. Childhood condylomata acuminatum: association with genital and cutaneous human papillomaviruses. Paediatr Dermatol 1993; 10: 101–106

41 Wickenden C, Hanna N, Taylor-Robinson D et al. Sexual-transmission of human papillomavirus in heterosexual and male homosexual couples studied by DNA hybridization. Genitourin Med 1988; 64: 34–38

42 Campion M J, Singer A, Clarkson P K, McCance D J Increased risk of cervical neoplasia in consorts of men with penile condylomata acuminata. Lancet 1985; i: 943–946

43 Campion M J, McCance D J, Mitchell H S et al. Subclinical penile human papillomavirus infection and dysplasia in consorts of women with cervical neoplasia. Genitourin Med 1988; 64: 90–99

44 Maitland N J, Bromidge T, Cox M F et al. Detection of human papillomavirus genes in human oral tissue biopsies and cultures by polymerase chain reaction. Br J Cancer 1989; 59: 698–703

45 Greenough A, Osborne J, Sutherland S. Congenital, perinatal and neotal infections. London: Churchill Livingstone, 1992

46 Kunitake T, Kitamura T, Guo J et al. Parent-to-child transmission is relatively common in the spread of human polyomavirus JC virus. J Clin Microbiol 1995; 33: 1448–1451

47 Reed B D, Zazove P, Gregoire L et al. Factors associated with human papillomavirus infection in women encountered in community based offices. Arch Fam Med 1993; 2: 1239–1248

48 Zazove P, Reed B D, Gregoire L et al. Presence of human papillomavirus infection of the uterine cervix as determined by different detection methods in a low risk community based population. Arch Fam Med 1993; 2: 1250–1258.

49 Wheeler C, Parmenter C A, Hunt W C et al. Determinants of genital human papillomavirus infection among cytologically normal women attending university. Sex Transm Dis 1993; 20: 286–289.

50 Agorastos T, Bonitos J, Lambropoulos F et al. Epidemiology of human papillomavirus infection in Greek asymptomatic women. Eur J Cancer Prev 1995; 4: 159–167

51 Hippelainen M I, Yliskoski M, Syrjanen S et al. Low concordance of genital human papillomavirus lesions and viral types in HPV infected women and their sexual partners. Sex Transm Dis 1994; 21: 76–82

52 Monsonego J, Zerat L, Catalan F, Coscas Y. Genital human papillomavirus infections: correlation of cytological, colposcopic and histological features with viral types in women and their male partners. Int J STD AIDS 1993; 4: 13–20

53 Ho L, Tay S-K, Chan S-Y, Bernard H U. Sequence variants of human papillomavirus type 16 from couples suggest sexual transmission with low infectivity and polyclonality in genital neoplasia. J Infect Dis 1993; 168: 803–809

54 Fairley C K, Chen S, Tabrizi S N et al. Absence of genital human papillomavirus DNA in virginal women. Int J STD AIDS 1992; 3: 414–417

55 Pao C C, Tsai P L, Chang Y L et al. Possible non-sexual transmission of genital human papillomavirus infections in young women. Eur J Clin Microbiol Infect Dis 1993; 12: 221–223

56 Jochmus-Kudielka I, Schneider A, Braun R et al. Antibodies against the human papillomavirus type 16 early proteins in human sera: correlation of anti-E7 reactivity with cervical cancer. J Natl Cancer Inst 1989; 81: 1698–1704

57 Ley C, Bauer H M, Reingold A et al. Determinants of genital human papillomavirus infection in young women. J Natl Cancer Inst 1991; 83: 997–1003

58 Gutman L T, St Claire K K, Everett V D et al. Cervico-vaginal and intraanal human papillomavirus infection of young girls with external genital warts. J Infect Dis 1994; 170: 339–344

59 Horn J E, McQuillan G M, Shah K V et al. Genital human papillomavirus infections in patients attending an inner city STD clinic. Sex Transm Dis 1991; 18: 183–187

60 Rock B, Naghasfar Z, Barnett Z et al. Genital tract papillomavirus infections in children. Arch Dermatol 1986; 122: 1129–1132

61 Matsumura N, Kumasaka K, Maki H et al. Giant condylomata acuminatum in a baby boy. J Dermatol 1992; 19: 432–435

62 Benton E C, MacKinlay G A, Barr B B B et al. Characterization of human papillomavirus DNA from genital warts in children. Br J Dermatol 1989; 121 (Suppl.): 34–36

63 Simon M, Khan T, Schneider A, Pirsig W. Laryngeal carcinoma in a 12 year old child: association with human papillomavirus types-18 and -33. Arch Otolaryngol Head Neck Surg 1994; 120: 277–282

64 Puranen M, Yliskoski M, Saarikoski S et al. Vertical transmission of human papillomavirus from infected mothers to their newborn babies and persistence of the virus in childhood. Am J Obstet Gynecol 1996; 174: 694–699

65 Roman A, Fife K. Human papillomavirus DNA associated with foreskins of normal newborns. J Infect Dis 1986; 153: 855–860

66 Muller M, Viscidi R P, Ulken V et al. Antibodies to the E4, E6 and E7 proteins of human papillomavirus type-16 in patients with HPV associated diseases and in the normal population. J Invest Dermatol 1995; 104: 138–141

67 Jenison S A, Yu X, Valentine J M et al. Evidence of prevalent genital-type human papillomavirus infections in adults and children. J Infect Dis 1990; 162: 60–69

68 Cason J, Kambo P K, Best J M, McCance D J. Detection of antibodies to a linear epitope on the major capsid protein of human papillomavirus type 16 in sera from patients with cervical intraepithelial neoplasia and children. Int J Cancer 1992; 50: 349–355

69 Marias D, Rose R C, Williamson A-L. Age distribution of antibodies to human papillomavirus in children, women with cervical intraepithelial neoplasia and blood donors from South Africa. J Med Virol 1997; 51: 126–131

70 Cason J, Kambo P K, Shergill B et al. Detection of class-specific antibodies to baculovirus derived human papillomavirus type 16 capsid proteins. In: Stanley M A. (ed) Immunology of human papillomaviruses. New York: Plenum, 1994; 155–160

71 Cason J, Kaye J N, Jewers R J et al. Perinatal infection of human papillomavirus types 16/18 in infants. J Med Virol 1995; 47: 209–218

72 Andersson-Ellstrom A, Dillner J, Hagmer B et al. No serological evidence for non-sexual spread of HPV-16. Lancet 1994; ii: 1435

73 Schneider A, Koutsky L A. Natural history and epidemiological features of genital HPV infections. In: Munoz N, Bosch F X, Shah K V, Meheus A. (eds) The epidemiology of cervical cancer and human papillomavirus. Lyon: International Agency for Research on Cancer, 1992; 25–52

74 Basta A, Strama M, Pitynski K et al. Human papilloma virus (HPV) infections of the uterine cervix, vagina and vulva in women of childbearing age. Ginekol Pol 1994; 65: 563–569

75 Schneider A, Hotz M, Gissmann L. Increased prevalence of human papillomaviruses in the lower genital tract of pregnant women. Int J Cancer 1987; 40: 198–201

76 Rando RF, Lindheim S, Hasty L et al. Increased frequency of detection of human papillomavirus DNA in exfoliated cervical cells during pregnancy. Am J Obstet Gynecol 1989; 161: 50–59

77 de Roda Husman A M, Walboomers J M, Hopman E et al. HPV prevalence in cytomorphologically normal cervical scrapes of pregnant women as determined by PCR: the age-related pattern. J Med Virol 1995; 46: 97–102

78 Sedlacek T V, Lindheim S, Eder C et al. Mechanism for human papillomavirus transmission at birth. Am J Obstet Gynecol 1989; 161: 55–59

79 Smith E M, Johnson S R, Cripe T P et al. Perinatal transmission of human papillomavirus and subsequent development of respiratory tract papillomatosis. Ann Otol Laryngol 1991; 100: 479–483

80 St Louis M E, Icenogle J P, Manzila T et al. Genital types of papillomavirus in children of women with HIV infection in Kinshasa, Zaire. Int J Cancer 1993; 54: 181–184

81 Pakarian F B, Kaye J M Cason J et al. Cancer-associated human papillomaviruses: perinatal transmission and persistence. Br J Obstet Gynaecol 1994; 101: 514–517

82 Kaye J N, Starkey W G, Kell B et al. Human papillomavirus type-16 in infants: use of DNA sequence analyses to determine the source of infection. J Gen Virol 1996; 77: 1139–1143

83 Fredericks B D, Balkin A, Daniel H W et al. Transmission of human papillomavirus from mother to child. Aust N Z J Obstet Gynaecol 1993; 33: 30–32

84 Smith E M, Johnson S R, Cripe T et al. Perinatal transmission and maternal risks of human papillomavirus infection. Cancer Detect Prev 1995; 19: 196–205

85 Kaye J N, Cason J, Pakarian F B et al. Viral load as a determinant for transmission of human papillomavirus type 16 from mother to child. J Med Virol 1994; 44: 415–421

86 Tseng C-J, Lin C-Y, Wang R-L et al. Possible transplacental transmission of human papillomaviruses. Am J Obstet Gynecol 1992; 166: 35–40

87 Armbruster-Moraes E, Ioshimoto LM, Leao E, Zugaib M. Presence of human papillomavirus DNA in amniotic fluids of pregnant women with cervical lesions. Gynecol Oncol 1994; 54: 152–158

88 Bauer H M, Ting X, Greer C F et al. Genital human papillomavirus infection in female university students as determined by a PCR based method. JAMA 1991; 265: 472–477

89 Hildesheim A, Schiffman M H, Gravitt P E et al. Persistence of type-specific human papillomavirus infection among cytologically normal women. J Infect Dis 1994; 169: 235–240

90 Borysiewicz L K, Fiander A, Nimako M et al. A recombinant vaccinia virus encoding human papillomavirus types 16 and 18, E6 and E7 proteins as immunotherapy for cervical carcinoma. Lancet 1996; 347: 1523–1527

Sue Smith   Alain Gregoire

Postnatal mental illness

Postnatal depression is the commonest serious complication of the postnatal period, yet one of the least talked about and anticipated. A woman has the greatest risk in her life of developing a new episode of a mood disorder during the first 90 days after having a baby. 10% of all newly delivered women will meet the criteria for depressive disorder, and 4 per 1000 will be admitted to psychiatric hospital, half of whom will be psychotic.

Whilst psychiatric disorders occurring during pregnancy and postnatally differ little in their symptoms from those occurring at other times, several aspects of their management pose a challenge.

The symptoms occur at a time when a great number of other emotional and physical demands are being made on the mother and at an early stage in the development of the relationship with her child and when separation of mother from her child, her family and social network may have damaging consequences which must be considered if admission to hospital is needed. There is evidence of long-term effects of postnatal depression on the social and cognitive development of the child which prompts the need for early intervention. Inability to care for the child, neglect or abuse necessitates assessment of parenting skills and possibly the use of childcare law. Suicide and infanticide, whilst uncommon, are tragic and may be avoidable. Use of drugs **in** pregnancy and lactation present special problems.

The most commonly described psychiatric problems associated with childbirth are the maternity blues, postnatal depression and puerperal psychosis. However, psychological symptoms during pregnancy also need to be considered as well as other psychiatric disorders occurring in the puerperium such as anxiety and obsessive compulsive disorders.

Dr Sue Smith, Consultant, Sully Hospital, Hayes Road, Sully, Vale of Glamorgan CF64 5YA, UK

Dr Alain Gregoire, Honorary Senior Lecturer and Director, Mental Health Service, The Old Manor Hospital, Wilton Road, Salisbury, Wiltshire SP2 7EP, UK

PREGNANCY

Even when planned and much wanted, pregnancy can be a time of anxiety about changes in role, ability to cope, fears of the baby not being 'perfect'. It may be particularly difficult if the baby was not planned or if there has been previous miscarriage or termination. Certain other situations also increase a woman's vulnerability. One study found 1 in 5 mothers attending an antenatal clinic had a psychiatric disorder of some sort.[1] Compared with non-pregnant controls, depression may not be more common, but symptoms may be more severe.[2] Care of women with pre-existing mental illness who become pregnant will need careful liaison between psychiatric and maternity services.

MATERNITY BLUES

At least 50% of women experience tearfulness, lability of mood, irritability, anxiety and sleeplessness some time during the first 10 days after childbirth, with a peak on days 4 or 5. Women who experience the most severe blues will often have been anxious during pregnancy. The blues often occurs at home and so is witnessed by the GP or health visitor. Whilst in most cases it is self-limiting, there is an increased rate of later postnatal depression.[3] Appropriate management consists of antenatal information, reassurance, support and encouraging support from family and friends. Identified aetiological factors include a history of premenstrual syndrome and a possible association with the fall in progesterone levels.

POSTNATAL DEPRESSION

10–15% of women experience postnatal depressive illness, which can last from weeks to years causing considerable suffering to the woman with wider effects on her family and her child (Table 16.1). Peak onset is at 4–6 weeks post partum but new episodes of depression can of course occur at any time. Mothers are often reluctant to tell anyone how they are feeling, a particularly common fear being that their baby may be taken away from them. They may interpret their feelings as rejection of the baby and fear they may harm it. Explanation and reassurance that they are not 'going mad' and that their condition is common can go a long way towards relieving symptoms.

Table 16.1 Common symptoms of postnatal depression

Low mood
Anxiety
Tiredness
Ambivalence about the baby
Feelings of inadequacy
Irritability
Reduced or absent libido

Table 16.2   Symptoms of puerperal psychosis

> Severe insomnia or early morning waking
> Great lability of mood
> Perplexity, disorientation
> Overactivity, overtalkativeness
> Persecutory beliefs
> Hallucinations
> Lack of insight

PUERPERAL PSYCHOSIS

This is rare, occurring after only 0.2% of births, but the onset is very sudden and produces symptoms which are more severe than psychoses occurring at other times (Table 16.2). Detection of risk factors antenatally allows primary care and maternity services to liaise with mental health services in planning preventative and rapid treatment strategies to reduce suffering for both the woman and her family. This opportunity for targeted primary prevention of severe illness is unique in psychiatry.

OTHER DISORDERS

Obsessive compulsive disorder

Obsessional symptoms are common in postnatal depression. Obsessive compulsive disorder in isolation is not very common, but often worsens during pregnancy. It may present for the first time during pregnancy or after childbirth. Specialist help should be sought, with behaviour therapy the treatment of choice, though SSRI antidepressants are also effective.

Eating disorders

Amennorhoea is common in anorexia nervosa, so becoming pregnant is likely to happen at a time when the illness is at least in remission. Women with previous anorexia may react badly to their changing body shape and postnatal weight loss may become excessive.

Bulimia nervosa may improve during pregnancy as women feel they have a reason to be larger. Symptoms often return post partum and women often worry about the effect their eating disorder has had on the baby.[4]

Post traumatic stress disorder

There have a been a number of reports of women experiencing symptoms typical of post traumatic stress when they have perceived childbirth as a dangerous or life-threatening event.[5] They experience repeated intrusive recollections of the labour, may have recurrent dreams, avoid stimuli associated with childbirth (such as going near a hospital) and complain of difficulty sleeping and irritability. These symptoms can be disabling so recognition is important and should allow the woman to recount the events and her accompanying feelings.

Anxiety and panic disorder

Specific anxiety symptoms of clinical significance may occur during pregnancy and in the post partum period. In one study, women in the third trimester of pregnancy were more likely to worry about dying than non-pregnant controls.[6] There is evidence that panic disorder may improve during pregnancy but worsen again in the post partum period.[7,8] There has been recent discussion in the literature about the possible relationship between maternal anxiety and adverse obstetric outcome.[9]

CONTRIBUTION OF HORMONES

Before considering treatment and management for specific symptoms, it is worth reviewing the current place of hormonal theories in the production and maintenance of puerperal psychiatric disorders. Support for the role of hormonal factors in puerperal psychosis comes from an interesting case report of psychosis following hydatidiform mole.[10]

Thyroid hormones

Disturbed thyroid function is associated with a variety of psychiatric symptoms. Lability of mood and anxiety symptoms can occur with hyperthyroidism; lethargy, mood changes and poor concentration with hypothyroidism. It has been estimated that about 10% of women with postnatal depression have post partum thyroid disturbance indicated by either abnormal T3 or T4 levels or by the presence of thyroid antibodies.[11] Long-term treatment of post partum thyroid dysfunction is not usually necessary. Antidepressants are often indicated as well.

Gonadal steroids

Receptors for progesterone and oestrogen are widely distributed throughout the central nervous system. They have multiple, complex and profound effects on brain structure and function including neurogenesis, synaptogenesis, neural growth, migration and differentiation and on brain gender dimorphism and behaviour.[12] The precipitous drop in levels in the days immediately following childbirth have been postulated as responsible for corresponding mood changes. However, no association between levels or changes in levels and postnatal depression or psychosis have been found. It may be that some women have an abnormal response to the normal changes.

Progesterone

Progesterone has an anaesthetic action. A recent study showed a modest association of progesterone changes in the early post partum period and the maternity blues,[13] but not depressive illness. Although the use of progesterone for prophylaxis and treatment of postnatal depression has been promoted, this is not supported by controlled trials.

Oestrogen

Oestrogen's effect on mental state has been demonstrated by a number of studies. The rapid changes in oestrogen levels during the menstrual cycle appear to be associated with an increase in mild depressive symptoms. Premenstrual relapse of psychotic symptoms has been described following recovery from puerperal psychosis[14] and abrupt oestrogen withdrawal in transexual men causes puerperal like psychoses.[15] Trials of oestradiol have shown improved mood in premenstrual syndrome and the menopause.[16,17] A recent study demonstrated a significant improvement in postnatal depression using oestrogen patches compared with placebo.[18]

Cortisol

Diurnal variation in cortisol levels persists during pregnancy while overall levels rise to 34 times their normal levels, returning to normal by 2 weeks post partum. Several studies have found positive dexamethasone suppression tests up to 6–8 weeks post partum irrespective of changes in mood. One study[19] found an association with lower evening cortisol and depression at 6 weeks post partum indicating the need for more research into the part the hypothalamic axis plays in post partum mood disorders and its complex interaction with gonadal steroids.

Oxytocin and prolactin

Indirect evidence supports a link between oxytocin and prolactin and psychiatric symptoms, but no evidence of an association with postnatal depression has been found.[20]

TREATMENT AND MANAGEMENT

Postnatal mental illness offers a unique potential for predictability. This is particularly so for puerperal psychosis. A past history of psychotic illness gives a woman a 1 in 2 chance of postnatal psychosis, a family history of psychotic illness a 1 in 4 chance. There is double the risk with the first baby, and also an

Table 16.3 Risk factors emerging consistently in the literature

Risk factor	Postnatal depression	Psychosis
Past psychiatric history	+	+
Family psychiatric history		+
Poor social support	+	+
Marital disharmony	+	
Lack of a confiding relationship	+	
Poor relationship with own parents	+	
Stressful life-events	+	
Unwanted pregnancy	+	
First baby		+
Older or younger mother	+	

increased risk following still birth. There are also a number of established risk factors associated with postnatal depression, but these are not predictive enough to be clinically useful (Table 16.3). Prediction offers the opportunity for prevention, which can be divided into primary, secondary and tertiary.[21] Various elements of health and social services may be involved at each level.

Primary prevention

This aims to reduce the incidence of a condition by eliminating factors causing it. Universal, selective and indicated measures should be considered. Universal measures involve education of the public at large via the media, schools and health professionals in general. Television can have a profound effect on the beliefs of the general population, for example via story lines in soap operas. Selective measures consider all people who may be at risk, in this case pregnant or newly delivered women. For example, there is great scope within the provision of antenatal classes to educate women and their partners about the importance of support in promoting psychological well-being, and to ensure they know how and where to ask for help.

Finally, indicated measures mean that women identified as vulnerable by possession of recognised risk factors should be particular targets for preventative measures.

Secondary prevention

This aims to reduce the prevalence of a disorder by early diagnosis and intervention acting to reduce the length of the disorder. One of the main reasons postulated for the failure to diagnose postnatal depression is the reluctance of women to talk about how they feel. Education through the primary preventative measures already mentioned should enable women to admit if something is wrong. Health visitors are ideally placed to detect depression, particularly if they have built a relationship with the mother before she has had the baby. The Edinburgh Postnatal Depression Scale is a well standardised and validated screening tool which is now used routinely by health visitors in many areas to detect depression in women which might otherwise have gone undetected.[22] Once detected, the various treatment options described below can be discussed with the woman.

Tertiary prevention

This aims to reduce the disability caused by a condition that cannot be completely prevented and overlaps with primary and secondary prevention. In the case of postnatal depression, treating the condition will reduce the disability. However, during the time of recovery, the needs of the baby, other children in the family and the partner need to be considered.

In the case of more severe postnatal illness requiring hospital admission, particularly puerperal psychosis, prompt and vigorous treatment, ideally in a dedicated mother and baby unit, should limit the longer term effects on the rest of the family.

Once a postnatal depression is detected, or a woman is deemed vulnerable, further management is considered in terms of pharmacological, psychological and social. The relative contribution of each of these approaches will vary depending on the symptoms, the situation and the views of the individual woman.

PHARMACOLOGY

In pregnancy

A woman may already be taking psychotropic medication when she becomes pregnant, and her reaction is often to want to stop the drug. Women who become depressed or continue to experience other longer standing psychiatric symptoms are similarly reluctant to take drugs of any sort. The risks of deterioration in mental state if the drugs are discontinued needs to be weighed up against the potential risks of continuation. Some manufacturers are keeping databases on clinical use of drugs in pregnancy (e.g. fluoxetine) which will help evaluate effects.

Tricyclic antidepressants

Experience over many years of use has shown no evidence of teratogenic effects when given in early pregnancy and, whilst there is some evidence of anticholinergic effects on the baby when taken in late pregnancy, mothers can be reassured that they are unlikely to harm their baby by taking them.

SSRI antidepressants

As these drugs are newer there is less known about the possible dangers of their use in pregnancy, but preliminary evidence suggests they are probably safe.

Lithium

First trimester exposure is associated with an increased risk of cardiac abnormalities, in particular Ebstein's anomaly. The risk is probably not high but, nevertheless, doctor and patient must balance this risk against the risk of the illness itself. If a woman continues to take lithium during pregnancy, fetal cardiac ultrasound is recommended at about 20 weeks.

Antipsychotic drugs

There is no evidence for teratogenicity with older compounds although there is little experience with newer ones. The risks associated with untreated psychosis are likely to be greater than any arising from treatment. Depot medication may be safer in that it reduces the peaks of serum concentration. Clozapine should not be continued.

Psychotropic medication in lactation

Breast-feeding is **not** incompatible with taking psychotropic medication and being told to stop doing so in order to take an antidepressant may add to distress. As in pregnancy, a risk versus benefit assessment will need to be made in discussion with the patient.

Tricyclics
Small amounts pass into breast-milk with no measurable effects on the baby so tricyclics can be safely used during lactation.

SSRI antidepressants
Lack of sufficient evidence leads to caution and advised avoidance during lactation. However, no significant adverse effects in babies have been reported.

Lithium
Great care should be exercised if the decision is made to continue both breast-feeding and lithium. Careful observation of the infant is required to pick up signs of toxicity, e.g. poor feeding, vomiting, appearing generally unwell.

Antipsychotic drugs
Small amounts pass into breast-milk, but can be continued while closely observing the baby for signs of sedation. The exceptions are newer antipsychotics.

ECT
In cases of severe depressive disorder or puerperal psychosis, ECT can be the quickest and most effective way of alleviating suffering with no risk of adverse effects on the infant.

PSYCHOLOGICAL

Psychological therapies can be used alone or as an adjunct to pharmacological treatment. There are various forms of therapy available within the NHS and in the private sector. Many GPs now employ practice counsellors. Resources vary from place to place, as do the special interests and expertises of different professionals. Common to all forms is the provision of a confiding relationship in which the patient is listened to, enabled to release emotions and given information as appropriate to the problem and the type of therapy being used.

Health visitors as the professionals who are most likely to have detected postnatal depression are similarly well placed to provide basic counselling, or supportive listening. One study has demonstrated the effectiveness of this approach.[23]

Cognitive behaviour therapy is gathering popularity and a recent study showed 6 sessions were as effective as treatment with an antidepressant for postnatal depression.[24] It is based on inducing changes in the patterns of thinking and behaviour which are associated with depression. For example, a depressed mother may avoid contact with other mothers and the resulting isolation can exacerbate the depression and her assumption that others do not want her company. These negative assumptions would be challenged and behaviour that would increase social contact encouraged.

SOCIAL

Attention to the social setting of a mother and the emotional and practical support available to her can go a long way toward preventing postnatal depression or at least alleviating some of the suffering associated with it. Woman are often worried by the mention of a social work referral and need to be reassured that the intention is to keep the family together not break it apart. In some areas, health visitors have set up support groups for postnatally depressed mums. Voluntary organisations such as MAMA (Meet-a-Mum Association) and the Association for Postnatal Illness play an important part in supporting depressed mums and in providing contacts for them.

ROLES OF PROFESSIONALS

The care of women with mental health problems associated with childbirth takes place in a wide variety of health care settings and the UK National Health Service provides a unique opportunity to organise collaborative interagency care. High levels of structured healthcare for pregnant women already exist leading to the opportunities for prevention, early detection and prompt intervention already described. Utilising these opportunities is a challenge for planners of healthcare and clinicians in every tier of the health service.

The role of the maternity services

It is the responsibility of the maternity services to be aware of the issues relating to the mental health of women in their care and to be involved in the prevention and treatment of these conditions in liaison with primary care and psychiatric services. They have a key role in helping women through a crucial transition and major life event and are in a position to help women and their partners manage difficulties as they arise.

The booking process provides the first opportunity for picking up women at risk, particularly those with a past or close family history of psychotic illness. A few standard questions on the booking form can facilitate this process, and provide a starting point for discussion of such matters which may otherwise not be addressed.

Routine antenatal care should involve facilitating support for women by involvement of their partners and family. Antenatal education in the form of parent craft classes must include information about postnatal depression and act as a starting point for interested or concerned women to discuss the facts in greater detail. There have been suggestions in other countries on how antenatal teaching could be improved.[25,26]

Table 16.4 The role of the maternity services

Ensuring an awareness and understanding of perinatal mental health issues amongst all staff
Working with primary care to develop prediction and prevention strategies for perinatal mental illness
Ensuring continuity of care between hospital care and primary care to ensure risk factors detected in one setting are communicated to the next
Liaison with Mental Health Services

During labour and in the delivery room, women need to be listened to and feel they are in control of events. Careful explanation of the process is essential as the experience, which may be routine to the midwife can be extremely frightening for a mother.

In the immediate post partum period, monitoring of a woman's psychological reaction to the birth and the timing of and severity of the 'blues' can help detect women who may be at risk of depression later on in the puerperium (Table 16.4).

The role of primary care

Pregnant and postnatal women have regular contact with primary care professionals during pregnancy and postnatally. This will normally provide a local and less threatening setting in which identification of problems and, in the majority of cases, management of them, should occur.

Detection of risk factors antenatally allows the primary care team to liaise with mental health and maternity services in planning, possibly allowing prevention of illness (Table 16.5).

Table 16.5 Role of primary care

Ensuring an awareness and understanding of perinatal mental health issues amongst all staff
Ensuring that an effective system is in place for the detection of postnatal depression
Agreeing a protocol amongst staff for the management of mental health problems
Developing prediction and prevention strategies for perinatal mental illness
Liaising with secondary care mental health services and specialist perinatal services and purchasing such services

Health visitors play a vital role in the early detection of postnatal depression and are in an ideal position to liaise with maternity and psychiatric services.

The role of the psychiatric services

Psychiatric services are generally organised by sectors, with particular GP practices and areas referring to specific multidisciplinary teams made up of a variety of professionals including psychiatrists, community psychiatric nurses, psychologists, social workers and occupational therapists. Women with chronic or recurrent serious mental illness face a considerable and predictable risk to their mental health by giving birth. New post partum psychiatric morbidity is also predictable in any area given the birth rate. In addition, the needs of mentally ill people who are parents are rarely considered by services. In one study, 10% of all new female referrals had a child under the age of 1 year; 25% had a child under the age of 5 years.[27]

Mental illness occurring around the time of childbirth is heterogeneous with a spectrum of severity and complexity. The needs of the baby and other

Table 16.6 The role of general adult Mental Health Services

> Ensuring an awareness and understanding of the special needs of mentally ill parents and their children amongst staff
>
> Ensuring service provision takes account of these needs
>
> Identifying a key professional to liaise closely with the perinatal service
>
> Co-operating with the perinatal service and primary care in prediction, prevention, detection and management of perinatal mental illness

children in the family must be considered as part of the management plan. Community Mental Health Teams are likely to be able to provide most of the secondary care that is required, but symptoms can often be severe and require vigorous treatment and, therefore, hospital admission (Table 16.6).

Due to financial and other constraints, increasing pressure is put on services to deal only with serious mental illness. The concept of serious mental illness is not an easy one to classify, but the majority of postnatal depressive illnesses do not fit into this category. So it often falls on primary care and even maternity services to deal with these conditions, which, nonetheless, can cause considerable suffering for the woman and her family. Advice could be sought from psychiatric services about these cases, and this is made easier in areas where a specialist perinatal service exists.

Specialist perinatal care

The needs of women with young babies requires a rather different organisation of service. Maternal mental illness and fears for the child lead to anxiety in families, social services and primary care. A higher proportion of referrals will be urgent and there is a greater demand for home-based treatment and Community Psychiatric Nursing support. Specialist perinatal services exist in many areas of the UK and provide several essential functions (Table 16.7).

Table 16.7 The role of specialist perinatal psychiatric services

> Provision of admission to a mother and baby unit or intensive community based treatment
>
> Liaison with primary care, maternity services, social services (adult and child) and local voluntary services
>
> Advice on management of pregnant women with pre-existing mental illness
>
> Establish systems for screening for postnatal depression
>
> Develop protocols for treating antenatal and postnatal mental illness in different settings
>
> Assessment of parenting capacity in mentally ill parents
>
> Education within undergraduate and postgraduate medicine; midwifery and primary healthcare staff training

CONCLUSIONS

Recurrence and first onset of psychiatric disorders are an important cause of ill health and disability in pregnancy and the puerperium. More research is needed to clarify the role of hormones, both in causation and treatment and to understand better the risks of using medication which need to be balanced against the risks of untreated illness. The many professionals already involved with women at this time need to be aware of the potential problems, risk factors and methods of prevention, early detection and treatment. Involvement of secondary care should only be necessary where there is actual or identified high risk of serious mental illness. Specialist perinatal psychiatric services, however, also have an educative role, working with primary care and maternity service to enable them to manage those with disorders at the less severe end of the spectrum which are a major cause of suffering for women and their families.

REFERENCES

1 O'Hara M W, Zekoski E M, Phillips E J. Controlled prospective study of postpartum mood disorders: comparison of childbearing and nonchildbearing women. J Abnorm Psychol 1990; 99: 3–15

2 Cox J L, Connor Y M, Kendell R E. Prospective study of the psychiatric disorders of childbirth. Br J Psychiatry 1982; 140: 111–117

3 Haanah P, Adams D, Lee A et al. Links between early postpartum mood and postnatal depression. Br J Psychiatry 1992; 160: 777–780

4 Lacey J H, Smith G. Bulimia nervosa: the impact of pregnancy on mother and baby. Br J Psychiatry 1987; 150: 777–781

5 Moleman N, van der Hart O, van der Kolk B A. The postpartum stream reaction: a neglected aetiological factor in postpartum psychiatric disorders. J Nerv Ment Dis 1982; 180: 271–272

6 Fava G A, Grandi S, Michelacci L et al. Hypochondriacal fears and beliefs during pregnancy. Acta Psychiatr Scand 1990; 82: 70–72

7 George D T, Ladenheim J A, Nutt D J. Effect of pregnancy on panic attacks. Am J Psychiatry 1987; 1448: 1078–1079

8 Metz A, Sichel D A, Goff D C. Postpartum panic disorder. J Clin Psychiatry 1988; 497: 278–279

9 Copper R L, Goldenberg R L, Das A. The preterm prediction study: maternal stress is associated with spontaneous preterm birth at less than thirty five weeks gestation. Am J Obstet Gynecol 1996; 175. 1286–1292

10 Hopker S W, Brockington I F. Psychosis following hydatidiform mole in a patient with recurrent puerperal psychosis. Br J Psychiatry 1991; 158: 122–123

11 Harris B. A hormonal component to postnatal depression. Br J Psychiatry 1993; 163: 403–405

12 Pilgrim C, Hutchinson J B. Developmental regulation of sex differences in the brain: can the role of gonadal steroids be redefined? Neuroscience 1994; 60: 843–855

13 Harris B, Lovett L, Newcombe R L, Read G F, Walker R, Riad Fahmy D. Cardiff puerperal mood and hormone study paper 2: the progesterone factor. BMJ 1994; 308: 949–953

14 Brockington I F, Keely A, Hall P, Deakin W. Premenstrual relapse of puerperal psychosis. J Affect Dis 1988; 14: 287–292

15 Faulk M. Psychosis in a transexual [letter]. Br J Psychiatry 1990; 156: 285

16 Watson N R, Studd J W W, Garnet T, Baker R J. A randomised placebo controlled study of transdermal patches for the treatment of premenstrual syndrome. Lancet 1989; ii: 730–732

17 Montgomery J C, Appleby L, Brincat M et al. Effect of oestrogen and testosterone implants on psychological disorders in the climacteric. Lancet 1987; 1: 297–299

18 Gregoire A J P, Kumar R, Everitt B, Henderson A F, Studd J W W. A controlled trial of transdermal oestrogen therapy for postnatal depression. Lancet 1995; 347: 930–933

19 Hams B, Lovett L, Smith J, Read G, Walker R, Newcombe R. Cardiff puerperal mood and hormone study III. Postnatal depression and its hormonal correlates across the postpartum period. Br J Psychiatry 1996; 168: 739–744

20 Nott P, Frankel M, Armitage C, Gelder M G. Hormonal changes and mood in the puerperium. Br J Psychiatry 1976; 128: 379–383

21 Caplan G. Principles of preventative psychiatry. New York: Basic Books, 1964

22 Cox J L, Holden J, Sagovsky R. Detection of postnatal depression: development of the 10-item Edinburgh Postnatal Depression Scale. Br J Psychiatry 1984; 150: 782–786

23 Holden J M, Sagovsky R, Cox J L. Counselling in a general practice setting: controlled study of intervention in treatment of postnatal depression. BMJ 1989; 298: 223–226

24 Appleby L, Warner R, Whitton A, Faragan B. A controlled study of fluoxetine and cognitive behavioural counselling in the treatment of postnatal depression. BMJ 1997; 314: 932–936

25 Van Hall E V, Bos G, van der Lugt B et al. A proposal for training requirements concerning the psychosomatic, psychological and psychosexual aspects of the speciality obstetrics and gynaecology. J Psychosom Obstet Gynaecol 1982; 1: 91–92

26 Chalmers B E, Hofmeyr G F. The gestation of a childbirth diploma. J Psychosom Obstet Gynaecology 1989; 10: 179-187

27 Oates M R. The development of an integrated community orientated service for severe postnatal illness. In: Kumar R, Brockington I. (eds) Motherhood and mental illness, vol 2. London: Wright, 1988

David W. Sturdee

HRT – which route?

In the affluent countries of the West, there are an ever increasing number of hormone replacement therapy (HRT) preparations available,[1] so that it is often difficult even for the menopause expert to decide what may be suitable for a particular individual patient. But the first decision to be made when prescribing HRT is what is the most suitable route of administration. For the majority of women requiring HRT for the relief of symptoms, it makes no difference which route is chosen and patient preference may be the most important determining factor. In reality, for most women starting HRT, oral tablets will be the best option, but there are some differences in the effects of the various routes which will indicate a specific preference. Preparations of HRT are available for delivery orally, transdermally, by subcutaneous implant or vaginally. In addition, sublingual and intranasal spray options are being evaluated.

ORAL

Oral oestrogen is the most suitable initial therapy for most women; in the UK, for women with a uterus who are taking HRT, over 80% take oral therapy.[2] Just over 100 years ago, when it was first realised that climacteric symptoms were related to ovarian failure, the first attempts at treatment involved the prescription of sheep's ovaries in a sandwich of unleavened bread.[3] The effectiveness of this therapy was not documented, but now we have a wide range of natural oestrogen preparations containing oestradiol, oestrone, conjugated equine oestrogens and the synthetic steroid tibolone, which has oestrogenic, androgenic and progestogenic activity. The particular merits and main disadvantages of oral administration are summarised in Table 17.1.

Mr David W. Sturdee, Consultant Gynaecologist and Senior Clinical Lecturer, Department of Obstetrics and Gynaecology, Solihull Hospital, Lode Lane, Solihull, West Midlands B91 2JL, UK

Table 17.1 Advantages and disadvantages of oral HRT administration

Advantages

Easy to take; most people are used to swallowing tablets

Tablets are usually cheaper than other routes of administration

Good control due to short half-life, so can be withdrawn quickly

Wide choice of preparations available

Disadvantages

A high dose of oestrogen is required to overcome the extensive metabolism in the intestine and liver before reaching the systemic circulation

Wide variation in absorption and metabolism during the first pass of intestine and liver

Alteration of some liver function and protein synthesis

Oral oestradiol is mainly converted to oestrone

Higher incidence of minor side effects than with other routes

Requires daily dosage

All tablets contain lactose

After oral administration of oestradiol, there is extensive metabolism in the wall of the small intestine, and further changes on reaching the liver, so that only about 10% reaches the systemic circulation as oestradiol, and much larger proportions as oestrone, oestrone sulphate or oestradiol glucuronide.[4] Following oral oestrone there is a similar result in the circulation, but, with any oestrogen preparation, up to 90% of the administered dose may be inactivated before reaching the systemic circulation.[5] Thus the dose of administered oestrogen has to be correspondingly higher than that given by non-oral routes to achieve the same effective blood levels. This so called 'first pass' effect constitutes the major difference between oral and non-oral administration of oestrogen and has various clinical implications. In particular, the measurement of serum oestradiol will not give a true reflection of the total circulating oestrogen pool that may be contributing to oestrogenic activity in target tissues. In the postmenopausal woman who is not taking HRT, oestrone is the dominant oestrogen and there is an oestradiol:oestrone ratio of about 0.2. Following oral oestrogen administration a similar ratio is maintained (Table 17.2).

The hepatic response to the high hormone concentrations emerging in the portal vein is to increase synthesis of 'oestrogen-sensitive' proteins such as sex

Table 17.2 Mean serum levels and ratios of oestradiol and oestrone before and during therapy with transdermal oestradiol, oral oestradiol and conjugated equine oestrogens (CEE). (Adapted from Powers et al[6] with permission.)

	Before treatment	Estraderm® 25 µg	50 µg	100 µg	Oestradiol oral 2 mg	CEE 1.25mg
Oestradiol (pmol/l)	27	84	143	272	242	114
Oestrone (pmol/l)	119	121	151	217	1226	558
Oestradiol:oestrone	0.23	0.7	0.95	1.25	0.2	0.2

hormone-binding globulin, corticosteroid-binding globulin, thyroxine-binding globulin, transferrin, caeruloplasmin, apolipoprotein A1, pregnancy zone protein, pregnancy associated α_2 glycoprotein,[7] renin substrate and various coagulation and fibrinolytic factors.[8] The biological rationale for many of these responses is incompletely understood. In particular, the changes in plasma levels of hormone binding globulins do not appear to be matched by any physiological effects.[9]

The increase in plasma levels of renin substrate, plasma renin activity and aldosterone excretion is particularly evident with conjugated equine oestrogens,[10] and while these changes might be expected to increase blood pressure, this has not been found with current oral therapies even in hypertensive women.[11,12]

All routes of administration of oestrogen lower serum cholesterol, and especially the low density lipoprotein fraction, but serum triglyceride, which may be an independent risk factor for cardiovascular disease,[13] is elevated with oral oestrogen,[14,15] whereas transdermal oestradiol causes a reduction.[15,16] The effect of oestrogens on carbohydrate metabolism is less clear-cut. The data have been extensively reviewed by Godsland.[17] Oral conjugated equine oestrogens 1.25 mg daily seem to cause an impairment of glucose tolerance, whereas this is improved by the lower 0.625 mg daily dose and by oestradiol preparations. There are less data on the effects of transdermal oestradiol but there seems to be a reduction in fasting plasma insulin levels and an improvement in insulin sensitivity.[18,19]

The semi-synthetic oestrogens, ethinyl oestradiol and mestranol, were developed primarily for oral contraception, and are generally considered less suitable for HRT. Ethinyl oestradiol is a stable compound due to the ethinyl group attached to the C17 position which prevents oxygenation and so ethinyl oestrone is not formed. Ethinyl oestradiol is also well absorbed from the intestine without undergoing metabolism, and passes unchanged to the liver.[20] Mestranol and ethinyl oestradiol are still used for HRT and are much cheaper than the more 'natural' preparations, but there is concern that their greater metabolic effects on the liver may result in an increased risk of venous and arterial thrombosis.[21,22]

TRANSDERMAL OESTROGEN

Oestrogen is absorbed well through skin and subcutaneous fat, as well as vaginal epithelium, nasal and sublingual mucosa. The main advantage of all these routes of administration is that metabolism in the intestine and liver is avoided. Pure oestradiol can, therefore, be administered directly into the systemic circulation causing a predominant rise in plasma oestradiol concentration, and an oestradiol:oestrone ratio similar to that found in premenopausal women (Table 17.2). Theoretically, therefore, transdermal should be preferable to oral oestradiol, but there is no clinical evidence of this.

Patches

The first oestradiol skin patch, Estraderm TTS®, contains a reservoir of oestradiol with an alcohol solvent behind a rate-limiting membrane and an

Table 17.3 The advantages and disadvantages of transdermal patches

Advantages	Disadvantages
Low dose pure oestradiol	Skin reactions
Avoids intestine and liver metabolism	More expensive than tablets
Physiological oestradiol:oestrone ratio	Not well tolerated in warm climates
Reduces serum triglyceride	Variable absorption
Few side effects	

Table 17.4 Selected metabolic effects of transdermal and oral oestrogen therapies. (Adapted from Crook,[9] with permission)

	Oral oestradiol	Transdermal oestradiol
Binding globulins, e.g. SHBG, CBG, TBG	↑	←→
Renin substrate	↑	←→
Antithrombin III	↓↓	←→
Plasminogen activator inhibitor-1	↓↓	←→
High density lipoproteins	↑	←→
Low density lipoproteins	↓	↓
Triglycerides	↑/←→	↓/←→
Lipoprotein (a)	↓	↓
Bile saturation	↑	←→

↑ = increase ←→ = no change ↓ = decrease.

adhesive layer. Satisfactory circulating oestradiol levels are achieved, but local skin reactions can be a troublesome side effect in up to 35% of women.[23,24] Newer transdermal systems consist of a single transparent matrix with an adhesive layer which contains oestradiol. The dose delivered is proportional to the surface area of the patch in contact with the skin. They cause less skin reaction and are cosmetically more acceptable than the alcohol-containing reservoir patch,[25] which they will supersede. An important disadvantage of the matrix patch, however, is that it cannot be re-applied after being taken off the skin, so it should not and need not be taken off prior to bathing. Most patches have to be changed twice weekly, but two systems will maintain satisfactory oestradiol levels over 7 days – FemSeven® and Progynova TS® which may improve compliance.

By avoiding the hepatic first pass, transdermal oestradiol has minimal effect on hepatic protein synthesis, but perhaps the most significant difference from the effects of oral oestrogen is the tendency to reduce rather than elevate serum triglyceride. This may be of clinical relevance for women who have hypertriglyceridaemia[26] in whom oral oestrogen should not be used because of their adverse effect. Severe hypertryglyceridaemia (> 13 mmol/l) and pancreatitis have been documented in overtly hypertriglyceridaemic women given oral conjugated equine oestrogens.[27] The advantages and disadvantages of transdermal patches are summarised in Table 17.3 and selected metabolic effects of transdermal and oral oestrogen therapies are compared in Table 17.4.

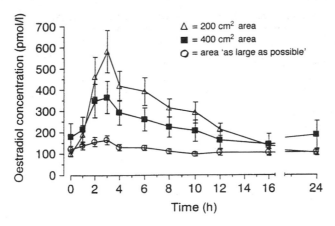

Fig. 17.1 Serum oestradiol concentrations (mean ± SEM) in 16 postmenopausal women after treatment with 1 mg oestradiol daily as transdermal gel for 14 days when the gel was applied on a 200 cm² area, 400 cm² area or an area as large as possible. From Järvinen[28] with permission.

Gel

An alternative transdermal administration is by application of a gel containing oestradiol. This has been available in France for over 20 years where it is the most popular method of HRT. It is a hydro-alcoholic gel containing 0.06% w/w 17β-oestradiol and, in the UK, it is packaged in a non-pressurised canister, oestrogel®. A measured dose of 0.75 mg oestradiol is dispensed and the usual recommended starting dose is two measures daily applied to arms or legs. A similar gel containing 1 mg 17β-oestradiol/g gel has recently been introduced in the UK as Sandrena®.

Absorption through the skin is rapid while the alcohol evaporates and effective blood levels are obtained. However, variation in the size of the application area may have impact on absorption and the subsequent levels of circulating oestradiol (Fig. 17.1).[28] Comparisons with oral and transdermal oestradiol by a patch have shown similar effects on symptoms and bone mineral density.[29]

This route of administration allows the woman a feeling of greater control over her therapy, and is gradually becoming more popular in the UK. There have been relatively few studies published on the effects of oestradiol gel,[30] but there is no reason to believe that the benefits will be different from those reported for patch therapy.

IMPLANTS

Pellets of crystalloid oestradiol have been available for subcutaneous implant for over 50 years[31–33] and for most of that time this was the only alternative to oral therapy. However, despite a long history and many advantages of this route of administration, it is not widely used, particularly outside the UK, and so data on long term benefits and possible risks are limited.

Insertion of the pellets requires a minor surgical procedure which may be one reason for limited popularity, though it is easy, takes only 3–4 min and is safe.

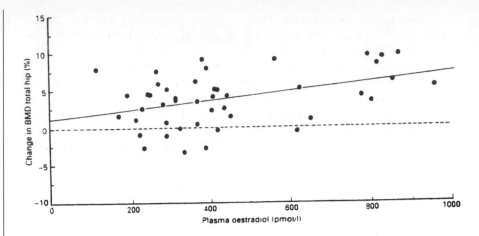

Fig. 17.2 The relation between the increase in bone mineral density at the proximal hip and post-treatment oestradiol levels. From Holland et al[36] with permission. $r = 0.25$; $P < 0.05$.

The technique has been described in detail by several authors.[32-34] Pellets of oestradiol are available in 25, 50 and 100 mg doses. The 50 mg dose is most commonly used for postmenopausal oestrogen replacement, and given at 6 monthly intervals produces a circulating level of approximately 400 pmol/l at one year.[35] For the prevention of osteoporosis, a level of at least 300 pmol/l is required and higher levels may achieve greater replacement of bone (Fig. 17.2).[36]

The elevation in circulating oestradiol varies considerably between individuals but it is usually greater than with the oral route. Inevitably, repeated implants will cause higher levels of oestradiol because of the residual effect of the previous implants, which may last for as long as two years.[37] It is, therefore, appropriate to monitor oestradiol levels especially if there is request for a repeat implant at shorter intervals than 6 months, to avoid supraphysiological levels. Symptoms returning despite an apparently adequate oestradiol level may be provoked by the falling level of oestradiol, but there is also evidence of a high incidence of psychological disturbance amongst such women.[38,39] There is no evidence, however, that supraphysiological levels of oestradiol are hazardous, but for women with a uterus there is a risk of endometrial hyperplasia from prolonged endometrial stimulation.[40] For this reason, and the need to take additional progestogen, repeated implants are probably less suitable for women

Table 17.5 The advantages and disadvantages of HRT implants

Advantages	Disadvantages
Pure oestradiol	Surgical procedure
Six monthly insertion	Unable to control absorption
High levels oestradiol in blood	Risk of supraphysiological blood levels
Avoids first pass effects	Difficult to remove pellet
Physiological oestradiol:oestrone ratio	Prolonged release of oestradiol
Testosterone can also be given	

with a uterus. The lower implant dose of 25 mg may reduce this risk[41] and is particularly suitable for older postmenopausal women for whom it will provide good protection from osteoporosis.[36,42]

Testosterone in a 100 mg pellet can also be given by implant to women who have an incomplete response to oestrogen alone, particularly if they are troubled by headaches, loss of energy, depression and especially loss of libido.[43–45] This is usually given at the same time as oestradiol. However, some authors have not found that supplementary testosterone is helpful for women with reduced sexual response alone.[46] The advantages and disadvantages of HRT implants are summarised in Table 17.5. Serum concentrations of oestradiol and oestrone after oral, transdermal and subcutaneous implant administration of oestradiol are summarised in Figure 17.3.

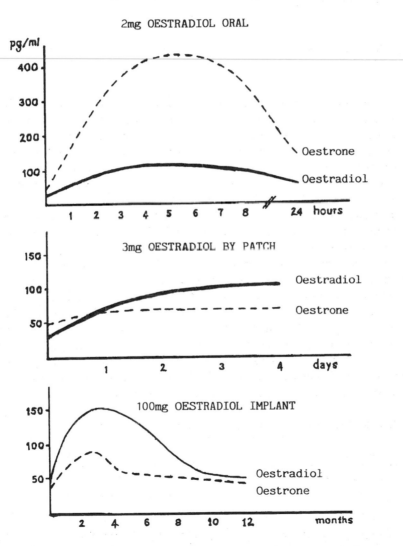

Fig. 17.3 Serum concentrations of oestradiol and oestrone after oral, transdermal and subcutaneous implant administration of oestradiol. Adapted from Kuhl[5] with permission.

ADDITIONAL PROGESTOGEN

The need to add progestogen to regimens of HRT for women with a uterus to protect the endometrium is well established and accepted. Until recently this has only been suitable by the oral route and many proprietary HRT preparations have contained 10–14 days either separately or combined in the daily tablet. Separate progestogen administration allows greater flexibility in type and dosage, but also has the potential hazard of permitting the woman to omit the progestogen if she considers it is the cause of unwanted side effects.

Progestogens are now also incorporated in some matrix patch preparations in either a 28 day sequential regimen, Nuvelle TS® and Evorel sequi®, or a continuous combined regimen, Evorel conti®.

Natural progesterone can also be administered via the vagina as a pessary, Cyclogest®, or a new gel, Crinone®. This route avoids the first pass hepatic and intestinal metabolic effects, and causes less side effects than with oral synthetic progestogens.

The only proven merit of additional progestogen is for prevention of endometrial hyperplasia and carcinoma. The administration of progestogen direct into the endometrial cavity in an intra-uterine device (IUD) provides a high local concentration with little systemic absorption, and, therefore, fewer of the unwanted side effects. The Levonorgestrol IUD, Mirena® which at present is only licensed for contraception in the UK, will maintain an atrophic endometrium and, in combination with oestrogen administered orally, transdermally or by implant, may provide an alternative method of continuous combined therapy (CCT).[47,48] This technique may become particularly suitable for the perimenopausal woman to help control dysfunctional bleeding and can then be continued during the transition to the postmenopause when bleeding problems can be so troublesome.

VAGINAL OESTROGEN

For older women in particular who are troubled by symptoms related to urogenital ageing, local oestrogen therapy is often more appropriate, but these problems are not well recognised or treated.[49] Local oestrogen administration will provide relief, but is often given for too short a time to have an adequate response. Systemic therapy does not always produce an improvement in vaginal symptoms, and for women with symptoms of systemic and local oestrogen deficiency, a combination of systemic and vaginal oestrogen may be necessary initially, until the vaginal epithelium has responded. For the older woman who does not wish to experience the effects of systemic oestrogen, the use of a natural oestrogen vaginal preparation can avoid significant systemic absorption.[50,51] There are several creams and pessaries and a vaginal tablet. A soft 5 cm diameter ring, Estring®, releases oestradiol locally over 3 months, and is more user-friendly.[52]

WHICH ROUTE?

Natural oestrogens given by any route provide comparable relief of climacteric symptoms with good patient acceptability, but for the majority of patients oral therapy will be the most suitable initial treatment. Review after 2–3 months may indicate a change of regimen or dose, depending on the symptomatic response and side effects. There are, however, certain situations for which a specific route of administration may be more suitable because of the particular effects outlined earlier.

Hypertension

Hypertension is a major risk factor for coronary artery and cerebrovascular disease. Synthetic oral oestrogen (ethinyl oestradiol) in oral contraceptive preparations can stimulate hepatic production of renin substrate and angiotensinogen with an increased risk of hypertension, vasoconstriction and platelet aggregation,[53,54] so that hypertension is generally considered to be a contra-indication for this method of contraception. In a few women, oral conjugated equine oestrogens may cause a similar effect[10,55–57] which can be identified at the first return visit after initiating HRT. However, despite the occasional patient in whom hypertension may be induced, oestrogen also causes vasodilatation[58,59] so that overall there is no evidence that HRT affects blood pressure.[60]

For those with hypertension, it would obviously be prudent to control this with appropriate therapy, but current oral HRT does not appear to increase blood pressure in hypertensive women.[11,12] Indeed in the Nurses' Health Study,[61] there is evidence that such women have an even greater reduction in the risk of myocardial infarction than those who are normotensive.

Nevertheless, by avoiding the hepatic first pass effect, non-oral oestrogens do not stimulate renin substrate synthesis[62,63] and so, on theoretical grounds, any risk of hypertension with oral therapy should be avoided.[9]

Thromboembolism

A previous history of venous thromboembolism (VTE) is usually considered to be a contra-indication to HRT. Recent studies have suggested that HRT increases the risk of VTE particularly in the first year of use by a factor of about three,[64–67] although put into perspective this equates to only one extra case of VTE in 5000 users per year. Several studies have shown that oral oestrogen increases coagulation activation[68–71] but causes other changes that might counteract this effect[72] and the addition of progestogen may also be beneficial.[73] Transdermal oestrogen, however, by avoiding the hepatic first pass effect, does not adversely affect coagulation.[74,75] The risk of VTE with transdermal HRT preparations is not yet known, as the number of subjects in the recent studies is so low. However, for a woman who has had a VTE or is for other reasons at increased risk, the transdermal route might be preferable.[72]

Other cardiovascular disease risk factors

Oral and non-oral routes of oestrogen therapy have beneficial effects on plasma and lipoproteins, but only oral oestrogen significantly elevates high-density lipoproteins, which are important in the protection from cardiovascular disease. However, non-oral therapy reduces triglyceride levels, a major predictor of cardiovascular disease in women. Transdermal therapy may reduce insulin resistance, whereas oral oestrogens and androgenic progestogens do not improve, and may slightly worsen glucose tolerance and insulin resistance, but the clinical implications are uncertain.[9,19,76]

Smoking is the most important health hazard in the Western world. It also results in an earlier menopause by 1–1.5 years[77] and reduces the circulating levels of oestradiol and oestrone in postmenopausal women taking long-term oral HRT.[78] Nevertheless, the Nurses' Health Study[61] has shown that smokers can achieve a considerable reduction in the risk of myocardial infarction with oral oestrogen. The levels of circulating oestrogen in smoking women are not reduced, however, when oestradiol is administered transdermally,[79] so for some women this may be a more suitable route in order to optimise the benefits.

Osteoporosis

All routes of HRT have a beneficial effect on bone, and at the appropriate dose will prevent bone loss. However, for those who have severe osteoporosis there may be a better response with some return of bone density by the use of oestradiol by implant, which tends to give higher circulating levels of oestradiol.[35] In the older woman, a 25 mg implant is usually sufficient.[36,42]

Loss of libido

If loss of libido does not respond to oestrogen with or without progestogen, testosterone which can only safely be given by implant may be helpful. This would usually be given in combination with oestradiol also by implant.

Uro-genital symptoms

Not infrequently the uro-genital tract may not respond satisfactorily to oestrogen administered systemically, and local insertion of oestrogen may provide a quicker and more effective response. Once the vaginal epithelium has thickened and the blood supply improved, the benefits can then be maintained with systemic therapy. Older women may prefer to take vaginal oestrogen only.

Gall bladder disease

If has long been recognised that oral oestrogen replacement therapy is associated with an increased risk of gallstones.[80,81] Oestrogen increases the free cholesterol pool in hepatic cells from which cholesterol is secreted into the bile, which becomes supersaturated. However, transdermal oestradiol, by avoiding the first pass through the liver, has no adverse effect on the biliary cholesterol saturation index and biliary salt composition.[82] This suggest that where there may be a particular risk of gallstone formation, and after non-surgical gallstone therapy, that the non-oral routes of HRT would be more suitable.

Side effects or poor response

Oral HRT is commonly associated with minor initial and short-lived side effects. However if these persist a change to a non-oral route will usually relieve the problem. Poor symptomatic response can be due to inadequate absorption from intestine or transdermally. For such women an implant of oestradiol will ensure good circulating blood levels.[35]

Lactose intolerance

People who are sensitive to lactose may experience variable gastrointestinal and some systemic effects when ingested. Lactose is present as a bulking agent in all the currently available oral oestrogen preparations, and all additional oral progestogen, except for the progestogen-only contraceptive pill Femulen® which contains ethynodiol diacetate 500 μg. The prevalence of adult-type hypolactasia, the cause of lactose intolerance, varies from less than 5% to almost 100% between different populations of the world. The lowest prevalence has been found in northwestern Europe, around the North Sea, and the highest prevalence in the Far East.[83]This problem is avoided by all the non-oral routes of administration.

SUMMARY AND CONCLUSIONS

All routes of administration of HRT are beneficial. For most women the oral route will be the simplest, cheapest and most suitable for initial therapy. Some previous and current medical conditions may indicate a preference, particularly for avoidance of the first pass hepatic effect, and this is now much easier with the recent rapid expansion in the number of non-oral therapies available. Future developments of intra-uterine devices releasing progestogen, vaginal rings and the oral selective oestrogen receptor modulators (SERMs) will further increase the options so that few women will not be able to find some suitable therapy. With life expectancy increasing, the need to improve compliance into old age will be even greater so that longevity can be matched by good quality of life as well.

REFERENCES

1 Sturdee D W. Newer HRT regimens. Br J Obstet Gynaecol 1997; 104: 1109–1115
2 Torgerson D J, Donaldson C, Russell I T, Reid D M. Hormone replacement therapy: compliance and cost after screening for osteoporosis. Eur J Obstet Gynecol Reprod Biol 1995; 59: 57–60
3 Richardson R G. The menopause – a neglected crisis. Queensborough: Abbot Laboratories, 1973
4 Longcope C, Gorbach S, Goldin B et al. The metabolism of estradiol: oral compared to intravenous administration. J Steroid Biochem 1985; 23: 1065–1070
5 Kuhl H. Pharmacokinetics of oestrogens and progestogens. Maturitas 1990; 12: 171–197
6 Powers M S, Schenkel L, Darley P E et al. Pharmacokinetics and pharmacodynamics of transdermal dosage forms of 17β-estradiol: comparison with conventional oral estrogens used for hormone replacement. Am J Obstet Gynecol 1985; 152: 1099–1106
7 Sturdee D W, Burnett D, Moore B, Bradwell A R. Pregnancy associated α$_2$-glycoprotein in postmenopausal women receiving hormone replacement therapy. Clin Chim Acta 1976; 72: 233–239
8 de Ziegler R W. Is the liver a target organ for estrogen? In: Sitruk-Ware R, Utian W H. (eds) The menopause and hormone replacement therapy. New York: Marcel Dekker, 1991: 201–206

9 Crook D. The metabolic consequences of treating postmenopausal women with non-oral hormone replacement therapy. Br J Obstet Gynaecol 1997: 104 (Suppl 16): 4–13

10 Pallas K G, Holzworth G J, Stern M P et al. The effect of conjugated estrogens on the renin-angiotensin system. J Clin Endocrinol Metab 1997; 44: 1061–1068

11 Lip G Y H, Beevers M, Churchill D, Beevers D G. Hormone replacement therapy and blood pressure in hypertensive women. J Hum Hypertens 1994; 8: 491–494

12 Sands R H, Studd J W W, Crook D et al. The effect of estrogen on blood pressure in hypertensive postmenopausal women. Menopause 1997; 4: 115–119

13 Castelli W P. The triglyceride issue: a view from Framingham. Am Heart J 1986; 112: 432–437

14 Stevenson J C, Crook D, Godsland I F, Lees B, Whitehead M I. Oral versus transdermal hormone replacement therapy. J Fertil 1993; 38 (Suppl 1): 30–35

15 The Writing Group for the PEPI Trial. Effects of estrogen/progestin regimens on heart disease risk factors in postmenopausal women. JAMA 1995; 273: 199–208

16 Basdevant A, De Lignières B, Guy-Grand B. Differential lipemic and hormonal responses to oral and parenteral 17β-estradiol in postmenopausal women. Am J Obstet Gynecol 1983; 147: 77–81

17 Godsland I F. Female sex hormones and gonadal steroids. J Intern Med 1996; 240 (Suppl 738): 3–60

18 Lindheim S R, Duffy D M, Kojima T et al. The route of administration influences the effect of estrogen on insulin sensitivity in postmenopausal women. Fertil Steril 1994; 62: 1176–1180

19 Cagnacci A, Soldani R, Carriero P et al. Effects of low doses of transdermal 17β-estradiol on carbohydrate metabolism in postmenopausal women. J Clin Endocrinol Metab 1992; 74: 1396–1400

20 Warren R J, Fotherby K. Plasma levels of ethinyloestradiol after administration of ethinyloestradiol or mestranol to human subjects. J Endocrinol 1973; 59: 369–370

21 von Schoultz B. Potency of different oestrogen preparations. In: Studd J W W, Whitehead M I. (eds) The menopause. Oxford: Blackwell, 1988; 130–137

22 Mashchak C A, Lobo R A, Dozano-Takano R et al. Comparison of pharmacodynamic properties of various estrogen formulations. Am J Obstet Gynecol 1982; 144: 511–518

23 Laufer L R, De Fazio J L, Lu J K H et al. Estrogen replacement therapy by transdermal estradiol administration. Am J Obstet Gynecol 1983; 146: 533–540

24 Cheang A, Sitruk-Ware R, Utian W H. A risk-benefit appraisal of transdermal estradiol therapy. Drug Safety 1993; 9: 365–379

25 The Transdermal Investigators Group. A randomised study to compare the effectiveness, tolerability and acceptability of two different transdermal estradiol replacement therapies. Int J Fertil 1993; 38: 5–11

26 Crook D, Stevenson J C. Transdermal hormone replacement therapy, serum lipids and lipoproteins. Br J Clin Pract 1996; Suppl 86: 17–21

27 Glueck C J, Lang J, Hamer T, Tracy T. Severe hypertriglyceridaemia and pancreatitis when estrogen replacement therapy is given to hypertriglyceridaemic women. J Lab Clin Med 1994; 123: 59–64

28 Järvinen A, Granander M, Nykänen S, Laine T, Geurts P, Viitanen A. Steady-state pharmacokinetics of oestradiol gel in post-menopausal women: effects of application area and washing. Br J Obstet Gynaecol 1997; 104 (Suppl 16): 14–18

29 Hirvonen E, Lamberg-Allardt C, Lankinen K S, Guerts P, Wilén-Rosenqvist G. Transdermal oestradiol gel in the treatment of the climacterium: a comparison with oral therapy. Br J Obstet Gynaecol 1997; 104 (Suppl 16): 19–25

30 Rees M. A new oestradiol gel: impact on climacteric symptoms, pharmacokinetic profile and metabolic effects. Br J Obstet Gynaecol 1997; 104 (Suppl 16): 1–3

31 Bishop P M F. A clinical experiment in oestrogen therapy. BMJ 1938; 1: 939–941

32 Greenblatt R B, Suran R R. Indications for hormonal pellets in the therapy of endocrine and gynecological disorders. Am J Obstet Gynecol 1949; 57: 294–301

33 Magos A L, Studd J W W. Hormonal implants in gynaecology. In: Studd J W W, (ed) Progress in Obstetrics and Gynaecology. London: Churchill Livingstone, 1990; 313–334

34 Studd J W W. Hormone implantation. Diplomate 1996; 3: 19–24

35 Studd J W W, Holland E F N, Leather A T, Smith R N J. The dose-response of percutaneous oestradiol implants on the skeletons of post-menopausal women. Br J Obstet Gynaecol 1994; 101: 787–791

36 Holland E F N, Leather A T, Studd J W W. The effect of 25 mg percutaneous oestradiol implants on the bone mass of postmenopausal women. Obstet Gynecol 1994; 83: 43–46

37 Hunter D J S, Akande E O, Carr P et al. Clinical and endocrinological effect of oestradiol implants at the time of hysterectomy and bilateral salpingo-oophorectomy. J Obstet Gynaecol Br Commonw 1973; 80: 827–835

38 Garnett T, Studd J W W, Henderson A, Watson N, Savvas M, Leather A T. Hormone implants and tachyphylaxis. Br J Obstet Gynaecol 1990; 97: 917–921

39 Pearce J, Horton K, Blake F et al. Psychological effect of continuation versus discontinuation of HRT by oestrogen implants; a placebo controlled study. J Psychosomat Res 1997; 42: 177–186

40 Paterson M E L, Wade-Evans T, Sturdee D W, Thom M H, Studd J W W. Endometrial disease after treatment with oestrogens and progestogens in the climacteric. BMJ 1980; 280: 822–824

41 Owen E J, Siddle N C, McGarrigle H T, Pugh M A. 25 mg oestradiol implants: the dosage of first choice for subcutaneous oestrogen replacement therapy? Br J Obstet Gynaecol 1992; 99: 671–675

42 Naessen T, Persson I, Thor L, Mallmin H, Ljunghal S, Bergstrom R. Maintained bone density at advanced ages after long term treatment with low dose oestradiol implants. Br J Obstet Gynaecol 1993; 100: 454–459

43 Burger H G, Hailes J, Nelson Y et al. Effect of combined implants of oestradiol and testosterone on libido in postmenopausal women. BMJ 1987; 1: 936–939

44 Studd J W W, Chakravarti S, Collins W P et al. Oestradiol and testosterone implants in the treatment of psychosexual problems in the postmenopausal woman. Br J Obstet Gynaecol 1977; 84: 314–315

45 Brincat M, Magos A, Studd J W W. Subcutaneous hormone implants for the control of climacteric symptoms: a prospective study. Lancet 1984; 1: 16–18

46 Dow M G T, Hart D M, Forrest C A. Hormonal treatments of sexual unresponsiveness in postmenopausal women: a comparative study. Br J Obstet Gynaecol 1983; 90: 361–366

47 Andersson K, Mattsson L-Å, Rybo G, Standberg G. Intrauterine release of levonorgestrel – a new way of adding progestogen in hormone replacement therapy. Obstet Gynecol 1992; 79: 963–967

48 Randaskoski T H, Lahti E I, Kauppila A J. Transdermal estrogen with a levonorgestrel-releasing intra-uterine device for climacteric complaints: clinical and endometrial responses. Am J Obstet Gynecol 1995; 172: 114–119

49 Barlow D H, Cardozo L D, Francis R M et al. Urogenital ageing and its effect on sexual health in older British women. Br J Obstet Gynaecol 1997; 104: 87–91

50 Schiff I, Tulchinsky D, Ryan K J. Vaginal absorption of estrone and 17β-estradiol. Fertil Steril 1977; 28: 1063–1067

51 Mettler L, Olsen P G. Long-term treatment of atrophic vaginitis with low-dose oestradiol vaginal tablets. Maturitas 1991; 14: 23–31

52 Smith P, Heimer G, Lindskog M, Ulmsten U. Estradiol-releasing vaginal ring for treatment of postmenopausal urogenital atrophy. Maturitas 1993; 16: 145–154

53 Crane M G, Harris J J, Winsor W. Hypertension, oral contraceptive agents and conjugated estrogens. Ann Intern Med 1971; 74: 13–21

54 Weir R J, Briggs E, Mack A et al. Blood pressure in women taking oral contraceptives. BMJ 1974; 1: 533–535

55 Pfeffer R, Kunaski T T, Charlton S K. Estrogen use and blood pressure in later life. Am J Epidemiol 1979; 110: 469–478

56 Wren B G, Routledge A D. The effect of type and dose of oestrogen on the blood pressure of postmenopausal women. Maturitas 1983; 5: 134–142

57 L'Hermite M. Risks of estrogens and progestogens. Maturitas 1990; 12: 215–246

58 Volterrani M, Rosano G, Coats A et al. Estrogen acutely increases peripheral blood flow in postmenopausal women. Am J Med 1995; 99: 119–122

59 Williams J K, Adams M R, Clarkson T B. Effects of oestrogens on vascular tone. J Cardiovasc Pharmacol 1996; 8 (Suppl 5): S29–S33

60 Nabulsi A A, Folsom A R, White A et al. Association of hormone replacement therapy with various cardiovascular risk factors in postmenopausal women. N Engl J Med 1996; 328: 1069–1075

61 Grodstein F, Stampfer M J, Manson J E et al. Postmenopausal estrogen and progestin use and the risk of cardiovascular disease. N Engl J Med 1996; 335: 453461

62 Hassager C, Riis B J, Strøm V, Guyenne T T, Christiansen C. The long-term effect of oral and percutaneous estradiol on plasma renin substrate and blood pressure. Circulation 1987; 76: 753–758

63 Oelkers W K. Effects of estrogens and progestogens on the renin-aldosterone system and blood pressure. Steroids 1996; 61: 166–171

64 Daly E, Vessey M P, Hawkins M M et al. Risk of venous thromboembolism in users of hormone replacement therapy. Lancet 1996; 348: 977–980

65 Jick H, Derby L E, Myers M W et al. Risk of hospital admission for idiopathic venous thromboembolism among users of postmenopausal oestrogens. Lancet 1996; 348: 981–983

66 Grodstein F, Stampfer M J, Goldhaber S Z et al. Prospective study of exogenous hormones and risk of pulmonary embolism in women. Lancet 1996; 348. 983–987

67 Gutthann S P, Rodriguez L A G, Casjeusague J et al. Hormone replacement therapy and risk of venous thromboembolism: population based case-control study. BMJ 1997; 314: 796–800

68 Lindberg U B, Crona N, Stigendal L et al. A comparison between effects of estradiol valerate and low-dose ethinyl estradiol on haemostasis variables. Thromb Haemost 1989; 61: 65–69

69 Caine Y G, Bauer K A, Barzegar S et al. Coagulation activation following oestrogen administration to postmenopausal women. Thromb Haemost 1992; 68: 392–395

70 Meade T W. Hormone replacement therapy and haemostatic function. Thromb Haemost 1997; 78: 765–769

71 Chae C U, Ridker P M, Manson J E. Postmenopausal hormone replacement therapy and cardiovascular disease. Thromb Haemost 1997; 78: 770–780

72 Lowe G D O. Effects of oestrogens on thromboembolism. In: Sturdee D W. (ed) HRT and thromboembolism. London: Royal Society of Medicine Press, 1997; 3–16

73 Medical Research Council. Randomised comparison of oestrogen versus oestrogen plus progesterone hormone replacement therapy in hysterectomised women. BMJ 1996; 312: 473–478

74 Fox J, George A J, Newton J R et al. Effect of transdermal oestradiol on the haemostatic balance of menopausal women. Maturitas 1993; 18: 55–64

75 Kroon U-B, Tengborn L, Rita H, Bäckström A-C. The effects of transdermal oestradiol and oral progestogens on haemostasis variables. Br J Obstet Gynaecol 1997; 104 (Suppl 16): 32–37

76 Godsland I F, Stevenson J C. Postmenopausal hormone replacement therapy and insulin metabolism: effects of route of administration and implications for heart disease and diabetes risk. Br J Clin Pract 1996; Suppl 86: 1–5

77 McKinlay S M, Bifano N L, McKinlay J B. Smoking and age at menopause in women. Ann Intern Med 1985; 103: 350–356

78 Jensen J, Christiansen C, Rodbro P. Cigarette smoking, estrogens and bone loss during postmenopausal replacement early after menopause. N Engl J Med 1985; 313: 973–975

79 Jensen J, Christiansen C. Effects of smoking on serum lipoproteins and bone mineral content during postmenopausal hormone replacement therapy. Am J Obstet Gynecol 1988; 159: 820–825

80 Boston Collaborative Drug Surveillance Program. Surgically confirmed gallbladder disease, venous thromboembolism and breast tumors in relation to postmenopausal estrogen therapy. N Engl J Med 1974; 290: 15–19

81 Pettiti D B, Sidney S, Perlmann J A. Increased risk of cholecystectomy in users of supplemental estrogen. Gastroenterology 1988; 94: 91–95

82 Van Erpecum K J, van Berge Henegouwen G P. Oestrogen replacement therapy and risk of hepatobiliary disease in postmenopausal women . Br J Clin Pract 1996; Suppl 86: 9–13

83 Sahi T. Genetics and epidemiology of adult-type hypolactasia. Scand J Gastroenterol 1994; 202 (Suppl): 7–20

Gautam Khastgir   John Studd

Hysterectomy and depression

Hysterectomy has long been reputed to produce an adverse psychological outcome.[1] This remains an intractable anxiety to many women even though the recent research findings do not support the earlier views. Such a sensitive issue has been exploited by feminists in their fight against hysterectomy which is yet another example of inaccurate and biased interpretation of research findings for a political motive.[2,3] A high incidence of post-hysterectomy depression shown in the earlier retrospective studies[4–17] is usually quoted, ignoring other contemporary papers that did not support that finding.[18–27] Similarly, more valid results of recent prospective studies,[28–35] showing an improvement in mood after hysterectomy among the majority of patients, are uniformly overlooked. It is, however, true that hysterectomy can precipitate recurrence of depression in patients with previous psychiatric illness and the incidence of depression after hysterectomy remains higher than in the general female population. Due to such diverse findings, much debate still continues with conflicting views about the effects of hysterectomy on mood.

How can depression be associated with hysterectomy? The loss of the uterus may cause an emotional crisis with concerns over loss of femininity, end of reproductive potential and diminished sexuality. With sensible counselling these misconceptions are unlikely to produce depression, except in individuals with a neurotic personality or psychological disturbance. Any pre-existing depression may also be aggravated by the stress of hysterectomy. Another possible explanation is that primary depression is masked as gynaecological complaints leading to hysterectomy. A contrary but more realistic view is that depression results from distressing gynaecological problems of bleeding and

Mr Gautam Khastgir, Subspecialty Senior Registrar in Reproductive Medicine, Academic Department of Obstetrics and Gynaecology, Chelsea and Westminster Hospital, 369 Fulham Road, London SW10 9NH, UK

Mr John Studd, Consultant Gynaecologist, Academic Department of Obstetrics and Gynaecology, Chelsea and Westminster Hospital, 369 Fulham Road, London SW10 9NH, UK

pain which improves dramatically following hysterectomy. Associated ovarian failure may induce depression that persists or manifests after hysterectomy without appropriate hormone replacement therapy (HRT). It may be difficult to tease out the cause and effect since hysterectomy and depression are both common in middle-aged women. In this chapter, the varying rates and causes of hysterectomy related depression have been analysed to identify the risk factors involved and steps that may be taken to improve the psychological outcome.

HISTORICAL BACKGROUND

The uterus has been implicated as having a great importance in the psychological make-up of women since antiquity. The origin of the term hysterectomy, from the Greek *hysteros* meaning uterus, and its etymological association with *hysteria* is well known. Hippocrates, Galen, Aretaeus and Celsius described hysteria as a disease of women and considered the diseased uterus to be the source of the illness.[36] For several centuries it had been the firm belief that both personality disorder and psychiatric illness were related to the uterus. Thus, the psychological significance of hysterectomy has been a source of controversy from the outset. As early as 1890, Kraft-Ebing noted that psychosis was more frequent after hysterectomy than any other major surgical procedure.[6] In the early part of this century, hysterectomy or bilateral oophorectomy was incorrectly recommended for relieving the psychosomatic symptoms.[37] The treatment often failed and led to an adverse psychological outcome in those vulnerable women. With present day indications, although hysterectomy results in an effective and permanent cure, the views on the psychological outcome remain conflicting.

POST-HYSTERECTOMY DEPRESSION

There have been many studies investigating the psychological state of patients who had a hysterectomy in the past. These earlier retrospective studies can be evenly divided into some suggesting a definite association between hysterectomy and depression, whereas others refute any such link. In those studies supporting an adverse psychological outcome, the incidence of post-hysterectomy depression varied between 30–70%.[4–17] No such effect or even beneficial outcome was shown in other contemporary studies, which reported a much lower depression rate of 4–15% after hysterectomy.[18–27]

Such discrepant findings can be explained by faulty research design and methodological limitations in those studies. Instead of using standardised psychiatric measures and diagnostic end-points, indirect evidence, such as referral to a psychiatrist,[10,13] prescribing of anti-depressant medication[12] or admission to mental hospital,[7,20,23] was taken into account. The follow-up period also varied largely, between 3 months[14,19] and three years.[12,13,15] Sampling was another limitation: some were too small for meaningful analysis or had a high attrition rate,[8,16,17] while others were heterogeneous including both benign and malignant indications.[7,10,16,27] However, the greatest limitation

Table 18.1 Summary of the studies on the psychological outcome of hysterectomy

Authors (Year)	Study type	Sample size	Assessment index	Duration of follow-up	Pre-hyster. depression rate (%)	Post-hyster. depression rate (%)	Non-hyster. control depression rate (%)
Richards (1973)[12]	Cross-sectional case-control	200	Use of antidepressant medications	36 months	–	33	7
Richards (1974)[13]	Cross-sectional case-control	56	Self-rating depression questionnaire	36 months	–	70	30
Gath et al (1982)[29]	Prospective with historical control	156	Psychiatric case status	18 months	58	29	12
Lalinec-Michaud (1984)[30]	Prospective with control	102	Self-rating depression scales	12 months	16	8	6
Ryan et al (1989)[31]	Prospective cohort	60	Psychiatric case status	14 months	55	32	–
Osborn and Gath (1990)[32]	Prospective cohort	54	Psychiatric case status	6 months	28	7	
Carlson et al (1994)[33]	Prospective cohort	418	Mental health index	12 months	44	14	–
Gath et al.(1995)[34]	Prospective cohort	190	Psychiatric case status	6 months	9	4	–

hyster. = hysterectomy

of all these studies was their retrospective nature. The diagnosis of depression after hysterectomy cannot exclude whether it was present beforehand. Thus without knowing the pre-operative mental state of the patients, it is unjustified to presume that hysterectomy caused their postoperative depression.

PRE-HYSTERECTOMY DEPRESSION

Recent well-designed prospective studies did not support the earlier views on psychologically detrimental effects of hysterectomy. Instead, they have uniformly shown that the incidence of psychological morbidity before hysterectomy (16–58%)[28–33] is higher than that in the general population (6–14%).[38,39] The abnormal psychological state was not just a short term anxiety or stress reaction to the impending operation, as depression rather than anxiety was the main problem.

After hysterectomy, the mood improved in the majority of patients and the incidence of psychological morbidity reduced by more than a half, suggesting a beneficial role.[29–33] The incidence of residual depression (8–32%) still remained higher than that in the general population, but was similar to some of the retrospective studies reaching a contradictory conclusion (Table 18.1). In some reports, the incidence of psychological morbidity did not change after hysterectomy, possibly due to the short duration of follow-up (3 months), high drop out rate (48%) and an overrepresentation of psychiatric patients in the studied population.[40–42]

In the prospective studies, standardised methods of psychological assessment, including structured psychiatric interviews and self-administered questionnaires of psychological rating, were adopted. The frequency of assessment was thought to influence the outcome favourably,[28,29] but such therapeutic benefits of the interview process has not been supported by others.[31] The improvement in the mood profile was noted during the initial follow-up at 4–6 months and was maintained even 14–18 months after hysterectomy. Figure

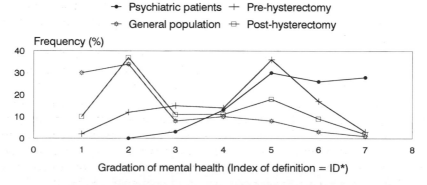

* ID: lower value indicates normal and higher value indicates abnormal mental state

Fig 18.1 Comparison of the mental health of patients before and after hysterectomy with that in normal populations and psychiatric patients. Adapted from Gath et al[29] with permission.

18.1 illustrates the distribution of mental health gradation (index of definition) as assessed by the Present State Examination in different populations. The incidence and severity of abnormal mental state in patients before hysterectomy were intermediate between the general population and the psychiatric patients. In the postoperative period, the mental state of the hysterectomy group was much closer to the general population, although still significantly different.

Several studies have highlighted the strong influence of the pre-existing psychological dysfunction on the outcome of hysterectomy. Depression that was present before hysterectomy was far more likely to persist or recur (31–64%) than for it to develop postoperatively (8–14%).[29,30,33,40] Such unfavourable psychological outcome of hysterectomy was limited to patients with predisposing personality features and a past history of psychiatric illness. In the majority of patients, depression was related to disabling gynaecological symptoms and thus hysterectomy resulted an excellent psychological outcome.[31,35] The cyclical depression associated with severe pre-menstrual syndrome (PMS) is related to ovarian function and is unlikely to be cured by hysterectomy with ovarian conservation.[43,44] Thus, past history of severe pre-menstrual syndrome (PMS) was present in a significant proportion of patients who became depressed after hysterectomy.[32,45]

PERI-MENOPAUSAL DEPRESSION

Associated decline in ovarian function has also been implicated with hysterectomy related depression.[33,46] Oestrogen deficiency symptoms such as hot-flushes, headache, fatigue, depression, loss of libido and urinary symptoms, collectively referred as *post-hysterectomy syndrome*, was reported in 70% of the patients after 3 years of hysterectomy.[13] This is partly attributable to hysterectomy-induced premature ovarian failure which affects 25–50% of the patients and usually develops within 2–5 years of surgery.[47,48] As hysterectomy is commonly performed in the peri-menopausal age,[49] these symptoms are likely to be present before surgery and may well be described as *pre-hysterectomy syndrome*. The problem is often incorrectly considered as a vague emotional reaction to hysterectomy, because the actual cause remains unrecognised due to the absence of characteristic menstrual irregularity of ovarian failure.[14,50]

Most prospective studies have been conducted at 1 year which was too early to identify the effect of hysterectomy induced ovarian failure on the psychological state.[30,32–35] With a relatively longer follow-up of 18 months, the post-hysterectomy depression rates have been comparatively higher.[29,31] In a long-term prospective study, depression was absent at 4 month but developed after 24 months of surgery.[51] These observations imply that depression is more likely to be due to a failure of the residual ovaries rather than an emotional reaction to hysterectomy. The hormonal basis has also been confirmed by a relatively lower incidence of post-hysterectomy depression (3.6%) in patients on long term HRT.[52] Among those who take HRT before hysterectomy, some suffer from progestogen induced cyclical depression.[53] Hysterectomy avoids the need of progestogens for endometrial protection and thereby improves the mood as well as the compliance to HRT.[54]

The incidence of depression is higher after bilateral oophorectomy than hysterectomy with ovarian conservation.[42,46,55,56] Depressive symptoms usually present early but also manifest as the most common long-term problem.[57–59] In some reports, concurrent bilateral oophorectomy has shown no increase in depression when compared to hysterectomy.[29,31,60] However, it is difficult to judge the role of ovarian hormones in these studies where patients had varied menopausal state and incidences of bilateral oophorectomy and HRT use were often unstated.

DOWNWARDS TREND IN HYSTERECTOMY RELATED DEPRESSION

A recent report compared the results of three prospective studies on the psychological outcome of hysterectomy performed by the Oxford group.[34] The incidence of pre-operative psychiatric morbidity had dropped from 58% to 9% during a period of 14 years. However, the general trend of reduction in the incidence of psychiatric morbidity and improvement in the mood after hysterectomy remain unchanged. The decreasing incidence of psychiatric morbidity was attributable to the alteration in patient selection for hysterectomy and the increased use of HRT in the last decade.

In the earlier study with a high psychological morbidity rate,[29] although a large proportion of patients was perimenopausal, only a few had HRT, but many were on psychotrophic drugs. Hysterectomy was perhaps unnecessary in some of these patients with primary depression who perceived the gynaecological symptoms more seriously. In perimenopausal patients, HRT would have relieved psychological symptoms and some of the symptoms that led to hysterectomy. These views were confirmed by the lower psychological morbidity rate in a recent study,[34] where most patients were premenopausal at hysterectomy and had medical treatment for menorrhagia. Women with emotional problems were treated with reassurance and explanation rather than hysterectomy. The failure of medical treatment for menorrhagia also helped women to accept hysterectomy as more justified and, thereby, caused fewer emotional upsets of losing the reproductive organs.

POSSIBLE CAUSES OF DEPRESSION

There are various theories to explain how depression could be associated with hysterectomy. Some of these assumptions have been proven incorrect in the light of current knowledge on the subject. It has also become apparent that the cause of depression may precede hysterectomy and can change postoperatively (Fig. 18.2). Depression developing after hysterectomy is more likely to be of hormonal rather than emotional in origin

Perceived loss of femininity

Earlier psychoanalytic studies have suggested that the uterus may have a symbolic importance to the concept of womanhood.[7,8,19,61,62] Hysterectomy is perceived by them as loss of *femininity* due to the cessation of menstrual and

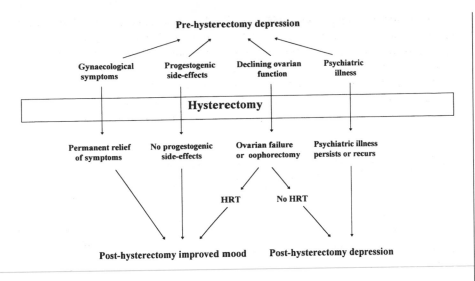

Fig. 18.2 Causes of depression before and after hysterectomy.

reproductive capacity. It may also be considered as an assault to the body image with a sense of mutilation.[7,15,20] In women with such views, the emotional trauma of hysterectomy results in loss of self-esteem and depression. The psychic influence of the uterus is not scientifically proven but remains as a strong myth based on misconceptions, although the social changes in the last few decades may have removed much significance of femininity and reproduction on women's self-esteem.[63,64] The emotional trauma with the loss of uterus has been refuted by similar psychological outcomes of hysterectomy, tubal ligation and cholecystectomy.[25,41] A prospective study on the psychological outcome also failed to show any influence of femininity, as these feelings remained unchanged in a large majority of women after hysterectomy.[45]

Crisis or stress response

Hysterectomy has been postulated as a stressful life event which may result in a *crisis* in emotional well-being.[14,15,61,65] The *crisis* can operate at different levels in the biological, psychological and social framework such as fear of ageing, loss of femininity and end of a relationship. Patients at an increased risk of such stress response syndrome are those with high level of anxiety, desire for further children, marital disruption or concerns over sexual function.[16] The theory has been refuted by the findings of a reduction in tension-anxiety after hysterectomy[41] and similar postsurgery stress disturbance rate as after tubal ligation and cholecystectomy.[25,41] Stress induced adverse psychological outcome may still occur in patients with a neurotic personality and a past history of depressive response to stress.[15] Patients with psychiatric illness are also more likely to present with crisis in the postoperative period[60]

Psycho-sexual problems

In early studies, the psychological morbidity following hysterectomies was related to the concept that the uterus was important for sexual fulfilment.[7,19,61,65]

The fear of impaired sex life and uncertainties about their relationship with their partner following hysterectomy have been suspected as causes of psychological morbidity.[15,66,67] Several prospective studies have shown that after hysterectomy there was either no change[28] or improvement[31,45] in the frequency and quality of sexual response in the majority of patients. The improved sexuality results from the absence of fear of unwanted pregnancy and cure of any gynaecological problem that may have been contributory to decreased libido before hysterectomy. Thus, it is the anxiety about the adverse effect on sexuality rather than any actual change which may result in depression. Pre-operative fear of sexual alteration was also found to be significantly associated with subsequent adverse sexual outcome.[16] The current psychological state is also an important predictor of sexual dysfunction which may be the effect rather than the cause of depression.[45]

Pre-existing psychiatric illness

A previous history of psychiatric illness has been shown to be an important predictor of depression after hysterectomy.[10,12,19,31,37,40,42,45,60] Hysterectomy is commonly performed in the middle life (late 30s to early 50s) when the incidence of emotional disorder is usually at its peak. Depressed and neurotic women are likely to perceive the menstrual symptoms more negatively and tolerate them less easily. They often present with gynaecological symptoms when the associated psychiatric illness may be confused with illness related altered mood – 'psychological conflict sailing under a gynaecological flag'.[48,68–70] Alternatively, a high stress level may lead to disturbance of the hypothalamic-pituitary-ovarian axis which in turn results in disturbed menstrual function. This view has been supported in a longitudinal study where the lasting psychological symptoms were related to poor gynaecological outcome but the reverse was not true.[71] Thus, hysterectomy in these patients is not the cause but the effect of depression. In a psychologically unstable woman, depression is also likely to develop or recur with the perceived emotional stress of hysterectomy. These facts partly explain the higher incidence of depression before hysterectomy and its persistence in some patients after surgery.

Gynaecological symptoms

The association between psychological and gynaecological problems has long being recognised. A high prevalence of psychological morbidity (29–62%) has been observed in gynaecological clinic populations, particularly in women with menorrhagia, pelvic pain and other conditions which led to hysterectomy.[72–75] Community surveys have also shown that both psychological morbidity and neurotic personality disorders are commonly associated with gynaecological symptoms.[76,77]. It should be no surprise that years of heavy painful periods, chronic pelvic pain, pre-menstrual syndrome and menstrual migraine make many women neurotic and depressed. The psychological morbidity correlates with the gynaecological symptoms and motivates the patients to accept hysterectomy'[31,77–79] The improvement in mood and drop in the incidence of psychiatric morbidity after hysterectomy is due to the relief of gynaecological symptoms. However, the cyclical psychological symptoms of pre-menstrual syndrome are related to ovarian activity and would therefore persist after hysterectomy with ovarian conservation.

Ovarian hormone deficiency

Ovarian failure is a likely cause of hysterectomy related psychological morbidity.[33,46] The peak incidence of hysterectomy is in the climacteric,[49] but it may induce premature ovarian failure in younger patients.[47,48] Thus, psychological symptoms due to declining oestrogen levels may be coincidental before hysterectomy but may also develop postoperatively.[44] Since depression often precedes other climacteric symptoms, it is not simply the consequence of hot flushes, sweats, insomnia and dyspareunia, although they may play a part.[46,80] The causal role of declining and fluctuating oestrogen level is supported by the occurrence of depression with similar hormonal changes in the pre-menstrual days and post partum months.[81,82] With bilateral oophorectomy, there is an abrupt decline in circulating oestrogen and testerone which commonly result in a long lasting depression, even when vasomotor symptoms are absent.[57–59] Ovarian hormonal deficiency remains uncontrolled in the majority of hysterectomised patient as the compliance with HRT is poor even after bilateral oophorectomy.[83,84] The lack of complete relief from depression after hysterectomy may also be due to inadequate oestrogen dosage and failure to replace testosterone after bilateral oophorectomy.

RISK FACTORS FOR DEPRESSION

Several risk factors emerged from earlier retrospective studies analysing the cause and effect relation between hysterectomy and depression (Table 18.2). The prospective studies did not support the influence of parity, marital status and socio-economic class on the psychological outcome of hysterectomy.[31,45] A higher rate of depression in younger patient was noted in only one prospective study.[60] Others suggested that older women were more prone to postoperative complications that may result in depression.[17,45] Depression was also common

Table 18.2 Possible risk factors for depression after hysterectomy

*Younger (< 40 years) and older age[12,14,17,20,23,30,45,62]
Desire to have children[6,10,14,20]
Single, divorced or separated[10,14,20]
*Low socio-economic status[55,60]
*Lower educational level[20,25,60]
Lack of support from family and friends[14]
Vulnerable to stressful life situations[14–16]
Fear and negative expectation about the outcome[55,67]
Threatened to lose one's femininity[7,15,19,61,62]
*Nervous and over anxious premorbid personality[7,15,16,37]
*Previous or present psychiatric illness[10,12,13,19,29–31,42,45,55]
Absence of organic pelvic pathology[10,12]

*Confirmed by the prospective studies.

in patients with limited education who had misconceptions regarding the role of uterus and were secretive about their fears and anxieties.[30,60] The difference in ethnic responses were due to cultural influences in relation to uterus, where some women put a greater emphasis on their reproductive abilities and have a stronger attachment to traditional roles.[17,60]

Hysterectomy performed as an emergency was commonly associated with anger and depression as these women did not get much time to psychologically adjust to the intervention.[30,60,85] In the prospective studies, neither the indication of hysterectomy nor the pathological diagnosis influenced the psychological outcome of hysterectomy. Although the route of hysterectomy influenced the physical recovery, the psychological well-being were similar. In the absence of an adequate HRT, simultaneous bilateral oophorectomy enhanced the risk of depression after hysterectomy.[42,46,55,56]

Patients who were very nervous, over- anxious and unable to cope with stress were particularly vulnerable to depression, both before and after hysterectomy.[7,15,16,37] The association between pre-operative anxiety scores and post-operative depression has been confirmed by multivariate analysis. It is also known that a high incidence of neuroticism and depression in women undergoing hysterectomy were responsible for the poor physical and psychological outcome.[30,42] The other predisposed group of women were those who regarded themselves as being low on instrumental traits, unassertive and dependent.[31] These women with predisposed personalities had considerable emotional stress with prolonged menorrhagia and severe premenstrual syndrome but continue to be depressed, although with a much lesser intensity, due to symptomatic relief after hysterectomy. Any misconception about adverse effects on physical activity, appearance, femininity and sexual life leading to a negative body and self image resulted in adverse psychological outcome.[15]

Pre-operative mental status and mood were significantly associated with psychological outcome following hysterectomy. Patients who are depressed before hysterectomy may remain depressed after the procedure, which explains the higher incidence of depression than in the general population both before and after the surgery.[29–31,42] A past history of referral to a psychiatrist, treatment for psychiatric symptoms and family history of psychiatric illness were also associated with poor psychological outcome.[10,12,13,19,29–31,42,45,55]

PREVENTIVE MEASURES

Careful patient selection

Hysterectomy is usually performed to improve the quality of life rather than as a life-saving measure. Thus, a detailed assessment of the severity of menstrual complaints, pelvic pain and pre-menstrual symptoms should be done to assess the need for hysterectomy. In the absence of a pathological diagnosis, such as fibroids or endometriosis, a careful case selection is more important to ensure that the decision of hysterectomy is justified. Detailed information on hysterectomy as well as its alternatives, both medical and surgical, allows patients to balance the benefits and risks of any treatment against the severity of the symptoms as perceived by them and, of course, make up their own mind. Such an informed choice would avoid any dissatisfaction or rare emotional trauma of losing the reproductive organs. However, adverse psychological effects may still be precipitated in patients with predisposing personality features, previous depressive response to stressful events and past history of psychiatric illness. Both general practitioners and gynaecologists should therefore be aware of the cause and effect link between psychiatric and gynaecological symptoms so that the primary illness is not overlooked.

Psychological evaluation

The emotional state of the patient after the decision of hysterectomy may identify those with an unstable or neurotic personality. The initial response in vulnerable women may be an outcry of anger or desperation. An assessment of the patient's mental status and inquiry of their personal or family psychiatric history should be a routine before taking the decision of hysterectomy. An awareness of the risk factors allows the clinician to exercise caution in recommending hysterectomy to such women, thereby reducing the likelihood of post-hysterectomy depression. In patients suspected of psychiatric risk factors, a simple questionnaire such as Hospital Anxiety and Depression (HAD) scale may be used as a screening test to detect an abnormal mental state.[86] If there is any cause for concern, these very rare selected patients should be referred to a psychiatrist or psychologist for opinion whether hysterectomy could be detrimental to their mental state. Some of these patients may need psychotherapeutic intervention before and after hysterectomy.

Psycho-sexual counselling

The attitude towards the decision of hysterectomy influences the psychological outcome. Thus patients themselves should be able to understand and accept the need for the treatment. Those with a negative view due to misconceptions regarding the adverse outcome of hysterectomy should have counselling and be offered other options. An opportunity for discussing their concerns and 'letting out' their feelings to a doctor, nurse or counsellor is often beneficial.[28,29] Some women find it helpful to meet other patients and share their experience within a support group. In the presence of fears, anxieties and uncertainties about the sexuality after hysterectomy, psycho-sexual counselling may help to improve the outcome.[31,45] Inclusion of their spouses, in explaining the improvement or unchanged sexuality after hysterectomy, could be most helpful as their support and reassurance are great boosts towards positive outlook.

ROLE OF HORMONE REPLACEMENT THERAPY

Routine assessment of ovarian function at the time of hysterectomy is important to detect any hormone deficiency as the possible cause of pre-existing depression. Pre-menopausal women undergoing hysterectomy with ovarian conservation should have long-term endocrinological monitoring to recognise any decline in ovarian function that could result in post-hysterectomy depression. If the

Table 18.3 Summary of the influence of HRT on the psychological outcome following hysterectomy and bilateral oophorectomy

Authors (Year)	Study type	Sample size	Type of HRT	Assessment index	Duration	Depression score
Dennerstein et al (1979)[89]	Prospective randomised double-blind crossover	49	Oral: (a) ethinyl oestradiol, (b) levonorgestrel, (c) placebo	Hamilton depression rating scale	12 months	Lowered with oestrogen but no such benefit with progestogen or placebo
Ditkoff et al (1981)[87]	Prospective randomised double-blind	36	Oral: conjugated oestrogen (a) 0.625 mg, (b) 1.25 mg, (c) placebo	Beck depression inventory	3 months	Lowered with oestrogen independent of dose but increased with placebo
Sherwin and Gelfand (1985)[90]	Prospective randomised double-blind crossover	43	Intramuscular injections: (a) oestrogen, (b) testosterone, (c) a and b, (d) placebo	Multiple adjective affective check list	7 months	Lowered with any form of active hormone therapy but none with placebo
Sherwin (1988)[93]	Prospective non-randomised cohort	44	Intramuscular injections: (a) oestrogen and testosterone, (b) oestrogen, (c) untreated	Multiple adjective affective check list. Profile of mood state	1 month	Lowered with all hormone therapy and affected by serum oestradiol levels
Best (1992)[88]	Prospective cohort	16	Subcutaneous implants: oestradiol 50 mg	Hamilton depression rating scale	6 weeks	Lowered much earlier than shown in other studies
Khastgir and Studd (1998)[52]	Cross-sectional	192	Subcutaneous implants: oestradiol 50 mg + testosterone 100 mg	Hospital anxiety and depression scale	3–5 years	Lowered for a longer period with 96% compliance to HRT

ovaries are removed or with the confirmation of compromised residual ovarian function, HRT should be started immediately. Before discharging the patient from the hospital, the gynaecologist should liaise with the primary care physician to decide who takes the responsibility for the monitoring of hormone levels and compliance with long term HRT.

Oestrogen replacement

Oestrogen improves mood by relieving vasomotor symptoms, insomnia and dyspareunia, but there is also a dose dependent mental tonic effect even in the absence of the climacteric symptoms.[28] A relatively higher dose of oestrogen may be required after hysterectomy to suppress the cyclical psychological symptoms of pre-menstrual syndrome.[27,70] Several randomised placebo controlled trials have convincingly shown that oestrogen improves the depression score and psychological symptoms after hysterectomy in peri- and post-menopausal patients (Table 18.3).[87,88] However, in pre-menopausal patients with residual ovaries, oestrogen may not influence mood within a year after hysterectomy.[28] This is due to the fact that it usually takes 2–5 years for the overt symptoms of ovarian failure to develop after hysterectomy. Oestrogen is also effective in lowering depression score after hysterectomy and bilateral oophorectomy at any age.[89]

Testosterone replacement

Testosterone acts synergistically with oestrogen in the treatment of hormone responsive depression (Table 18.3).[90] The therapeutic effect of testosterone on mood is partly due to the anabolic and energising properties. It also improves sexual desire and enjoyment which indirectly influence the mood.[91,92] In a prospective cross-over study following hysterectomy and bilateral oophorectomy, the depression score with testosterone with or without oestrogen

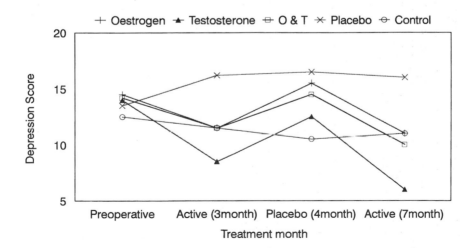

Fig. 18.3 Changes in mean depression score after hysterectomy and bilateral oophorectomy with different hormone replacement therapy and placebo, compared to a control group (hysterectomy with ovarian conservation). Adapted from Sherwin and Gelfand[90] with permission.

replacement was lower than that with oestrogen-alone and placebo (Fig. 18.3).[90] Long-term assessment of the psychological state two years after hysterectomy confirmed that combined oestrogen-testosterone replacement remained more effective than oestrogen alone.[93] With the routine use of combined oestradiol and testosterone implants after hysterectomy and bilateral oophorectomy, the incidence of depression dropped from 35.6% pre-operatively to 3.6%, 3–5 years after surgery.[52] Such therapeutic efficacy of oestrogen and testosterone on mood reiterates the hormonal basis of post-hysterectomy depression.

CONCLUSIONS

The higher incidence of depression in patients who subsequently have a hysterectomy is the psychological response to prolonged gynaecological problems. Hence, the therapeutic effect of hysterectomy include both the cure of physical symptoms and improvement of resultant depression. In patients with pre-existing psychiatric illness, depression is unlikely to settle after hyster-ectomy and in those with over-anxious neurotic personality, the emotional stress of surgery may precipitate depression. Ovarian failure is the more plausible cause of depression, but it is often overlooked and remains untreated after hysterectomy. With appropriate case selection, psychiatric evaluation and adequate preoperative counselling many cases of post-hysterectomy depression may be prevented. The practice of regular endocrinological monitoring after hysterectomy to detect the need for oestrogen replacement and a near-routine replacement of combined oestrogen and testosterone replacement after bilateral oophorectomy should also be adopted to avoid post-hysterectomy depression.

REFERENCES

1 Polivy J. Psychological reaction to hysterectomy: a critical review. Am J Obstet Gynecol 1974; 118: 417–426
2 Greer G. The change: women, ageing and the menopause. London: Penguin Books, 1992
3 Hufnagel V, Golant S. No more hysterectomies. Wellingborough, Northamptonshire: Thorsons, 1990
4 Menzer D, Morris T, Gates P et al. Patterns of emotional recovery from hysterectomy. Psychosom Med 1957; 19: 379–382
5 Stengel E, Zeitlyn B B, Rayner E H. Post-operative psychosis. J Ment Sci 1958; 104: 389–402
6 Ackner B. Emotional aspects of hysterectomy: a followup study of 50 patients under the age of 40. Adv Psychosom Med 1960; 1: 248–252
7 Hollender M H. A study of patients admitted to a psychiatric hospital after pelvic operations. Am J Obstet Gynecol 1960; 79: 498–503
8 Barglow P, Gunther M, Johnson A, Meltzer H J. Hysterectomy and tubal ligation: a psychiatric comparison. Obstet Gynecol 1965; 25: 520–527
9 Munday L N, Cox L W. Hysterectomy for benign lesions. Med J Aust 1967; 17: 759–760
10 Barker M G. Psychiatric illness after hysterectomy. BMJ 1968; 2: 91–95
11 Steiner M, Aleksandrowicz D R. Psychiatric sequelae to gynaecological operation. Isr Ann Psychiatry 1970; 8: 186–188
12 Richards D H. Depression after hysterectomy. Lancet 1973; 2: 430–433
13 Richards D H. A post-hysterectomy syndrome. Lancet 1974; 2: 983–985
14 Raphael B. Parameters of health outcome following hysterectomy. Bulletin of Postgraduate Committee in Medicine, University of Sydney 1974; 30: 214–220

15 Roeske N. Quality of life and the factors effecting the response to hysterectomy. J Fam Pract 1978; 3: 214–218

16 Kaltreider N B, Wallace A, Horowitz M D. A field study of the stress response syndrome: young women after hysterectomy. JAMA 1979; 242: 1499–1503

17 Gould D. Recovery from hysterectomy. Practitioner 1986; 230: 756–757

18 Dodds D T, Potgieter C R, Turner P J, Scheeper G P J. The physical and emotional results of hysterectomy. S Afr Med J 1961; 35: 53–54

19 Melody G F. Depressive reactions following hysterectomy. Am J Obstet Gynecol 1962; 83: 410–413

20 Patterson R M, Craig J B. Misconception concerning the psychological effects of hysterectomy. Am J Obstet Gynecol 1963; 85: 104–111

21 Hawkins J, Williams D. Total abdominal hysterectomy: 100 consecutive unselected operations. J Obstet Gynecol Br Commonw 1963; 70: 20–28

22 Ellison R M. Psychiatric complications following sterilization in women. Med J Aust 1964; 2: 625–628

23 Bragg R L. Risk of admission to mental hospital following hysterectomy and cholecystectomy. Am J Public Health 1965; 55: 1403–1410

24 Mills W G. Depression after hysterectomy. Lancet 1973; ii: 672

25 Hampton P T, Tarnasky W G. Hysterectomy and tubal ligation: a comparison of the psychological aftermath. Am J Obstet Gynecol 1974; 119: 949–952

26 Kav-Venaki S, Zakham L. Psychological effects of hysterectomy in premenopausal women. J Psychosom Obstet Gynecol 1983; 2: 76–78

27 Filiberti A, Regazzoni M, Garavoglia M et al. Problems after hysterectomy. A comparative content analysis of 60 interviews with cancer and non-cancer hysterectomised women. Eur J Gynaecol Oncol 1991; 12: 445 449

28 Coppen A, Bishop M, Beard R J, Barnard G J R, Collins W P. Hysterectomy, hormones and behavior. A prospective study. Lancet 1981; i: 126–128

29 Gath D, Cooper P, Day A. Hysterectomy and psychiatric disorder: I. Levels of psychiatric morbidity before and after hysterectomy. Br J Psychol 1982; 140: 335–342

30 Lalinec-Michaud M, Engelsmann F. Depression and hysterectomy: a prospective study. Psychosomatics 1984; 25: 550–558

31 Ryan M M, Dennerstein L, Pepperell R. Psychological aspects of hysterectomy: a prospective study. Br J Psychol 1989; 154: 516–522

32 Osborn M, Gath D. Psychological and physical determinants of premenstrual syndrome before and after hysterectomy. Psychol Med 1990; 20: 565–572

33 Carlson K J, Miller B A, Fowler F J. The Maine women's health study: I. Outcomes of hysterectomy. Obstet Gynecol 1994; 83: 556–565

34 Gath D, Rose N, Bond A, Day A, Garrod A, Hodges S. Hysterectomy and psychiatric disorder; are the levels of psychiatric morbidity falling? Psychol Med 1995; 25: 277–283

35 Alexander A D, Naji A A, Pinion S B et al. Randomised trial comparing hysterectomy and endometrial ablation for dysfunctional uterine bleeding: psychiatric and psychosocial aspects. BMJ 1996; 312: 280–284

36 Ananth J. Hysterectomy and depression. Obstet Gynecol 1978; 52: 724–730

37 Lindemann E. Observations on psychiatric sequelae of surgical operations in women. Am J Psychiatry 1941; 98: 132–135

38 Babbington P, Hurry J, Tennant C et al. Epidemiology of mental disorder in Camberwell. Psychol Med 1981; 11: 561–579

39 Henderson S, Bryne A G, Duncan-Jones P. Neurosis and the social environment. Sydney: Academic Press, 1981

40 Moore J T, Tolley D H. Depression following hysterectomy. Psychosomatics 1976; 17: 86–89

41 Meikle S, Brody H, Pysh F. An investigation into the psychological effects of hysterectomy. J Nerv Ment Dis 1977; 164: 36–41

42 Martin R L, Roberts W V, Cayton P J. Psychiatric status after hysterectomy: one year followup. JAMA 1980; 244: 350–353

43 Studd J W W. Prophylactic oophorectomy. Br J Obstet Gynaecol 1989; 96: 506–509

44 Khastgir G, Studd J W W. Hysterectomy, ovarian failure and depression. Menopause 1998; 5: 113–122

45 Gath D, Cooper P, Bond A, Edmonds G. Hysterectomy and psychiatric disorder: II. Demographic, psychiatric and physical factors in relation to psychiatric outcome. Br J Psychol 1982; 140: 342–350

46 Perlstein T B. Hormone and depression: what are the facts about pre-menstrual syndrome, menopause and hormone replacement therapy? Am J Obstet Gynecol 1995; 173: 646–653

47 Riedel H H, Lehman-Willenbrock E, Semm K. Ovarian failure phenomenon after hysterectomy. J Reprod Med 1986; 31: 597–600

48 Siddle N, Sarrel P, Whitehead M. The effect of hysterectomy on the age at ovarian failure: identification of a subgroup of women with premature loss of ovarian function and literature review. Fertil Steril 1987; 47: 94–100

49 Pokras R, Hufnagel V. Hysterectomy in the United States 1965–84. Am J Public Health 1988; 78: 852–853

50 Roos C. Hysterectomies in one Canadian province: a new look at risks and benefits. Am J Public Health 1984; 74: 39–45

51 Bernhard L A. Consequence of hysterectomy in the lives of women. Health Care Women Int 1992; 13: 281–291

52 Khastgir G, Studd J W W. A survey of patient's attitude, experience and satisfaction with hysterectomy, oophorectomy and hormone replacement by oestradiol and testosterone implants. Obstet Gynecol 1998; In press

53 Magos A L, Brewester E, Singh R, O'Dowd T, Brincat M, Studd J W W. The effects of norethisterone in postmenopausal women on oestrogen replacement therapy: a model for the premenstrual syndrome. Br J Obstet Gynaecol 1986; 93: 1290–1296

54 Studd J W W. Continuation rates with cyclical and continuous regimen of oral oestrogen and progestogens. Menopause 1996; 3: 181–182

55 Chynoweth R, Abrahams M J. Psychological complications of hysterectomy. Aust N Z J Obstet Gynaecol 1977; 17: 40–44

56 Rauramo L, Lagerspetz K, Engblom P, Punnonen R. The effect of castration and oral oestrogen therapy on some psychological function. Acta Obstet Gynecol 1976; 54: 3–15

57 Studd J W W, Chakravarti S, Collin W P. Plasma hormone profile after the menopause and bilateral oophorectomy. Postgrad Med J 1979; 54: 25–30

58 Chakravarti S, Collins W P, Newton J R, Oram D H, Studd J W W. Endocrine changes and symptomatology following oophorectomy in pre-menopausal women. Br J Obstet Gynaecol 1977; 84: 769–775

59 Sherwin B B, Gelfand M M. Differential symptom response to parenteral oestrogen and/or testosterone administration in the surgical menopause. Am J Obstet Gynecol 1985; 151: 153–160

60 Lalinec-Michaud M, Engelsmann F. Psychological profile of depressed women undergoing hysterectomy. J Psychosom Obstet Gynecol 1988; 8: 53–66

61 Drellich M G, Bieber I. The psychological importance of the uterus and its functions: some psychoanalytic implications of hysterectomy. J Nerv Ment Dis 1958; 126: 322–336

62 Wolf S R. Emotional reactions to hysterectomy. Postgrad Med 1970; 47: 165–169

63 Bem S L. The measurement of psychological androgeny. J Consult Clin Psychol 1974; 42: 155–162

64 Wiedeger P. Menstruation and the menopause. New York: Knopf, 1976

65 Kroger W S. Psychosomatic obstetric, gynaecology and endocrinology, including diseases of metabolism. Thomas, Springfield, 1957

66 Amias A G. Sexual life after gynaecological operations. BMJ 1975; 2: 608–609

67 Dennerstein L, Wood C, Burrows G D. Sexual response following hysterectomy and oophorectomy. Obstet Gynecol 1977; 49: 92–96

68 Roger F S. Emotional factors in gynaecology. Am J Obstet Gynecol 1950; 59: 321–325

69 Munro A. Psychiatric illness in gynaecological outpatients: a preliminary study. Br J Psychol 1969; 115: 807–812

70 Swales P J, Sheikh J I. Hysterectomy in patients with panic disorder. Am J Psychiatry 1992; 149: 846–847

71 Slade P, Anderson K J. Gynaecological symptoms and psychological distress: a longitudinal study of their relationship. J Psychosom Obstet Gynecol 1992; 13: 51–63

72 Ballinger C B. Psychiatric morbidity and the menopause: survey of a gynaecological out-patient clinic. Br J Psychol 1977; 131: 83–89

73 Bond M R. Psychological and psychiatric aspect of pain. Anaesthesis 1978; 33: 355–360

74 Bryne P. Psychiatric morbidity in a gynaecology clinic: an epidemiological study. Br J Psychol 1984; 144: 28–34

75 Greenberg M. The meaning of menorrhagia: an investigation into the association between the complaint of menorrhagia and depression. J Psychosom Res 1983; 27: 209–214

76 Ballinger C B. Psychiatric morbidity and the menopause: screening of general population sample. BMJ 1975; 294: 213–218

77 Gath D, Osborne M, Bunngary G et al. Psychiatric disorder and gynaecological symptoms in middle aged women: a community survey. BMJ 1987; 294: 213–218

78 Slater J R. Gynaecological symptoms and psychological distress in potential hysterectomy patients. J Psychosom Res 1985; 29: 155–159

79 Studd J W W. Hysterectomy and menorrhagia. Baillière's Clin Obstet Gynaecol 1989; 3: 415–424

80 Bungay G T, Vessey M P, McPherson C K. Study of symptoms in middle life with special reference to the menopause. BMJ 1980; ii: 181–183

81 Nolen-Hoeksema S. Sex difference in unipolar depression: evidence and theory. Psychol Bull 1987; 101, 259–282

82 Studd J W W, Smith R N J. Oestrogen and depression in women. Menopause 1994; 1: 33–37

83 Spector T D. Use of oestrogen replacement therapy in high risk groups in the United Kingdom. BMJ 1989; 299: 1434–1435

84 Speroff T, Dawson N V, Speroff L, Haber R J. A risk-benefit analysis of elective bilateral oophorectomy: effect of changes in compliance with oestrogen therapy on outcome. Am J Obstet Gynecol 1991; 164: 165–174

85 Tang G W K. Reaction to emergency hysterectomy. Obstet Gynecol 1985; 65: 206–210

86 Zigmond A S, Snaith R P. The Hospital Anxiety and Depression Scale. Acta Psychiatr Scand 1983; 67: 361–370

87 Dikoff E C, Crary W G, Christo M, Lobo R A. Oestrogen improves psychological function in postmenopausal women. Obstet Gynecol 1991; 78: 991–995

88 Best N, Rees M, Barlow D. Effect of oestradiol implant on nonadrenergic function and mood in menopausal patients. Psychoneuroendocrinology 1992; 17: 87–93

89 Dennerstein L, Burrows G D, Hyman G, Sharpe K. Hormone therapy and affect. Maturiatus 1979; 1: 247–254

90 Sherwin B B, Gelfand M M. Sex steroids and affect in the surgical menopause: a double blind cross over study. Psychoneuroendocrinology 1985; 10: 325–335

91 Sherwin B B, Gelfand M M, Brender W. Androgen enhances sexual motivation in females: a prospective, crossover study of sex steroid administration in the surgical menopause. Psychosom Med 1985; 47: 339–350

92 Sherwin B B, Gelfand M M. The role of androgen in the maintenance of sexual functioning in oophorectomised women. Psychosom Med 1987; 49: 397–409

93 Sherwin B B. Affective changes with estrogen and androgen replacement therapy in surgically menopausal women. J Affect Disord 1988; 14: 177–187

Austin Ugwumadu Patrick Neven

Current and future applications of antioestrogens

Oestrogen is an ambivalent steroid hormone. On the one hand it protects postmenopausal women against cardiovascular diseases,[1,2] osteoporosis,[3] tooth loss,[4] Alzheimer's disease and related neurodegenerative dementias.[5] On the other hand, it is implicated in the development of breast and uterine cancers. 'Antioestrogens' are a series of synthetic compounds that block the proliferative actions of oestrogen in reproductive tissues and related cell lines. They were extensively researched in the 1940s and 50s, driven by their anticipated application in contraception. Current antioestrogens however, are developed either to mimic the beneficial effects of oestrogen and/or block the adverse ones but most of them display similar biologically paradoxical effects as does the natural hormone oestrogen. The molecular basis for this contradictory profile of biological effects seems to derive from divergent intracellular signalling pathways and target genes. This process heralds a new era of exciting pharmacological precision with the potential for selective and tissue specific hormonotherapy, a truly significant progress in gynaecology.

The triphenylethylene derivative, tamoxifen, developed by Imperial Chemical Industries (ICI, UK) in 1966 is the most widely used and studied antioestrogen. It became highly successful and still is the endocrine treatment of choice for all stages of breast cancer especially in postmenopausal women with oestrogen receptor (ER) positive tumours. Being a tumoristatic agent, tamoxifen requires prolonged administration to achieve optimal results. Apart from a clear reduction in the risk of contralateral breast cancer, tamoxifen also protects against cardiovascular diseases and osteoporosis not only in postmenopausal breast cancer patients but also in healthy women.[6-11] Its oestrogen antagonist actions control breast cancer growth but the partial agonist activity may cause proliferative and neoplastic uterine lesions such as

Mr Austin H. N. Ugwumadu, Research Fellow/Honorary Senior Registrar, Department of Obstetrics and Gynaecology, St George's Hospital Medical School, Cranmer Terrace, London SW17 0RE, UK

Dr Patrick Neven, Consultant Gynaecologist, Department of Obstetrics and Gynaecology, Algemene Kliniek St Jan, Broekstraat 114, 1000 Brussels, Belgium

hyperplasia,[12] polyposis,[13] carcinoma,[14,15] sarcomas[16,17] and fibroid growth[18,19] in the long-term. This capability of tamoxifen to evoke a heterogeneous and often contrasting set of responses from classic oestrogen sensitive organs signalled the feasibility of selective oestrogen antagonism/agonism and indeed accelerated the race for the development of the 'ideal oestrogen' (selective and target organ specific without unwanted effects in distant non-target tissues). Since cardiovascular disease, breast cancer and osteoporosis are the leading causes of long-term morbidity, mortality and escalating health costs in postmenopausal women, the reduction of their risk factors demonstrated by tamoxifen has generated a considerable interest in the use of 'antioestrogens' as agents of disease prevention in healthy postmenopausal women.

This chapter will concentrate on the gynaecological sequelae and the wider health benefits of tamoxifen's application to breast cancer therapy and prevention and explore the potential role of the novel class of antioestrogens referred to as *selective (o)estrogen receptor modulators* (SERM) exemplified by raloxifen. Members of this family show great potential as non hormonal alternatives to existing oestrogen replacement therapy with better risk:benefit ratio and without the requirement for progestogens, nor the anxieties about breast cancer risk. The reader is referred to appropriate texts for other applications of antioestrogens, such as in the treatment of anovulatory infertility.

CLASSIFICATION AND BIOCHEMISTRY OF ANTIOESTROGENS

The major classes of synthetic antioestrogens include: (i) the triphenylethylenes (TPE); (ii) the benzothiophenes; and (iii) 'pure' antioestrogens. Others are: (iv) the dihydronaphthylene derivatives; and (v) the benzophyrans.

The triphenylethylenes (TPE)

The TPE derivatives are non steroidal oestrogen analogues containing an ethylene core to which three phenyl rings are attached. They were developed by successive chemical modifications of the stilbene nucleus which yielded the first oestrogen mimetic diethylstilbestrol (DES) in 1938. Further modifications of DES resulted in compounds with antioestrogenic properties, such as clomiphene, and the relatively more potent tamoxifen, although both are still weak oestrogen agonists. The widespread clinical use of tamoxifen has highlighted its adverse oestrogenic effects on the uterus and focused attention on the newer and potentially safer but still unproven analogues such as toremifene, droloxifen and idoxifen (Fig 19.1).

The benzothiophenes

These are sulphur containing non steroidal compounds (Fig. 19.1). The chief member of this family is raloxifen, previously known as keoxifen, LY139481

Fig. 19.1 (see page opposite) Chemical structures of representative antioestrogens. (**A**) triphenylethylene derivatives: (**B**) benzothiophene derivatives: (**C**) pure antioestrogens: (**D**) dihydronaphthylene derivatives: (**E**) benzophyrans.

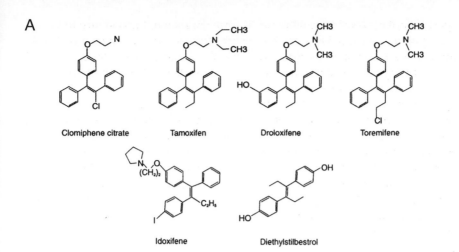

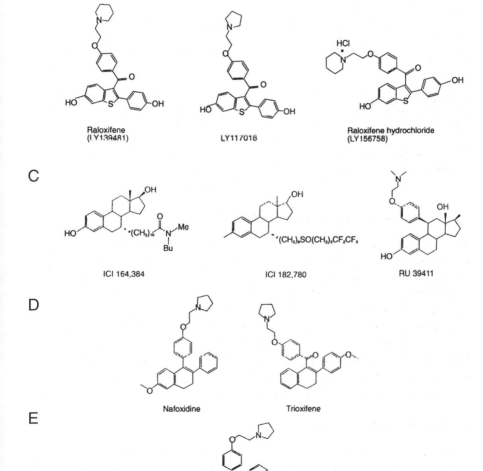

Fig. 19.1

and LY156758 for the hydrochloride salt form. Raloxifen binds avidly to the ER and has tissue specific effects that are distinct from oestradiol and tamoxifen. In animal models, raloxifen produced profound antioestrogenic effects on breast and uterine tissues whilst exerting potent osteoblastic and hypolipidaemic effects.[18,19] In postmenopausal women, it increased bone mineral density, lowered serum lipids without stimulating the endometrium.[20,21] Drug designers at Eli Lilly have developed a more potent variation of raloxifen called SERM 111 with greater antioestrogenic effects on the breast and uterus. Two trials of SERM 111 are in progress testing its efficacy in chemoprevention and treatment of breast cancer. A third trial addresses the prevention of osteoporosis.

'Pure' antioestrogens

The 7α-alkylamine derivatives such as ICI164384 and ICI182780 and the 11β-amidoalkyl 17β-oestradiol derivative RU51625 are synthetic steroids structurally identical to oestradiol but for the substituted groups at the 7- and 11- positions, respectively (Fig. 19.1). ICI182780 has replaced ICI164384[22] and lacks the ability to activate transcription of oestrogen responsive genes and elicit transcriptional hormone responses, presumably because of its side chain.[23] It achieves complete blockade of the trophic actions of oestrogen, which none of the prior clinically available antioestrogens was capable of. Preliminary animal studies show that the pure antioestrogens did not alter gonadotrophic concentrations in intact rats but significantly reduced uterine size, suggesting a selective peripheral action that could be highly beneficial in premenopausal women where antiuterotrophic effects and breast cancer inhibition can be achieved without disturbing the hypothalamic pituitary ovarian axis.[24] Their clinical usefulness, however, will depend on the wider antioestrogenic effects exerted on the skeleton, the cardiovascular system and on serum lipids. Two experimental studies in female rats found contradictory bone density effects of treatment with ICI182780.[24,25] Its efficacy using the long acting intramuscular formulation was proven in a pilot trial in women with advanced tamoxifen-resistant breast cancer and no significant adverse effects were observed.[26] Overall, very scanty data exist on the long term safety of the pure antioestrogens.

MECHANISMS OF OESTROGEN AND ANTIOESTROGENIC ACTION

The ER subtypes and multiple alternative signaling pathways

The ER is a nuclear transcription factor with binding domains for DNA and ligands. It also contains two special domains with transcription activating functions [AF-1 and AF-2].[27] AF-1 is constitutive and independent of oestrogen binding while AF-2 is specific for oestrogen.[27] When oestradiol engages the ligand binding domain of the ER, the receptor dimerizes and undergoes conformational changes enabling the AF domains to interact with the *(o)estrogen response element* (ERE), a specific DNA sequence within the promoter regions of oestrogen responsive genes which is responsible for the regulation of gene transcription (Fig. 19.2). All antioestrogens seem to exert some degree of ligand dependent conformational change in the ER.[28] For example, the binding of tamoxifen to the ER may activate AF-1 (which is constitutive) but inhibit AF-2 (oestradiol specific) and prevent gene transcription at the ERE. However, in some tissues, AF-1 activation is sufficient to elicit transcription and oestrogenic effects may follow in such tissues.[29]

The paradoxical effects of tamoxifen implied the existence and differential distribution of tissue specific ER subtypes such that individual organ responses depended on which native ER subtypes were activated. Recently, a second ER (ER-β) was demonstrated, first in the rat[30] and subsequently in man[31] and mouse.[32] The original ER first isolated by Elwood Jensen in 1958 is now renamed ER-α. These ER isoforms have similar binding affinities for oestradiol but display differential tissue expression and distribution.[30,33] The classical, albeit simplistic model of oestrogen action through a unitary nuclear ER is now challenged by recent advances in the development of the antioestrogens. It is evident now that selective ER modulation results from divergent and alternative molecular signaling pathways from a cell's ER to its genes.[34] Whereas oestradiol, tamoxifen and raloxifene act as agonists on bone, tamoxifen and raloxifene antagonise breast tissue while tamoxifen stimulates uterine tissue. This selective and tissue specific activity is biologically feasible because of the existence of distinct oestrogen dependent genes that do not have an ERE-like sequence within their promoter regions but contain other conserved DNA sequences such as the AP-1 site[35,36] and the *raloxifen response element* (RRE).[34] Furthermore, ER-α and -β may signal in opposite ways depending on the ligand and the response element. Oestradiol stimulated transcription through ER-α and ER-β in a classical ERE but inhibited transcription through the ER-β at an AP-1 site[37] suggesting that ER-α and -β may have different roles in gene regulation with the ER-β serving to turn off regulatory genes which have AP-1 sites in their promotor regions. In contrast, the antioestrogens tamoxifen, raloxifene and ICI164384 stimulated transcription through ER-β at an AP-1 site.[37] If those genes regulated by ER-β at an AP-1 site are identified and their native cells characterised we may be closer to unraveling the ultimate control mechanism of gene transcription in target cells. Presumably, other genes exist which may be activated by oestrogen by-products through alternative pathways (Fig. 19.2).

Regulation of growth factors

Tamoxifen and its analogues may also be useful in a wide range of other diseases, including autoimmune disorders,[38] osteoporosis,[39] atherosclerosis[40] and myocardial infarction. Since some 10% of ER negative breast cancers and other malignancies where hormone dependence is not well established respond to tamoxifen therapy,[41] it raises the question whether nonsteroidal antioestrogens modulate other molecular targets or could simply antagonising the ER function account for all of these diverse effects? One cellular target of interest is the multifunctional cytokine, transforming growth factor-β (TGF-β), a family of polypeptides involved in the inhibition of epithelial cell

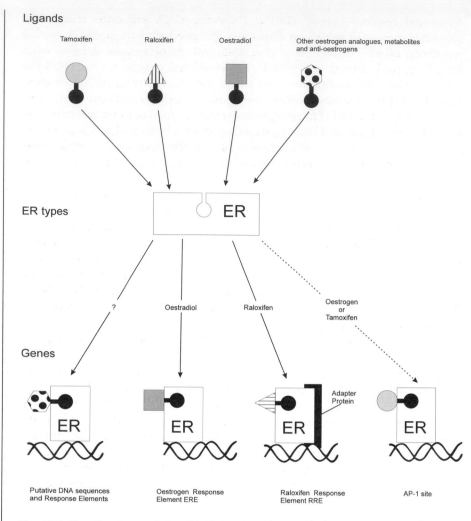

Fig. 19.2 The ER subtype, the multiple/divergent signaling pathways and gene recognition model. The resulting biologic effect will depend on the activated gene, the host organ and the function of the gene product.

proliferation and maintenance of normal pattern of gene expression in a wide variety of tissues. Loss of response to TGF-β by cells is associated with subsequent malignant transformation.[42] Tamoxifen up-regulates the production of TGF-β_1 by breast cancer cells in vitro and in vivo[43,44] and appears to exert at least part of its antitumour effect by elevation of this cytokine. Although other studies dispute this view,[45] tamoxifen is potentially still useful in a broader range of cancers where TGF-β regulation may alter the clinical course favourably. TGF-βs are present in the stromal and epithelial elements of the normal endometrium,[46] where they are under complex and differential steroid hormone regulation. Although tamoxifen and oestradiol reduce TGF-β_ in cultured human endometrial adenocarcinoma cells under oestrogen depleted conditions,[47] in breast cancer cells tamoxifen stimulates the production of TGF-β,[43,44] again demonstrating a tissue specific effect. Since tamoxifen exerts oestrogenic effects on the postmenopausal uterus, studies are now underway to test the hypothesis that this effect may be due to an initial down-regulation of TGF-β in the uterine tissues of women treated with tamoxifen. Such an inhibitory effect on TGF-β expression may result in a negative apoptotic effect and positive signal for proliferation of endometrial cells. The details of the modulatory processes of the different isoforms of the TGF-β family are far more complex than is outlined here and outside the scope of this chapter. There is, however, evidence to suggest that TGF-β suppresses early tumour development, but also enhances growth and proliferation of established malignancies, probably through angiogenesis and reduction of immune surveillance.[45]

Insulin-like growth factors (IGF) and their binding proteins (IGFBP) are expressed in the human endometrium[46] and regulated by steroid hormones.[47] Some members of this family may have a role in the proliferative actions of tamoxifen in the human endometrium. In the rat, tamoxifen suppresses uterine IGFBP-3 leading to increased IGF activity with resultant mitogenesis and growth.[47] In the human uterus, tamoxifen therapy increases the mRNA for IGFBP-2 but had no demonstrable effect on the mRNA for endometrial IGF-1.[48] These findings may suggest a possible role for IGFBP-2 in the genesis of proliferative uterine lesions.

In bone, TGF-β plays an essential role in the maintenance of normal bone density by regulating the balance between the bone producing osteoblasts and the bone resorbing osteoclasts.[37] Mutations in the TGF-β_1 locus has been correlated with low bone density in postmenopausal women.[49] Oestrogen itself has a complex mode of action on bone which is partly a receptor mediated effect on osteoblasts and osteoclasts and partly through inhibition of locally acting cytokines, such as IL-1 and IL-6, which promote osteoclast maturation and activity.[50] Overall, it would seem that the up-regulation of TGF-β production is a more plausible mechanism of the beneficial effect of tamoxifen and related TPEs on bone, rather than the direct modulation of ER function.

Genotoxicity and DNA-adduct formation

DNA-adducts are covalent modifications of DNA induced by metabolically activated chemical carcinogens and are believed to be a crucial step in chemical carcinogenesis. In the rat, tamoxifen is metabolised to α-hydroxytamoxifen (α(OH)T) which binds to DNA to form potent genotoxic DNA-adducts with carcinogenic effects on the rat liver.[54] Furthermore, tamoxifen induced chromosomal changes within the rat hepatocytes, including mutations in the tumour suppressor gene p53. A similar mechanism of induction of endometrial cancer in humans was postulated, but we found no DNA-adducts in human endometrium exposed to tamoxifen.[55] Although human endometrial explants formed α(OH)T, rats generated 20–40 times more with a tenth of the dose. The lowest dose of α(OH)T required to form detectable DNA-adducts was 10 000 times higher than the levels circulating in patients.[55] Humans are, therefore, less efficient at producing α(OH)T than rats and the levels produced are too low to form adducts in amounts sufficient to cause genotoxic damage as in the rat. Another study, however, demonstrated very weak signals for putative DNA adducts in tamoxifen exposed human endometrial tissue albeit using a different methodology.[56] The levels of adduct detected in this study are exceedingly low and at the very lowest limits of detection, even using this very highly sensitive technique. Species differences in the metabolism of tamoxifen may explain the dissimilar findings in the human endometrium compared to the rodent liver.

Other mechanisms

The structure and function of ERs can be attenuated by tamoxifen.[57] A resultant rogue ER could misinterpret cellular signals and produce oestrogenic effects in response to an antioestrogen. Metabolic products of tamoxifen such as the isomer *cis*-4-hydroxytamoxifen may act as an oestrogen agonist[58] and has been suggested to explain agonist activity in patients on tamoxifen. Some actions of antioestrogens – such as antagonism of calmodulin dependent cAMP phosphodiesterase and inhibition of protein kinase C and various chloride channels – do not involve transcription and protein synthesis.[59] Tamoxifen also increases the serum levels of sex hormone binding globulin (SHBG) which binds circulating oestradiol and decreases the availability of the free hormone.[60] In premenopausal women, however, the increased SHBG may be counteracted by elevated oestradiol levels with a net oestrogenic effect.

EFFECTS OF TAMOXIFEN ON ORGAN SYSTEMS

Breast

Tamoxifen antagonises the action of oestrogen on the breast by competitive binding to the ER resulting in growth inhibition of the mammary tissue. It also exerts a direct antigrowth effect even in the absence of oestrogen or its receptors. In breast cancer tissue, tamoxifen blocks oestrogen induced cancer growth, alters the production of local growth factors[61] and/or suppresses tumour angiogenesis.[62] This multistep inhibitory effect on breast cancer tissue is successfully exploited in clinical practice resulting in a response rate of 50% and 80% in ER only positive and oestrogen/progesterone receptor positive breast cancers, respectively.[41] In the latest worldwide overview of adjuvant tamoxifen for breast cancer, recurrence was reduced by 50% and mortality by 25%.[6]

Reproductive tract

In premenopausal women, tamoxifen produces predominantly antioestrogenic effects in the uterus and vagina despite circulating supraphysiological oestradiol levels.[63] In postmenopausal women, however, it acts as an oestrogen mimetic, stimulating the myometrium,[12] endometrium[13] and the vagina[64] with resultant increase in organ volume and water content. Adenomyosis,[65,66] probably induced de novo, reactivation of dormant/de novo endometriosis[67] and growth of fibroids[17] have all been reported in postmenopausal women on tamoxifen. Although atypical hyperplasia occurs commonly in deep foci of ectopic endometrium without a correspondingly higher incidence of primary adenocarcinoma at these sites, chronic and persistent oestrogenic effect exerted by tamoxifen may alter this balance. Perhaps clinicians supervising women on tamoxifen should modify their attitude towards growing uteri either from myomas or suspected adenomyosis as these lesions may not run their usually benign courses. Tamoxifen also stimulates the mucinous endocervical cells to proliferate and identical rest cells in the endometrium to undergo metaplastic changes.[68] In theory, neoplastic changes in these cells could occur and some retrospective studies suggest that these processes explain their observed increase in the incidence of mucinous and clear cell endometrial carcinoma in women treated with tamoxifen.[68,69] Data from randomised and controlled studies however, have not confirmed an excess of these tumours in women treated with tamoxifen compared to controls[15,70,71,72] nor shown an increase in death rates from carcinoma other than that of the breast in women treated with tamoxifen.[6,15,70]

Hypothalamic pituitary ovarian axis

At the hypothalamic level, tamoxifen exerts an antioestrogenic effect in premenopausal women with a 2–3-fold increase in steroidogenesis while gonadotrophin levels are either maintained or marginally increased.[73] This is contrary to an expected fall in gonadotrophin levels if tamoxifen was acting as an oestrogen. Irregular cycles are common during adjuvant tamoxifen therapy in premenopausal women and amenorrhoea may occur in up to 25%.[74] Of treated premenopausal women, 10% may also have ovarian cysts[75] and complications in such cysts may require surgical intervention.[76,77] In postmenopausal women, tamoxifen lowers serum gonadotrophin levels, an oestrogenic effect, although the levels remain within the postmenopausal range.[78]

Liver and steroid binding proteins

Hepatic synthesis of sex hormone, thyroxine and corticotrophin binding globulins are increased by tamoxifen in postmenopausal women.[79] Since thyroid stimulating hormone and free thyroxine levels are unaffected, there is usually no clinical manifestation of altered thyroid function. Primary hepatocellular carcinoma has been associated with tamoxifen treatment in man and in experimental animal models.[14,54] Data pooled from three major adjuvant tamoxifen studies in Scandinavia revealed an increase in stomach and colorectal cancers, although the authors point out that these findings are early and tentative[71] and yet to be confirmed by other studies.

Cardiovascular system and serum lipids

Like oestrogen, tamoxifen lowers total cholesterol and LDL-cholesterol in postmenopausal women.[80,81] There may be a marginal increase in triglycerides but levels are maintained within normal limits. It also lowers lipoprotein-a, a known risk factor for cardiovascular disease.[81] These favourable lipid changes may translate into a reduction in cardiovascular morbidity observed in women treated with tamoxifen.[9] A meta-analysis of randomised trials of cholesterol reduction in the prevention of coronary artery disease suggests a 2% reduction in the frequency of cardiac events for every 1% reduction in serum cholesterol.[82] In a randomised placebo controlled trial of tamoxifen therapy for 2 years in 46 healthy postmenopausal women, a 12% decline in total cholesterol was observed which translates into a 24% reduction in cardio-vascular events.[83] Tamoxifen inhibits the formation of lipid filled vascular lesions in experimental animals[40] and in man causes a slight reduction in antithrombin 111,[74] with a theoretical risk of thromboembolism. However, in the NSABP-B4 trial, serious thromboembolic events (deep vein thrombosis requiring hospitalisation, life threatening pulmonary embolism and death) were increased 4.7 times in the tamoxifen treated group compared to the placebo group. The Eastern Co-operative Oncology Group also reported a comparable 5.7-fold elevation in the risk of thromboembolic events.[84] Although the evidence linking tamoxifen to thromboembolic events is still accumulating, clinicians should maintain a high index of suspicion especially in those women with predisposing factors.

Skeleton

Contrary to initial fears that the antioestrogenic effects of tamoxifen may induce or accelerate existing osteoporosis, bone density is preserved in treated postmenopausal women.[8] Bone preservation however, has mainly been confirmed in the lumbar spine. More studies in healthy postmenopausal women are required to establish peripheral bone protection by tamoxifen since it is femoral neck fractures that are associated with significant morbidity and mortality unlike spinal osteoporosis. Besides, breast cancer may breach the integrity of bone and further confound the findings. At present, only preliminary evidence exists suggesting that tamoxifen may protect cortical bone which predominates in the femur and prevent femoral fractures.[85] The mechanism of cancellous bone protection by tamoxifen is unclear but thought to be through activation of the gene that codes for TGF-β_3 a key protein in maintaining the integrity of bone in living animals.[48] The situation is less clear in premenopausal women and the data in this group are conflicting.[86,87]

SELECTIVE (O)ESTROGEN RECEPTOR MODULATORS (SERM)

These are compounds that engage the ER and exert oestrogen agonist effects in desired target tissues, such as bone and the cardiovascular system, together with oestrogen antagonism (or clinically neutral effect) in reproductive tissues, such as the uterus and breast. Although tamoxifen exhibited this differential activity in human tissues (first generation SERM), the benzothiophene derivative, raloxifen, comes closer to the definition of the 'ideal oestrogen'. In vitro, raloxifen displayed activity against breast cancer models comparable to tamoxifen, selectively inhibited uterine tissues and simultaneously maintained bone density and favourable serum lipids profile.[18] In clinical trials, raloxifen exhibited similar attributes but failed to control postmenopausal vasomotor symptoms.[20,21]

Effects of raloxifen on organ systems

Breast

Raloxifen was originally developed for the treatment of breast cancer. It produced potent inhibition of oestradiol binding to the ER[88] and proliferation of the human MCF-7 breast cancer cell line.[89] Tamoxifen is more efficacious than raloxifen in in vivo systems despite comparable activities in vitro probably because of the in vivo generation of the active metabolite $\alpha(OH)T$.[89] Although raloxifen showed no antitumour activity after 4 weeks in its sole trial of breast cancer treatment in humans, the volunteers in that study had primary or secondary resistance to tamoxifen.[90] In a recent trial, daily raloxifen 60 mg and 120 mg achieved a 3-fold reduction in the incidence of breast cancer over a 36 months follow-up period.[21]

Uterus

In contrast to tamoxifen, raloxifen produces a complete or near complete blockade of oestrogenic effect in the uterus of castrated rats.[18] This unique effect on the uterus was underlined by histological evidence in one study using castrated rats as control. Raloxifen produced a 1.2–1.5-fold statistically insignificant and dose independent increase in epithelial cell height and endometrial thickness.[91] Moreover, there was no stromal eosinophillic infiltration. Tamoxifen, on the other hand, produced a 2–5-fold increase in these parameters.[92] In chemoprevention trials, tamoxifen raised endometrial cancer risk by 4-fold in postmenopausal women,[85] raloxifene, on the other hand, halved endometrial cancer risk compared to a placebo group.[21]

Serum lipids

Raloxifene reduced serum lipoproteins in the rat[92] and in postmenopausal women.[85] However, clinical reduction in cardiovascular disease is yet to be confirmed. Moreover, raloxifene did not elevate the serum levels of the protective HDL cholesterol lipid fraction nor significantly alter serum triglyceride in a recent trial.[20] As with tamoxifen and exogenous oestrogen, raloxifen seem to exert this effect by an up-regulation of the liver LDL-receptors leading to increased metabolic clearance of LDL-cholesterol.[93]

Bone

In postmenopausal women treated with raloxifene, biochemical markers for bone metabolism are similar to those observed with exogenous oestrogen. In castrated rats, raloxifen maintained bone density without a significant increase in uterine weight or histologic parameters such as epithelial cell height and stromal eosinophilia.[94] Delmans et al[20] have very recently confirmed a modest (2–2.5%) increase in bone mineral density [BMD] in 601 postmenopausal women randomly assigned to receive raloxifen or placebo for 2 years. BMD of course, is a surrogate marker of bone strength and at present, there is very scanty data on whether raloxifene reduces fractures in postmenopausal women. Equally, BMD measurements may grossly underestimate the capacity of raloxifene to reduce fracture risk.[95] Nevertheless, raloxifen is now licensed for osteoporosis prevention in postmenopausal women in the USA. The exact mechanism of action of raloxifene on bone is currently under investigation. It is however, known to activate the gene that codes for TGF-β_3.[96]

THE BREAST CANCER PREVENTION TRIALS (BCPT)

The global incidence of breast cancer is rising while mortality rates remain unchanged despite advances in therapeutic modalities.[97] By the year 2000 there will be approximately one million new diagnoses and over 400 000 deaths per annum. Primary prevention strategies have failed because we lack a clear understanding of the mechanisms through which the risk factors operate. Tamoxifen showed potential as a candidate chemopreventive agent against breast cancer and may even offer wider health benefits. It decreased the incidence of contralateral breast cancer by 47%, prolonged disease free survival[6,7] and achieved a 25% overall reduction in mortality.[6] Furthermore, it reduced the risk of myocardial infarction by 20% and prevented osteoporosis,[8,9] with only a 2-fold increase in the risk of endometrial cancer. Above all, tamoxifen is cheap and reputed to have few side effects. This favourable clinical profile and the dismal breast cancer statistics prompted world-wide trials to test the efficacy of tamoxifen as chemoprophylaxis for breast cancer in healthy women at increased risk according to the Gail et al[98] risk model. Because the trial began before the discovery of the BRCA1 and BRCA2 genes, women with these mutations were not specifically selected. The BCPT commenced in April 1992 and aimed to recruit 16 000 at risk women aged 35 and above from 300 centers across the USA and Canada. Other centers are in Italy [only hysterectomised women] and in a long list of countries participating in the International Breast Intervention Study (IBIS) including the UK, Australia, Germany, the Netherlands, Belgium and Switzerland. The prolonged period of administration of tamoxifen required to achieve results raised anxiety levels about its long-term effects.

The estimated 2-fold increase in endometrial carcinoma used in calculating the net benefit of tamoxifen was provided by its manufacturers. The mechanism of tamoxifen's action on the endometrium was presumed to be identical to that of oestradiol and the associated endometrial cancer similarly regarded as indolent and benign with good prognosis. Tamoxifen may produce or exacerbate menopausal symptoms and lower overall quality of life and compliance. However, none of these relatively lesser adverse effects was taken into account in the calculation of the risk-benefit equation of tamoxifen for the BCPT. Furthermore, uterine sarcomas and retinopathies are reported increasingly in women on tamoxifen.[71,99,100]

In April 1998, investigators at the National Cancer Institute halted the USA–BCPT 14 months earlier than expected after they found a 45% reduction in the incidence of breast cancer in women treated with tamoxifen compared to placebo. A total of 13 388 predominantly white women participated in the trial. Follow up was only for 4 years and at press time the findings have only been published on the internet (http://cancertrials.nci.nih.gov.). In the group randomised to take tamoxifen there were 85 cases of invasive breast cancer, 31 of noninvasive carcinoma *in situ* compared to 154 invasive and 59 *in situ* lesions in the placebo group. Despite the excitement generated by these results, they do not provide sufficient evidence to warrant the routine use of tamoxifen for breast cancer prevention in healthy women. Interim analysis of the UK–BCPT101 and preliminary findings in the Italian arm of IBIS102 did not corroborate the American findings. Differences in the study populations, sample sizes and definitions of risk have been suggested to account for the conflicting findings. The reduction in the incidence of breast cancer does not necessarily translate into a reduction in mortality. Will tamoxifen prevent oestrogen dependent cancers but select out resistant tumours with less favourable histological and biological characteristics? The anticipated

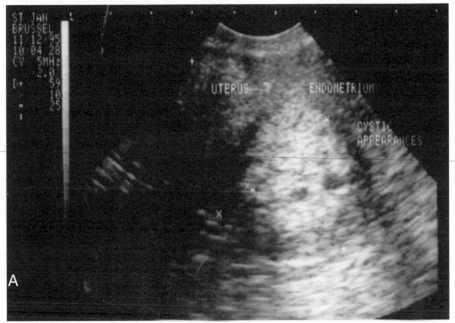

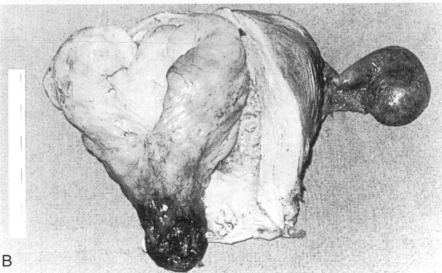

Fig. 19.3 (A) Transvaginal scan of an asymptomatic postmenopausal woman on tamoxifen 20 mg daily for 5 years showing ET of 25 mm with cystic pattern. Hysteroscopy demonstrated an endometrial polyp which on histology was a polyp cancer. **(B)** Giant adenomyomatous endometrial polyp and adenomyosis in a postmenopausal woman on tamoxifen 40 mg daily for 7 years. Reproduced with the permission of the *British Journal of Obstetrics and Gynaecology* from Ugwumadu et al.[65]

reduction in heart attacks did not materialise in the USA–BCPT although fewer women in the tamoxifen group suffered fractures of the hip, wrist and spine. There were 33 cases of endometrial cancer, 30 cases of DVT and 17 of pulmonary embolism in the tamoxifen group compared to 14, 19 and 6 cases respectively in the placebo group.

The optimal duration of tamoxifen prophylaxis and its long-term effects/results are still unknown. In adjuvant therapy the beneficial effect of tamoxifen is lost after 5 years and longer therapy increases its detrimental effects. Termination of the trial may also have jeopardised a unique opportunity to examine the interaction between tamoxifen and HRT in a potential 40% of the participants who were premenopausal. However, outside the USA and certainly in the UK, women are encouraged to remain in the trial until these questions are resolved. In spite of its adverse effects, evidence from randomised comparisons do not provide proof beyond reasonable doubt that tamoxifen is contraindicated in any group of women. At present, the BCPTs are scientifically justified although the ethical and safety debate may persist. Whereas gynaecological surveillance to identify women at risk of uterine pathology would seem desirable, uncertainties surround the test characteristics and cost effectiveness of the available methods of endometrial monitoring.

GYNAECOLOGICAL SURVEILLANCE AND PREVENTION OF UTERINE LESIONS

Pelvic ultrasound

Transvaginal ultrasound scan

Conventional transvaginal scan (TVS) as a tool for endometrial assessment in asymptomatic women on tamoxifen is of limited value and could be frankly misleading. It is not sufficiently sensitive to detect endometrial polyps which may complicate up to 40% of long-term tamoxifen therapy. The polyps have unusual histological features and have been suggested to represent inter-mediate stage lesions between hyperplasia and carcinoma (Fig. 19.3A,B).[103] Tamoxifen also exerts a unique but false endometrial hyperechogenicity, multiple and heterogeneous sonoluscent areas and blurring of the endometrial/myometrial junction.[104] These changes probably result from stromal and proximal myometrial oedema and the presence of numerous irregularly distributed myometrial microcysts attributed to foci of active adenomyosis (Figs 19.4A,B & 19.5).[104] Overall, this sonographic appearance makes accurate measurement of the endometrial thickness (ET) impossible and, although the changes do not necessarily imply epithelial disease, they are sufficiently misleading to preclude the application of previously described cut-off values for ET to patients on tamoxifen. Moreover, it provokes anxiety and unnecessary biopsies in affected patients. It is now clear from sonohystero-graphic and hysteroscopic examinations that this characteristic sonographic 'honeycomb' appearance is due to changes involving the subendometrial and myometrial elements of the uterus.[105] Bourne obtained and studied full thickness endometrial resection biopsy from 73 tamoxifen treated patients with ET > 8 mm on TVS and found atypical hyperplasia or endometrial carcinoma in 16% of his cases, none of which was detected by prior outpatient endometrial biopsy.[106] Of these women, 84% had ET measurements suggestive of carcinoma but in fact had no pathology.[106] Another study examined the correlation between the anatomical, pathological and sonographic findings in 2 specific cases and confirmed that these changes represent benign cystic endometrial atrophy and cystic foci of reactivated adenomyosis.[104] A study of 72 asymptomatic postmenopausal women on tamoxifen showed a poor correlation between ET and histological findings.[107] In women with ET 6–46

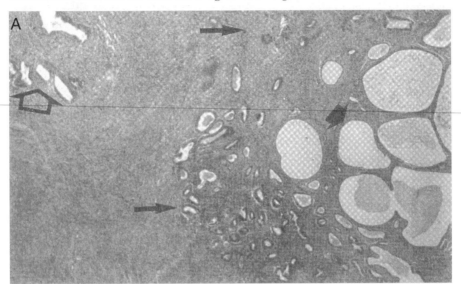

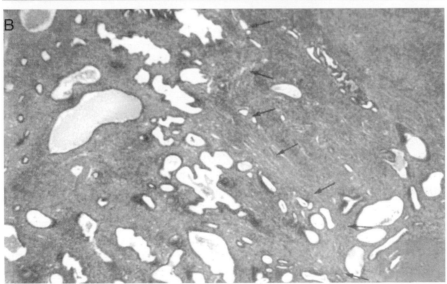

Fig. 19.4 **(A)** Cystic atrophy of the endometrium (black arrow head). Endometrium-myometrium junction (arrow). Intramyometrial cysts (hollow arrow head). **(B)** Irregular and blurred endometrial-myometrial junction (arrows). Cystic endometrial atrophy and adenomyosal cysts could be seen on the left and right sides of the picture respectively. Reproduced with the permission of *Ultrasound in Obstetrics and Gynecology* from Perrot et al.[104]

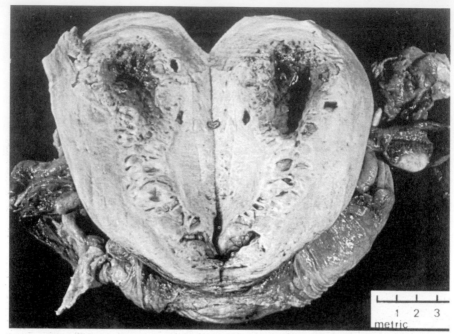

1 2 3
metric

Fig. 19.5 Postmenopausal uterus of an 85 year-old woman treated with tamoxifen. The uterus is enlarged and shows diffuse endometrial thickening with numerous cystic spaces. Reproduced with the permission of the *Journal of Clinical Pathology* from Ismail.[103]

mm, approximately 70% yielded no tissue on biopsy using suction aspiration, 24% had only small fragments of proliferative endometrium.[107] Although Lahti et al detected all significant endometrial pathology in asymptomatic women on tamoxifen using TVS and an ET > 5 mm, the false positive rate was so high that 50% of their subjects would have had unnecessary endometrial biopsies.[108] These studies consistently demonstrate the inability of the traditional TVS to discriminate between the benign and pathological endometrium in asymptomatic women on tamoxifen and sonographic findings in this group of women should be interpreted with caution.

Saline infusion sonography (SIS), hysterosonography, hydrosonography or hysterosalpingo-contrast-sonography (HyCoSo)

This technique was first described by Randolph et al in 1986 when they injected saline into the uterine cavity through a thin flexible cervical catheter and observed the intracavitory contours using the abdominal ultrasound probe.[109] Parsons and Lense in 1993[110] described the transvaginal approach which was subsequently applied to the investigation of a tamoxifen treated patient by Bourne and his colleagues in 1994.[111] The procedure delineates the uterine cavity accurately providing a contrast medium as well as a distending agent and facilitates a more precise ET measurement. (Fig. 19.6A,B) Its superiority over traditional TVS in the diagnosis of endometrial polyps and distinguishing endometrial from subendometrial/myometrial lesions is now well established. Using saline infusion sonography, Goldstein demonstrated that the ultrasound changes suggestive of endometrial thickening in his series of women on tamoxifen were in fact localised to the subendometrium[105] and further hysteroscopic evaluation revealed smooth atrophic endometria, scanty material on curettage and inactive endometrium on histological examination.

Transvaginal Doppler studies

Tamoxifen induces significant reductions of the impedance to blood flow in the endometrial and subendometrial vasculature regardless of the presence or absence of pathology.[112] This is probably due to dilatation of the existing vascular

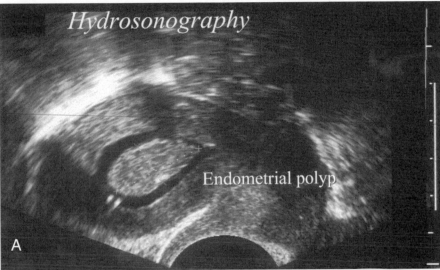

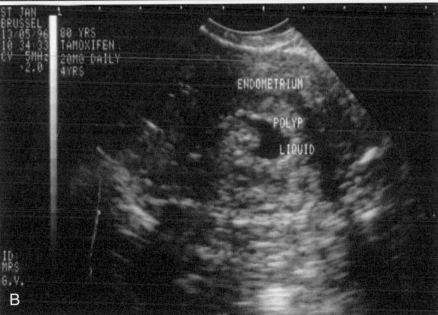

Fig. 19.6 (**A**) Hydro-hysterosonography demonstrating an endometrial polyp (courtesy of Dr Elisabeth Krampl). (**B**) Saline infusion sonography (SIS) showing an endometrial polyp on a background of thickened endometrium 20 mm. The patient was an asymptomatic 80 year-old woman on tamoxifen 20 mg daily for 4 years. The polyp was resected at hysteroscopy and found to be benign on histology.

bed. Nevertheless, the size of reduction in impedance (mean resistance index, RI = 0.39 ± 0.10 range 0.32–0.54) in 6 out of 8 tamoxifen treated women (with ET > 5 mm and benign endometrial polyps),[112] compared favourably to that seen in endometrial malignancy RI < 0.4.[113] Intriguingly, hysteroscopic resection of the polyps restored the RIs to values similar to those of patients with thin and normal endometria.[112] Tamoxifen also exerts profound reductions in impedance to blood flow in the uterine arteries of treated subjects compared to controls on placebo.[12] The reductions in RI observed in the uterine artery, subendometrial and myometrial vasculature of patients on tamoxifen therapy do not necessarily imply disease and similar alterations have been documented in women on HRT.[114] Again, a different cut off value of RI is required for women on tamoxifen. Although tamoxifen treated women are more likely to have thickened and cystic endometrium with altered uterine vascularity, the significance of these findings is still unclear and the value of TVS, SIS and colour Doppler flow studies as endometrial surveillance tests in women on tamoxifen therapy requires further investigation.

Pipelle aspiration biopsy and dilatation and curettage

Suction aspiration biopsy (Pipelle, Vabra, etc.) and D&C are effectively blind and may fail to sample endometrial polyps. In one study, D&C performed prior to hysterectomy failed to sample even 50% of the cavity in 60% of the cases examined.[115] In another study, D&C also performed prior to hysterectomy missed 5.7% of endometrial hyperplasia and carcinoma.[116] Pipelle frequently yields inadequate tissue for histology and may explain some of the discrepancies in apparent disease prevalence reported in women on tamoxifen. These limitations weaken their value as reliable methods of evaluating the endometrial cavity exposed to tamoxifen. In a study of 111 randomised participants in the UK-BCPT, TVS followed by endometrial biopsy showed 39% of histologically abnormal endometrium in patients on tamoxifen compared to 10% in the placebo group,[12] but the findings were based on endometrial cytology which is also an unreliable method of endometrial sampling. Moreover, follow-up in this study was only for 22–24 months and more sinister lesions may evolve in the longer term. The high frequency of histological abnormalities reported was also suggested to be metaplastic changes induced by tamoxifen.[117]

Hysteroscopy and biopsy

Hysteroscopy and directed biopsy, by reducing the risk of sampling error may be a more reliable tool of endometrial evaluation.[118] It is of particular value in the diagnosis of localised lesions and endometrial polyps which commonly complicate long-term tamoxifen. Hysteroscopy is user friendly and allows direct visualisation of the endometrial cavity with biopsy option in an outpatient setting. However, it also assumes that the operator will recognise areas of endometrial abnormalities and, in the UK, some gynaecologists are still reluctant to use it routinely. At present, opinion is divided on the optimal frequency of hysteroscopic examinations and on the typically pale smooth but pseudopolypoid and glandulocystic appearance of the endometrial cavity exposed to tamoxifen. Besides, a policy of mass hysteroscopic screening of all volunteers in the BCPT and indeed adjuvant therapy has considerable resource implications. It would seem reasonable to screen all perimenopausal and postmenopausal women prior to tamoxifen therapy to exclude pre-existing endometrial disease which may potentially become accelerated by tamoxifen.

Any role for progestogens?

Progestogens are effective in preventing endometrial hyperplasia and carcinoma in women on oestrogen replacement and so have been proposed and in some cases used to treat/prevent endometrial lesions in women on tamoxifen therapy.[14,69] At present, there is no scientific evidence to support this approach, the basis of which is the presumption that tamoxifen and oestradiol have identical mechanisms of action on the endometrium. Moreover, in a recent study, supplementary progestogen therapy failed to alter the frequency of endometrial hyperplasia in women on tamoxifen.[119] Furthermore, endometrial cancers occurring in women on tamoxifen have been reported to be morphologically similar to those occurring after synthetic gestagen therapy and different from those arising from unopposed oestrogen therapy.[68]

Even in low doses, progestogens seem to blunt the anti-tumour action of tamoxifen on breast tissue.[120,121] The addition of progestogen to tamoxifen may, therefore, sacrifice its efficacy on the breast in pursuit of an unproven endometrial protection. Its adverse effects on lipid profile may also lower overall life expectancy. It is unknown which progestogen if any, what route of administration, dosage or duration of treatment and whether continuous or intermittent therapy is best. Although Levonorgestrel bearing IUCD is effective in treating all types of endometrial hyperplasia,[122] there is no evidence that it is equally efficacious against similar lesions mediated by tamoxifen.

CONCLUSIONS

'Antioestrogens' are poised to assume clinical roles far removed from their original goal of simply antagonising the actions of oestrogen. By displaying selective tissue oestrogen agonist and antagonist activity, the novel class of SERM compounds are designed to mimic the beneficial actions of the oestrogen while simultaneously blocking its adverse effects and they show immense promise as agents for postmenopausal disease prevention. Although tamoxifen therapy has fringe benefits in the prevention of bone loss and cardiovascular disease, wider clinical application for these indications is controversial because of its agonist activities in non target organs. Raloxifen, however, has a selective tissue pharmacological profile that may overcome this concern. Many other compounds are being tested in phase II and phase III trials.

In the prevention trials, the risk:benefit equation of tamoxifen therapy is different for the healthy volunteers and between pre- and postmenopausal women. For a breast cancer patient, hysterectomy and continued adjuvant tamoxifen may be appropriate if atypical endometrial hyperplasia occurs. However, a healthy subject participating in the chemoprophylaxis trials presents a different dilemma. Such women should receive appropriate treatment and be withdrawn from the trial since no data exist on the optimal management approach.

It is unknown, but unlikely, that an asymptomatic but thickened and cystic endometrium inevitably turns malignant. Saline infusion sonography enhances the diagnostic accuracy of TVS and to discriminate between endometrial and subendometrial lesions. Although out-patient hysteroscopy is particularly useful in the diagnosis of endometrial polyps, we await data on its large scale application to asymptomatic women on tamoxifen and its cost effectiveness. Women with normal pretreatment endometrium on 20 mg daily of tamoxifen for 5 years have very low risk of endometrial cancer. However, bleeding at any time during tamoxifen therapy should be thoroughly investigated.[123] The international meeting of the Flemish Gynaecological Oncology Group held in Belgium in December 1997 reached a consensus to screen all prospective tamoxifen receipients prior to treatment using TVS with SIS or hysteroscopy if the endometrium is thickened.[124] If the cavity is normal with ET < 5 mm, further screening may be withheld for 2–3 years[125] after which annual TVS with SIS or hysteroscopy may be resumed.[124] Unless prospective studies show progestogens to be efficacious in controlling the proliferative effects of tamoxifen on the endometrium, they should not be used. The intrinsic progestogenic action of tamoxifen observed on the human endometrium[67,126,127] weakens the potential value of these studies and further confuses our limited understanding of this fascinating substance.

THE FUTURE

The potential clinical and research applications of SERMs is considerable. The possibility now exists to prevent and treat osteoporosis, breast cancer, cardiovascular and probably central nervous system diseases without incurring other health risks. Molecular mimicry will enable the development of drugs with only the moiety that engages and activates precise and specific receptors without side effects in non target tissues. If, for example, the cardioprotective effect of oestrogen is localised to a part of the molecule distinct from the part that exerts its sexual role, then selective modulation may enable a 'designer oestrogen' extend its cardioprotective benefits to men without fear of emasculating them! HRT as we know it today consists of arbitrary doses of oestradiol and occasionally, token testosterone supplements. But the sex steroid precursors produced cyclically in variable but balanced quantities by the ovary may exert as yet unrecognised metabolic functions by activating DNA sequences other than the ERE as exemplified by 17-episterol.[34] The recognition and exploitation of these putative genes and their functions will 'fine tune' our concept and application of HRT.

Extensive and long-term trials are required to establish the efficacy of the newer 'antioestrogens' with respect to the skeleton, the cardiovascular system, alleviation of menopausal symptoms and their overall safety. Their clinical utility though, will depend on their design and tissue selectivity. The search is on for that member of the SERM class with a pharmacological profile that approximates the 'ideal oestrogen'.

ACKNOWLEDGEMENTS

We are grateful to Dr Graham Davies, Clinical Research Physician at Eli Lilly Industries Limited, Mr Kamlesh Patel of Novo Nordisk Pharmaceuticals and their staff for their help and support during the preparation of the manuscript and to Mr Bobert G N Thonet FRCS FRCOG consultant obstetrician and gynaecologist for his invaluable comments and suggestions.

REFERENCES

1 Stampfer M J, Colditz G A. Estrogen replacement therapy and coronary disease: a quantitative assessment of the epidemiological evidence. Prev Med 1991; 20: 47–63

2 Grady D, Rubin S M, Petitti D B et al. Hormone therapy to prevent disease and prolong life in postmenopausal women. Ann Intern Med 1992; 117: 1016–1037

3 Felson D T, Zhang Y, Hannan M T, Kiel D P, Wilson P W F, Andersen J J. The effect of postmenopausal estrogen therapy on bone density in elderly women. N Engl J Med 1993; 329: 1141–1146

4 Paganini-Hill A. The benefits of estrogen replacement therapy on oral health. The leisure world cohort. Arch Intern Med 1995; 155: 2325–2329

5 Paganini-Hill A, Henderson V W. Estrogen deficiency and risk of Alzheimer's disease in women. Am J Epidemiol 1994; 140: 256–261

6 Early Breast Cancer Trialists' Collaborative Group. Tamoxifen for early breast cancer: an overview of the randomized trials. Lancet 1998; 351: 1451–1467

7 Baum M, Houghton J, Riley D. Results of the Cancer Research Campaign adjuvant trial for perioperative cyclophosphamide and long term tamoxifen in early breast cancer reported at the tenth year of follow-up. Acta Oncol 1992; 31: 251–257

8 Wright C D P, Mansell R E, Gazet J C, Compston J E. Effect of long term tamoxifen treatment on bone turnover in women with breast cancer. BMJ 1993; 306: 429–430

9 McDonald C C, Alexander F E, Whyte B W, Forrest A P, Stewart H J. Cardiac and vascular morbidity in women receiving adjuvant tamoxifen for breast cancer in a randomised trial. BMJ 1995; 311: 977–980

10 Grey A B, Stapleton J P, Evans M C, Reid I R. The effect of the antiestrogen tamoxifen on cardiovascular risk factors in normal postmenopausal women. J Clin Endocrinol Metab 1995; 80: 3191–3195

11 Kenny A M, Prestwood K M, Pilbeam C P, Raisz L G. The short-term effects of tamoxifen on bone turnover in older women. J Clin Endocrinol Metab 1995; 80: 3287–3291

12 Kedar R P, Bourne T H, Powles T J et al. Effects of tamoxifen on uterus and ovaries of postmenopausal women in a randomised breast cancer prevention trial. Lancet 1994; 343: 1318–1321

13 Neven P, De Muylder X, Vanderick G, De Muylder E. Hysteroscopic follow-up during tamoxifen treatment. Eur J Obstet Gynaecol Reprod Biol 1990; 35: 235–238

14 Fornander T, Cedermark B, Mattson A et al. Adjuvant tamoxifen in early breast cancer: occurrence of new primary cancers. Lancet 1989; i: 117–120

15 Fisher B, Constantino J P, Redmond C K et al. Endometrial cancer in tamoxifen treated breast cancer patients: findings from National Surgical Adjuvant Breast and Bowel Project (NSABP) B-14. J Natl Cancer Inst 1994; 86: 527–537

16 Clement P B, Oliva E, Young R H. Mullerian adenosarcoma of the uterine corpus associated with tamoxifen therapy. A report of six cases and a review of tamoxifen-associated endometrial lesions. Int J Gynecol Pathol 1996; 15: 222–229

17 Ugwumadu A H N, Harding K. Uterine leiomyomata and endometrial proliferation in postmenopausal women treated with the anti-oestrogen tamoxifen. Eur J Obstet Gynecol 1994; 54: 153–156

18 Bryant H U, Turner C H, Frolick C A et al. Long term effects of raloxifen (LY139478 HCl) on bone, cholesterol and uterus in ovariectomised rats [abstract]. Bone 1995; 16 (Suppl): 116S

19 Bryant H U, Glasebrook A L, Yang Na N, Sato M. A pharmacological review of raloxifene. J Bone Miner Metab 1996; 14: 1–9

20 Delmas PD, Bjarnason NH, Mitlak BH. et al. Effects of raloxifene on bone mineral density, serum cholesterol concentrations, and uterine endometrium in postmenopausal women. N Engl J Med 1997; 337: 1641–1647

21 Cummings SR, Norton L, Eckert S. et al. Raloxifene reduces the risk of breast cancer and may decrease the risk of endometrial cancer in postmenopausal women. Two-year findings from the Multiple Outcomes of Raloxifene Evaluation (MORE) trial. Proc Am Soc Clin Oncol 1998; 17: 3

22 Wakeling A E, Bowler J. Novel antioestrogens without agonist activity. J Steroid Biochem 1988; 31: 645–653

23 Fawell S E, White R, Hoare S, Sydenham M, Page M, Parker M G. Inhibition of estrogen receptor DNA binding by the pure antiestrogen ICI164384 appears to be mediated by impaired receptor dimerization. Proc Natl Acad Sci USA 1990; 87: 6883–6687

24 Wakeling A E. The future of new pure antioestrogens in clinical breast cancer. Breast Cancer Res Treat 1993; 25: 1–9

25 Gallagher A. Chambers T J, Tobias J H. The estrogen antagonist ICI183780 reduces cancellous volume in female rats.   Endocrinology 1993; 133: 2787–2791

26 Howell A, DeFriend D, Robertson J et al. Response to a specific antioestrogen (ICI182780) in tamoxifen-resistant breast cancer. Lancet 1995; 345: 29–30

27 Parker M G, Fawell S E, Lees J A, White R, Emmans C E, Danielian P. Function of estrogen receptor as a transcription factor: a target for antiestrogens. In: Brugge J, Curran E, McCormick F. (eds) Origins of human cancer: a comprehensive review. New York: Cold Spring Harbour Laboratory Press, 1991; 667–674

28 Brzozowski A M, Pike A C W, Dauter Z et al. Molecular basis of agonism and antagonism in the oestrogen receptor. Nature 1997; 389: 735–738

29 Berry M, Metzger D, Chambon P. Role of the two activating domains of the oestrogen receptor in the cell-type and promoter context dependent agonistic activity of the antioestrogen 4-hydroxytamoxifen. EMBO J 1990; 9: 2811–2818

30 Kuiper G G. Enmark E. Pelto-Huikko M. Nilsson S. Gustafsson J A. Cloning of a novel receptor expressed in rat prostate and ovary. Proc Natl Acad Sci USA 1996; 93: 5925–5930

31 Mosselman S, Polman J, Dijkema R. ER beta: identification and characterization of a novel human estrogen receptor. FEBS Lett 1996; 392: 49–53

32 Tremblay GB, Tremblay A, Copeland NG. et al. Cloning, chromosomal localization, and functional analysis of the murine estrogen receptor beta. Mol Endocrinol 1997; 11: 353–365

33 Kuiper GG, Carlsson B, Grandien K. et al. Comparison of the ligand binding specificity and transcript tissue distribution of estrogen receptors alpha and beta. Endocrinology 1997; 138: 863–870

34 Yang Na N, Venugopalan M, Hardikar S, Glasebrook A. Identification of an estrogen response element activated by metabolites of 17β-estradiol and raloxifen. Science 1996; 253: 1222–1224

35 Umayahara Y, Kawamori R, Watada H et al. Estrogen regulation of the insulin-like growth 1 gene transcription involves an AP-1 enhancer. J Biol Chem 1994; 269: 16433–16442

36 Webb P, Lopez G N, Uht R M, Kushner P J. Tamoxifen activation of the estrogen receptor/AP-1 pathway: potential origin for the cell specific estrogen-like effects of antiestrogen. Mol Endocrinol 1995; 9: 443–456

37 Paech K, Webb P, Kuiper GG. et al Differential ligand activation of estrogen receptors ERalpha and ERbeta at AP1 sites. Science 1997; 277: 1508-1510.

38 Santambrogio L, Hochwald GM, Saxena B, L, et al. Studies on the mechanisms by which transforming growth factor-β protects against allergic encephalomyelitis-antagonism between TGF-β and tumour necrosis factor. J Immunol 1993; 151: 1116–1127

39 Ward R L, Morgan G, Dalley D, Kelly P J. Tamoxifen reduces bone turnover and prevents lumbar spine and proximal femoral bone loss in early postmenopausal women. Bone Miner 1993: 22; 87–94

40 Grainger D J, Witchel C M, Metcalfe J C. Tamoxifen elevates transforming growth factor-β and suppresses diet induced formation of lipid lesions in mouse aorta. Nat Med 1995; 1: 1067–1072

41 Jordan V C, Wolf M F, Mirecki D M, Whitford D A, Welshons W V. Hormone receptor assays: clinical usefulness in the management of carcinoma of the breast. CRC Crit Rev Clin Lab Sci 1988; 26: 97–152

42 Markowitz S, Wang J, Myeroff L, et al. Inactivation of the type 2 TGF-β receptor in colon cancer cells with microsatellite instability. Science 1995; 268: 1336–1338

43 Jeng M H, Tendijke P, Iwata K K, Jordan V C. Regulation of the levels of three TGF-β mRNAs by estrogen and their effects on the proliferation of human breast cancer cells. Mol Cell Endocrinol 1993; 92: 115–123

44 Butta A, MacLennan K, Flanders KC, et al. Induction of transforming growth factor-β_1 in human breast cancer in vivo following tamoxifen treatment. Cancer Res 1992; 52: 4261–4264

45 Torre-Amione G, Beauchamp RD, Koeppen H, et al. A highly immunogenic tumour transfected with a murine transforming factor type β_1 cDNA escapes immune surveillance. Proc Natl Acad Sci USA 1990; 87: 1486–1490

46 Chegini N, Zhao Yong, Williams R S, Flanders K C. Human uterine tissue throughout the menstrual cycle expresses transforming growth factor-β_1, (TGFβ$_1$), TGFβ$_2$, TGFβ$_3$ and TGFβ Type 11 receptor messenger ribonucleic acid and protein and contains [^{125}I]-TGFβ$_1$ binding sites. Endocrinology 1994; 135: 439–449

47 Anzai Y, Gong Y, Holinka C F et al. Effects of transforming growth factors and regulation of their mRNA levels in two human endometrial adenocarcinoma cell lines. J Steroid Biochem Mol Biol 1992; 42: 449–455

48 Grainger D J, Metcalfe J C. Tamoxifen: teaching an old drug new tricks? Nat Med 1996; 2: 381–385

49 Kleinman D, Karas M, Danilenko M et al. Stimulation of endometrial cancer cell growth by tamoxifen is associated with increased insulin-like growth factor (IGF)-I induced tyrosine phosphorylation and reduction in IGF binding proteins. Endocrinology 1996; 137: 1089–1095

50 Huynh H, Pollak M. Uterotrophic actions of estradiol and tamoxifen are associated with inhibition of uterine insulin-like growth factor binding protein 3 gene expression. Cancer Res 1994; 54: 3115–3119

51 Laatikainen T J, Tomas E I, Voutilainen R J. The expression of insulin-like growth factor and its binding protein mRNA in the endometrium of postmenopausal patients with breast cancer receiving tamoxifen. Cancer 1995; 76: 1406–1410

52 Langdahl B L, Brixen K, Jensen H K, Gregersen N, Eriksen E F. Mutations in the TGF-β_1 gene are correlated to low bone mass and increased bone turnover. J Bone Miner Res 1995; 10: (Abstract)185

53 Eriksen E F, Colvard D S, Berg N J et al. Evidence of estrogen in normal human osteoblast-like cells. Science 1988; 241: 84–86

54 Han X, Liehr J G. Induction of covalent DNA adducts in rodents by tamoxifen. Cancer Res 1992; 52: 1360–1363

55 Carmichael P L, Ugwumadu A H N, Neven P, Hewer A J, Poon G K, Phillips D H. Lack of genotoxicity of tamoxifen in human endometrium. Cancer Res 1996; 56: 1475–1479

56 Hemminki K, Rajanierri H, Lindahl B, Moberger B. Tamoxifen induced DNA adducts in endometrial samples from breast cancer patients. Cancer Res 1996; 56: 4374–4377

57 Katzenellenbogen B S. Antiestrogen resistance: mechanisms by which breast cancer cells undermine the effectiveness of endocrine therapy. J Natl Cancer Inst 1991; 83: 1434–1435

58 Osborne C K, Coronado E, Allred B C, Wiebe V, DeGregorie M. Acquired tamoxifen resistance: correlation with reduced breast tumour levels of tamoxifen and isomerization of trans-4-hydroxytamoxifen. J Natl Cancer Inst 1991; 83: 1477–1482

59 Weiss D J, Gurpide E. Non-genomic effects of estrogens and antiestrogens. J Steroid Biochem 1988; 31: 671–676

60 Jordan V C, Fritz N F, Tormey D C. Long term adjuvant therapy with tamoxifen: effects on sex hormone binding globulin and antithrombin 111. Cancer Res 1987; 47: 4517–4519

61 Jordan V C. Molecular mechanisms of antioestrogen action in breast cancer. Breast Cancer Res Treat 1994; 31: 41–52

62 Haran E F, Maretzek A F, Goldberg I, Horowitz A, Degani H. Tamoxifen enhances cell death in implanted MCF7 breast cancer by inhibiting endothelium growth. Cancer Res 1994; 54: 5511–5514

63 Boccardo F, Bruzzi L, Rubbagotti A et al. Estrogen-like action of tamoxifen on vaginal epithelium in breast cancer patients. Oncology 1981; 38: 281–285

64 Lahti E, Vuopala S, Kauppila A et al. Maturation of vaginal and endometrial epithelium in postmenopausal breast cancer patients receiving long-term tamoxifen. Gynecol Oncol 1994; 55: 410–414

65 Ugwumadu A H N, Bower D, Ho P K H. Tamoxifen induced adenomyosis and adenomyomatous endometrial polyp. Br J Obstet Gynaecol 1993; 100: 386–388

66 Cohen I, Beyth Y, Tepper R et al. Adenomyosis in postmenopausal breast cancer patients treated with tamoxifen: a new entity? Gynecol Oncol 1995; 58: 86–91

67 Ford M R W, Turner M J, Wood C et al. Endometriosis developing during tamoxifen therapy. Am J Obstet Gynecol 1988; 158: 119

68 Dallenbach-Hellweg G, Hahn U. Mucinous and clear cell adenocarcinomas of the endometrium in patients receiving antiestrogens (tamoxifen) and gestagens. Int J Gynecol Pathol 1995; 14: 7–15

69 Margriples U, Naftolin F, Schwartz P E, Carcangiu M L. High-grade endometrial carcinoma in tamoxifen-treated breast cancer patients. J Clin Oncol 1993; 11: 485–490

70 Van Leeuwen F E, Benraadt J, Coebergh J W W et al. Risk of endometrial cancer after tamoxifen treatment of breast cancer. Lancet 1994; 343: 448–452

71 Rutqvist L E, Johansson H, Signomklao T et al. Adjuvant tamoxifen therapy for early stage breast cancer and second primary malignancies. J Natl Cancer Inst 1995; 87: 645–651

72 Barakat R R, Wong G, Curtin J P, Vlamis V, Hoskins W J. Tamoxifen use in breast cancer patients who subsequently develop corpus cancer is not associated with a higher incidence of adverse histologic features. Gynecol Oncol 1994; 55: 164–168

73 Groom G V, Griffiths K. Effects of the antioestrogen tamoxifen on the plasma levels of luteinizing hormone, follicle stimulating hormone, prolactin, estradiol and progesterone in normal premenopausal women. J Endocrinol 1976; 70: 421–428

74 Sunderland M C, Osborne C K. Tamoxifen in premenopausal women with metastatic breast cancer: a review. J Clin Oncol 1991; 9: 1283–1297

75 Sawka C A, Pritchard K I, Paterson A H G et al. Role and mechanism of action of tamoxifen in premenopausal women with metastatic breast carcinoma. Cancer Res 1986; 46: 3152–3156

76 Barbieri R L, Ferracci A L, Droesch J N, Rochelson B L. Ovarian torsion in a premenopausal woman treated with tamoxifen for breast cancer. Fertil Steril 1993; 59: 459–460

77 Jolles C J, Smotkin D, Ford K L, Jones K P. Cystic ovarian necrosis complicating tamoxifen therapy for breast cancer in a premenopausal woman. J Reprod Med 1990; 46: 3152–3156

78 Jordan V C, Fritz N F, Tormey D C. Endocrine effects of adjuvant chemotherapy and long-term tamoxifen administration on node-positive patients with breast cancer. Cancer Res 1987; 47: 624–630

79 Mamby C C, Love R R, Kee K E. Thyroid function test changes with adjuvant tamoxifen therapy in postmenopausal women with breast cancer. J Clin Oncol 1995; 13: 854–857

80 Love R R, Wiebe D A, Feyzi J M et al Effects of tamoxifen on cardiovascular risk factors in postmenopausal women after 5 years of treatment. J Natl Cancer Inst 1994; 86: 1534–1539

81 Shewmon D A, Stock J L, Rosen C J et al. Tamoxifen and estrogen lower circulating lipoprotein (a) concentration in healthy postmenopausal women. Arterioscler Thromb 1994; 14: 1586–1593

82 Law M R, Wald N J, Thompson S G. By how much and how quickly does reduction in serum cholesterol concentration lower risk of ischaemic heart disease? BMJ 1994; 308: 367–373

83 Grey A B, Stapleton J P, Evans M C, Reid I R. The effect of the antiestrogen tamoxifen on cardiovascular risk factors in normal postmenopausal women. J Clin Endocrinol Metab 1995; 80: 3191–3195

84 Saphner T, Tromey D C, Gray R. Venous and arterial thrombosis in patients who received adjuvant therapy for breast cancer. J Clin Oncol 1991; 9: 286–294

85 Wickerham DL, Costantino JC, Fisher B. et al. The initial results from NSABP protocol P1: A clinical trial to determine the worth of tamoxifen for preventing breast cancer in women at increased risk. Proc Am Soc Clin Oncol 1998; 17: 3A

86 Powles T J, Hinkish T, Kanis J A, Tidy A, Ashley S. Effect of tamoxifen on bone mineral density measured by dual energy X-ray absorptiometry in healthy premenopausal and postmenopausal women. J Clin Oncol 1996; 14: 78–84

87   Love R R. Tamoxifen in healthy premenopausal women and postmenopausal women: different risks and benefits. J Natl Cancer Inst 1994; 86: 62–63

88   Black L J, Jones C D, Falcone J F. Antagonism of estrogen action with a new benzothiophene derived antiestrogen. Life Sci 1983; 32: 1031–1036

89   Wakeling A E, Valcaccia B, Newboult E et al. Non-steroidal antiestrogen-receptor binding and biological response in rat uterus, rat mammary carcinoma and human breast cancer cells. J Steroid Biochem 1984; 20: 111–120

90   Buzdar A U, Marcus C, Holmes F, Hug V, Hortobagyi G. Phase II evaluation of LY156758 in metastatic breast cancer. Oncology 1988; 45: 344–345

91   Jones C D, Jevinker M G, Pike A J et al. Antiestrogens. LY156758 a remarkably effective estrogen antagonist with only minimal intrinsic estrogenicity. J Med Chem 1984; 27: 1057–1066

92   Bryant H U, Turner C H, Frolick C A et al. Long term effects of raloxifen (LY139478 HCl) on bone, cholesterol and uterus in ovariectomised rats [abstract]. Bone 1995; 16 (Suppl): 116S

93   Brown M S, Goldstein J L. The estradiol-stimulated lipoprotein receptor of rat liver. J Biol Chem 1980; 225: 10464–10471

94   Black L J, Sato M, Rowley E R et al. Raloxifen (LY139478 HCl) prevents bone loss and reduces serum cholesterol without causing uterine hypertrophy in ovariectomized rats. J Clin Invest 1994; 93: 63–69

95   Cummings SR, Black DM, Vogt TM. Changes in BMD substantially underestimate the anti-fracture effects of alendronate and other antiresorptive drugs. J Bone Mineral Res 1996; 11(Suppl 1); S102

96   Yang Na N, Hardikar S, Kim J, Sato M. Raloxifen, an antiestrogen, simulates the effects of estrogen on inhibiting bone resorption through regulating TGF-β_3 expression in bone [abstract]. J Bone Miner Res 1993; 8 (Suppl): S118

97   Bush T L, Helzlsouer K J. Tamoxifen for the primary prevention of breast cancer: a review and critique of the concept of the trial. Epidemiol Rev 1993; 15: 233–243

98   Gail M H, Brinton L A, Byar D P et al. Projecting individualized probabilities of developing breast cancer for white females who are being examined annually. J Natl Cancer Inst 1989; 81: 1879–1886

99   Altaras M, Aviram R, Cohen I et al. Role of prolonged stimulation of tamoxifen therapy in the etiology of endometrial sarcomas. Gynecol Oncol 1993; 49: 255–258

100 Pavlidis N A, Petris C, Briassoulis E et al Clear evidence that long-term low-dose tamoxifen treatment can induce ocular toxicity. Cancer 1992; 69: 2961–2964

101 Powles T, Eeles R, Ashley S. et al. Interim analysis of the incidence of breast cancer in the Royal Marsden Hospital tamoxifen randomised chemoprevention trial. Lancet 1998; 352: 98–101

102 Veronesi U, Maisonneuve P, Costa A. et al. Prevention of breast cancer with tamoxifen: preliminary findings from the Italian trial among hysterectomised women. Lancet 1998; 352: 93-97

103 Ismail S M. Pathology of endometrium treated with tamoxifen. J Clin Pathol 1994; 47: 827–833

104 Perrot N, Guyot B, Antoine M, Uzan S. The effects of tamoxifen on the endometrium. Ultrasound Obstet Gynecol 1994; 4: 83–84

105 Goldstein S R. Unusual ultrasonographic appearance of the uterus in patients receiving tamoxifen. Am J Obstet Gynecol 1994; 170: 447–451

106 Bourne T. Evaluating the endometrium of postmenopausal women with transvaginal ultrasound [opinion]. Ultrasound Obstet Gynecol 1995; 6: 75–80

107 Cohen I, Rosen D J D, Tepper R et al. Ultrasonographic evaluation of the endometrium with correlation to endometrial sampling in postmenopausal women patients treated with tamoxifen. J Ultrasound Med 1993; 5: 275–280

108 Lahti E, Blanco G, Kaupilla A et al. Endometrial changes in postmenopausal breast cancer patients receiving tamoxifen. Obstet Gynecol 1993; 81: 660–664

109 Randolph J, Ying Y, Maier D et al. Comparison of real time ultrasonography, hystrosalpingography and laparoscopy/hysteroscopy in the evaluation of uterine abnormalities and tubal patency. Fertil Steril 1986; 46: 828–832

110 Parsons A, Lense J. Sonohysterography for endometrial abnormalities: preliminary results. J Clin Ultrasound 1993; 21: 87–95

111 Bourne T, Lawton F, Leather A et al. Use of intracavity saline instillation and transvaginal ultrasonography to detect tamoxifen associated endometrial polyps. Ultrasound Obstet Gynecol 1994; 4: 73–75

112 Achiron R, Lipitz S, Sivan E et al. Changes mimicking endometrial neoplasia in postmenopausal, tamoxifen-treated women with breast cancer: a transvaginal Doppler study. Ultrasound Obstet Gynecol 1995; 6: 116–120

113 Kurjak A, Shalan H, Sosic A et al. Endometrial carcinoma in postmenopausal women: evaluation by transvaginal color Doppler ultrasonography. Am J Obstet Gynecol 1994; 169: 1597–1603

114 Bourne T H, Hillard T, Whitehead M I, Crook D, Campbell S. Oestrogens, arterial status and postmenopausal women. Lancet 1990; 335: 1470–1471

115 Stock R, Kanbour A. Prehysterectomy curettage. Obstet Gynecol 1975; 45: 537–541

116 Stovall T, Solomon S, Ling F. Endometrial sampling prior to hysterectomy. Obstet Gynecol 1989; 73: 405–409

117 Ismail S M. Effects of tamoxifen on uterus. Lancet 1994; 334: 662–663

118 Neven P, De Muylder X, Van Belle Y, Vanderick G, De Muylder E. Tamoxifen and the uterus and the endometrium. Lancet 1989; i: 375

119 De Muylder X, Neven P, De Somer M, Van Belle Y, Vanderick G, De Muylder E. Endometrial lesions in patients undergoing tamoxifen therapy. Int J Gynecol Obstet 1991; 36: 127–130

120 Robinson S P, Jordan V C. Reversal of the antitumor effect of tamoxifen by progesterone in the 7,12-dimethylbenzanthracene rat mammary carcinoma model. Cancer Res 1987; 47: 5386–5390

121 Mourisden H T, Ellemann K, Mattson W et al. Therapeutic effect of tamoxifen vs tamoxifen and medroxyprogesterone acetate in advanced breast cancer in postmenopausal women. Cancer Treat Rep 1979; 63: 171–175

122 Anderson K, Mattson L A, Rybo G, Stadberg E. Intrauterine release of levonorgestrel: a new way of adding progestogen in hormone replacement therapy. Obstet Gynecol 1992; 79: 963–967

123 ACOG Committee opinion. Tamoxifen and endometrial cancer. Int J Gynecol Obstet 1996; 53: 197-199

124 Neven P, Vergote I. Should tamoxifen users be screened for endometrial lesions? Lancet 1998; 351: 155-157

125 Neven P, De Muylder X, Van Belle Y, Van Hooff I, Vanderick G. Longitudinal hysteroscopic follow-up during tamoxifen treatment [letter]. Lancet 1998; 351: 36

126 Corley D, Rowe J, Curtis M T et al. Postmenopausal bleeding from unusual polyps endometrial polyps in women on chronic tamoxifen therapy. Obstet Gynecol 1992; 79: 111–116

127 Ugwumadu A H N, Lapsley M. Intrinsic progestogenic effect of tamoxifen on the postmenopausal endometrium. J Obstet Gynaecol 1997; 17: 594–595

A. J. S. Watson S. D. Maguiness

Diagnostic and therapeutic aspects of tubal patency testing

One in six couples present to a health practitioner complaining of infertility and, of these, 14% have a tubal factor.[1] The assessment of patency of the fallopian tubes is an essential part of any infertility work-up. Presently, laparoscopic chromotubation and hysterosalpingography are the most commonly used techniques,[2] but many others have been used and new ones are being described. This review is intended to cover all these methods and, where possible, they will be compared with each other. The confirmation of tubal patency does not necessarily mean that there is normal function.[3-5] As it is believed by many practitioners that there is an enhancement in fecundity after tubal flushing,[6] the possible therapeutic aspect to tubal patency testing will be discussed.

There are essentially 3 categories of tubal patency test. These are: (i) where a test medium is flushed through the cervix into the tubes via the uterine cavity; (ii) direct cannulation of the fallopian tube; and (iii) tests dependent on the transport of particles.

TESTS WHERE MEDIUM IS INTRODUCED TRANSCERVICALLY

The most commonly used investigations all depend on the detection in some way of media in the peritoneal cavity instilled through the cervix. Various methods of passing the substance through the cervix have been described, including Leech Williams cannulas which screw into the cervix; Everard Williams cannulae; and suction cannula,[7] which can be time consuming in

Mr A.J.S. Watson, Senior Registrar, Department of Gynaecology, The Princess Royal Hospital, Saltshouse Road, Hull HU8 9HE, UK

Mr S.D. Maguiness, Consultant, Department of Gynaecology, The Princess Royal Hospital, Saltshouse Road, Hull HU8 9HE, UK

their application and may be impossible to use on an abnormally shaped cervix. The use of a tenculum enables the uterus to be manipulated. Placement of this on the cervix is a cause of pain for some patients which can be reduced by asking the patient to cough vigorously on insertion.[8] Some authorities suggest the use of a paediatric foley catheter,[9] or a special catheter with an intra-uterine balloon.[10] These minimise the need for tenaculum use, but are associated with significant discomfort when the balloon is inflated.

Flushing solutions through the cervix into the fallopian tubes and beyond puts the patient at risk of pelvic inflammatory disease (PID), especially if there is evidence of tubal disease when the test is performed or if there is immunological evidence of *Chlamydia trachomatis*.[11] To minimise this, it has been advocated that prophylactic antibiotics should be given to patients felt to be at risk of post procedure PID.[12]

There is an inherent problem with this form of tubal patency test in that a mobile flap of thickened endometrium adjacent to the tubal ostium can prevent passage into the oviduct of the substance being used to confirm patency. This false negative result can also be due to spasm of the tubal ostia. Various agents such as isoxupine,[13] glucagon,[14] and terbutaline[15] have been tried unsuccessfully to overcome this problem of spasm. Patients who are operated upon for bilateral proximal tubal blockage are confirmed to have tubal occlusion in only 50% of cases when the excised portion of tube is examined histologically.[16] Recently, amorphous material has been described within the tubes which have been found to be aggregates of histiocytes.[17,18] It may be that the difference in false negative rates between various methods of investigating tubal patency simply reflects differing abilities to dislodge these 'plugs'.[6]

Laparoscopic chromotubation (the laparoscopy and dye test)

Endoscopic tubal patency testing was first made popular with the use of the culdoscope but this method has fallen from general use. Laparoscopic chromotubation was first widely used in the early 1970s,[19] and is the main form of tubal assessment in many centres.[1]

Technique
The method of inserting the laparoscope is described in detail elsewhere.[20] Methylene blue dye is transcervically injected into the uterine cavity. Patency of the tube is demonstrated by observing the dye passing into the peritoneal cavity.

Advantages
An assessment of peritubal and other pelvic pathology such as endometriosis can be made. A definitive diagnosis of the presence or absence of adhesions is possible. The procedure can be combined with salpingoscopy and/or hysteroscopy. An adhesiolysis or tubal reconstructive surgery can be performed at the time of investigative surgery. Correct timing of the investigation will enable evidence of ovulation to be obtained by visualisation of a corpus luteum. There is no exposure to radiation.

Table 20.1 Comparison of oil- and water-soluble contrast media at HSG

	Oil-soluble	Water-soluble
Uterine image	Sharp	Less sharp
Ampullary rugae image	Difficult to define	Easier to define
Viscosity	Viscous	Less Viscous
Absorption	Months	Hours
Pain	Minimal	Significant
Granuloma formation	Rare	Very rare
Embolisation	Rare anaphylaxis	No major sequlae
Pregnancy rates after HSG	Doubled	No effect

Disadvantages

This is an invasive test requiring a general anaesthetic with its associated risks. There is a small risk of visceral damage on insertion. It is not always possible to determine the actual site of occlusion in any tube.

Hysterosalpingography

Initial descriptions involved the use of collargol as a contrast medium,[21] but the technique only became popular between the world wars after the introduction of the oily medium lipiodol which causes less abdominal discomfort than the previously used silver based media. There are safety issues associated with the use of lipiodol due to the rare occurrence of pulmonary embolism of intravasated media with associated anaphylaxis.[22] A small number of fatalities have been reported over the years.[23] The medium is very viscous and fills the tubes slowly which necessitates a 24 h film to be performed in a number of cases.[24] Absorption is slow and can take several months. High concentrations of the medium (for instance when trapped within hydrosalpinges) can lead to a granulomatous reaction in the irritated epithelium.[25] Advocates of oily media have advocated flushing of the lipiodol through the tubes with Hartmann's solution to minimise this risk and to reduce the need for a 24 h film.[26] The radiological properties of oil soluble contrast media are such that subtle signs are more difficult to determine than with the more modern media.[27] For these various reasons, water soluble contrast media were introduced in the 1950s. The original water soluble media were hyperosmolar and were associated with a significant amount of pain both during and after the procedure [28]. A recent development in this field is the introduction of non-ionic media which are associated with significantly less pain than the earlier aqueous media.[29] A comparison of the radiological properties of oil and water soluble contrast media is given in Table 20.1.

Technique

Radiological screening is utilised as the medium is instilled; therefore, the procedure can be stopped if intravasation is noted, thus preventing serious sequlae such as embolisation. One or more X-rays are taken so that the investigation can be recorded. Karande[5] measured perfusion pressure and found a lower pregnancy rate when tubal patency was associated with a measured pressure greater than 350 mmHg.

Table 20.2 Cumulative results of studies comparing laparoscopic hydrotubation and HSG to determine tubal patency n = 2473 [31]

	Hysterosalpingogram	
	Both tubes patent	One/both tubes occluded
Lap/dye		
Both patent	1416 (57.3%)	269 (10.9%)
One or both tubes blocked	221 (8.9%)	567 (22.9%)

Advantages
This is a relatively cheap and simple means of tubal patency testing. Evidence of pathology within the uterine cavity can be noted.[30] The position of any tubal occlusion can be noted, and unilateral patency can be differentiated from bilateral patency. The degree of damage to the fallopian endothelium and the presence of peritubal adhesions are assessable. There is no need for general anaesthesia.

Disadvantages
The pelvis including the ovaries is exposed to radiation. This could be a significant problem if the patient had an early pregnancy. Most patients experience some abdominal pain which peaks 5 min after starting the procedure and usually settles within 30 min. These symptoms can be minimised with premedication with a non-steroid anti-inflammatory drug 2 h before the HSG.[8]

Comparison with laparoscopic chromotubation
Although hysterosalpingography is no longer the test most commonly used in clinical practice to assess tubal patency, it can still be regarded as a gold standard, as other investigations tend to be compared with it in the literature. Only a minority of the numerous studies comparing laparoscopic and hysterosalpingographic findings are prospective trials. A recent analysis of 2473 patients from 14 studies revealed an 80.2% agreement between the two different procedures (see Table 20.2).[31] The positive predictive value of bilateral tubal patency was 86% for HSG compared with laparoscopy and 84% for laparoscopy compared with HSG. However, the predictive value of one or both tubes being occluded was 68% for HSG compared with laparoscopy and 72% for laparoscopy compared with HSG.

The high predictive value of a finding of bilateral tubal patency at HSG has lead some to suggest that HSG should be used as an initially screening test for those with infertility with a history that does not suggest tubal pathology.[32] Those 16% of patients with findings suggesting unilateral, or bilateral occlusion[31] could then proceed to laparoscopic chromotubation with sufficient theatre time allocated for laparoscopic tubal surgery to be performed at the same time.

Therapeutic aspects of hysterosalpingography

There are numerous uncontrolled reports of an increased pregnancy rate after tubal patency testing, especially when oil-soluble contrast media is employed.[23]

In fact, repeated tubal flushing was once a recognised treatment for infertility with both oily[33] and aqueous media.[34] A meta-analysis of 829 patients from 6 randomised controlled trials (RCTs) comparing pregnancy rates after HSG with the oil-soluble contrast medium lipiodol and water based media showed a significant benefit with lipiodol (odds ratio 2.09, 95% confidence intervals 1.52–2.86).[35] Various reasons for this near doubling of fecundity have been suggested. There are no RCTs comparing HSG and no treatment and, thus, the observation could in theory be due to a detrimental effect of the water based media. However, 2 non-randomised comparative groups suggest that this is not so.[36,37] Subgroup analysis shows that there is no benefit to patients with tubal infertility suggesting that the therapeutic benefit is not due to an antiseptic effect of the high iodine content of lipiodol. There appears to be most benefit to patients with unexplained infertility (odds ratio 2.67, 95% confidence intervals 1.95–3.81). One possible explanation is that the oily media is more efficient at flushing out plugs.[6] There is now a significant body of animal[37] and in vitro work[39,40] that suggests that the effect may in fact be immunological in basis. Although oily media are now rarely used at HSG, there may be a place for it in the treatment of unexplained infertility.[6]

Methylene blue test

Technique
Methylene blue injected into the uterine cavity can be detected in the Pouch of Douglas by culdocentesis if there is tubal patency.[41]

Advantages
This is a simple low-tech procedure. General anaesthesia and radiation exposure are avoided.

Disadvantages
It is impossible to differentiate between unilateral and bilateral patency. There is a failure rate of performing culdocentesis effectively.

Gas hydrotubation (Rubin's test)

Named after the author of an early description of its use, this was a commonly used investigation prior to the development of hysterosalpingography.[42]

Technique
The original technique was of the passage of 250–300 ml of gas (normally carbon dioxide) through the cervix. Tubal patency was confirmed by the patient complaining of abdominal and shoulder tip pain due to irritation of the peritoneum by the gas. Auscultation over each iliac fossa would reveal bubbling sounds as the gas escaped the tubes. An erect abdominal X-ray revealed subdiapragmatic gas. An adaptation of this technique is to measure the pressure of the insufflating gas using kymography.[43] The pressure measured rises until the gas escapes into the abdominal cavity when it will suddenly fall. With this technique only 30 ml of gas is needed reducing intra and post-procedural pain.

Advantages
This is a simple low tech procedure.

Disadvantages
Technical problems occur with leakage of the gas from the apparatus and out of the cervix. The hyperinflation of hydrosalpinges have been described.[44] It is not possible to differentiate between unilateral and bilateral patency.

Comparison with other techniques
Sobrero et al[45] noted that 59.2% of 500 patients investigated with Rubin's test and hysterosalpingography gave similar results. However, 14% of patients with a normal gas insufflation test revealed some abnormality on their HSG. In a prospective study, the World Health Organization found that, compared with HSG, tubal insufflation had a false positive rate of 42% and a false negative rate of 24% in 363 cases.[46] The same study found that, compared to laparoscopic chromotubation, gas insufflation had a 35% false positive rate and a 38% false negative rate in 180 cases.

Phenolsulphonaphthalein (PSP) test: the Speck test

PSP is absorbed rapidly from the peritoneal cavity but poorly from the reproductive tract.

Technique
A saline solution of PSP is infused into the uterus. The presence of the chemical in urine will suggest tubal patency and can shown by the urine developing a pink colour on adding 10% NaOH.[47]

Advantages
This is a simple, low-tech procedure.

Disadvantages
PSP can be absorbed from the mucosa of hydrosalpinges giving a false positive result of tubal patency. It is impossible to differentiate between unilateral and bilateral patency.

Comparison with other techniques
Gromadski found no significant difference in the results of the PSP test compared with gas insufflation.[48] Speck himself found agreement in 18 of 24 patients investigated with these two tests.[49] However, the diagnosis agreed in only 6 of 10 patients investigated with both the PSP test and HSG.

Investigations of tubal patency using ultrasound

Both transabdominal[7,50] and transvaginal[10,51] ultrasound have been described as modes of assessment of tubal patency. Dextran[52] and isotonic saline[10,51] have both been described as media. Recent work has been published using SH U 454 (Marketed as Echovist, Shearing AG, Germany). This consists of a vial containing 3 g of galactose microparticle granules which, when mixed with the dilutent in another vial, forms a milky echogenic suspension of galactose microparticles and tiny air bubbles.[53]

Technique

Initial transabdominal scanning techniques depended on the detection of insufflated normal saline as fluid accumulating in the Pouch of Douglas.[7] A technique has been described where the pelvis is filled with 300 ml normal saline and the mobility in the tubes can then be assessed by transvaginal scan.[54] Hysterosalpingo contrast synography (HyCoSy) consists of the detection of the flow of a media in the tube. Tufekci suggested that patency could be considered present if forward flow of the medium was noted for at least 5 s between the pars intermuralis and isthmus tubae without interruption in the absence of hydrosalpinges or the detection of turbulence around the fimbrae in the Pouch of Douglas.[51] Deichert found that HyCoSy with normal saline gave total agreement with the findings at HSG or laparoscopic chromotubation in only 1 of 8 patients.[55] He found partial agreement in 5 patients and disagreement in 2. When Echovist was used, 22 of 34 patients had complete agreement compared with HSG or laparoscopic chromotubation. There was partial agreement in 11 patients and there were no disagreements. It thus seems that the use of Echovist improves the accuracy of the test. Doppler ultrasound detects movement and is thus a useful adjunct to transvaginal techniques.[53,56]

Advantages

There is no radiation exposure or need for general anaesthesia. Uterine abnormalities, such as fibroids or septae, can be detected at the time of the investigation.[57] Distending the uterus with normal saline, and to a lesser extent Echovist, enables the configuration of the uterine cavity easier to visualise.[10,50] The ovaries can be assessed.

Disadvantages

The presence of fluid in the Pouch of Douglas may be due to hydrosalpinges, oedematous bowel, or pre-existing fluid and its detection does not differentiate between unilateral and bilateral patency. HyCoSy with Echovist is contraindicated in patients with galactosaemia.[55] A significant degree of operator transvaginal scanning skill is required to perform the investigation accurately.[2] Turbulence within a hydrosalpinx can be misdiagnosed as indicating tubal patency.[2] Transvaginal Doppler ultrasound machines are presently expensive.

Comparison with other techniques

Data from a large multicentre study[58] are summarised in Table 20.3. The concordance between HyCoSy with Echovist and laparoscopic chromotubation was 86.6% in 438 tubes. The concordance of HyCoSy with HSG was 83.8% in 136 tubes.

Radiolabelled gas

Technique

A solution of xenon 133 in 10 ml of saline is infused over 1 min transcervically into the uterine cavity. The detection of radioactivity over the adnexae with a gamma camera suggests tubal patency.

Table 20.3 Results of multicentre study comparing HyCoSy with laparoscopy and HSG[58]

Comparison of laparoscopic chromotubation and HyCoSy		
	HyCoSy	
	Not Patent	Patent
Lap and dye		
Not Patent	77	15
Patent	45	301
Comparison of HSG and HyCoSy		
	HyCoSy	
	Not Patent	Patent
HSG		
Not Patent	29	7
Patent	15	85

Advantages
There is no need for general anaesthesia.

Disadvantages
The pelvis is exposed to radiation.

Comparison with other techniques
In a study involving 30 patients, identical results were obtained with this technique compared with HSG.[59]

DIRECT CANNULATION OF THE FALLOPIAN TUBES

When cornual occlusion is found, only 'about half' of patients undergoing corrective surgery have histological confirmation of the diagnosis.[16] For the remainder, the finding is due to spasm, a mobile flap of endometrium, or tubal plugs of debris. It is thus very important to confirm the diagnosis prior to initiating treatment. In addition, even occluded tubes can now be corrected with techniques utilising direct cornual cannulation with consequent financial savings.[60] The main described complication for these procedures is isthmic perforation which seems to have no immediate significant sequelae.[4,61,62]

Direct cannulation can be performed hysteroscopically,[17,62,63] under radiological control,[4,64] or under tactile control with ultrasonic confirmation of successful recannulation.[60,65]

Technique
Hysteroscopic techniques require general anaesthesia especially if laparoscopic chromotubation is performed to confirm patency at the end. The other means of proximal tubal recannulation require sedation and analgesia,[65] but can normally be performed as an out-patient procedure.

Using an operating hysteroscope, a 0.97 mm guidewire with a flexible tip is passed through the ostium. When the wire is seen laparoscopically to be in the ampulla, it is withdrawn and chromotubation then performed to confirm successful recannulation.[62] Using this technique, Deaton showed there were 4 pregnancies from 7 patients who initially had bilateral proximal occlusion [62].

To perform selective salpingography, a 5.5 Fr preformed catheter is introduced into the uterine cavity via an HSG catheter. Under direct fluoroscopy, the ostium is cannulated and a contrast media gently injected to confirm tubal occlusion. A 0.38 mm wire with a soft platinum tip is then gently introduced into the tube. A 3 Fr catheter is then passed over the guide wire through the obstruction.[60] Using a similar method, Hovsepian et al managed to recannulate 45 of 63 tubes.[66] There were 25 successful procedures in 29 patients with either bilateral proximally obstructed tubes or unilateral in a patient with only one tube. Nine (36%) of these patients conceived. There were 3 live births, and 2 ectopics in this group. Hayashi et al were disappointed that, although they achieved patency in 96% of 42 patients with bilateral proximal occlusion, only 3 live pregnancies occurred.[4] Thurmond, in a recent study, achieved with this technique an intra-uterine pregnancy rate of 20.7% in 19 patients with bilateral occlusion due to salpingitis isthmica nodosa.[67]

A combination of HSG and selective salpingography has been used to differentiate between failing intra-uterine pregnancies and tubal ectopics.[68]

To perform tubal recatheterisation under purely tactile control requires a high degree of skill.[65] The use of transvaginal scanning with a contrast media allows determination of success. Because there is no radiation, multiple attempts at recannulation can be performed without undue worry of time scale.

TESTS DEPENDENT ON PARTICULAR TRANSPORT

Investigations where particular transport is used to determine tubal patency can be divided into ascending tests, where the particles are placed at the cervix and patency is suggested by finding them in the abdominal cavity, and descending tests. where the opposite is true. It is unknown how the transport occurs but the epithelial cilia may have a role.

Microsphere migration

This ascending test depends on active transport of radiolabelled microspheres from the cervical mucus through the upper genital tract.

Technique
A suspension of human albumin particles measuring 15–35 µg labelled with technetium 99 is injected into the cervical mucus with a blunt needle.[69] Care is taken to ensure that the suspension is not injected through the os, as it would be impossible to determine whether tubal filling was by active transport or by hydrostatic pressure. The test is most accurate around the time of ovulation.[70] A gamma camera measures radioactivity. Serial imaging for up to 4 h may be required. Patency is indicated on imaging by adnexal hot spots.

Advantages
Gives an indication of function as well as patency of the tubes. General anaesthesia is not required. The procedure is pain free.

Disadvantages
Radiation exposure was initially measured to be approximately 25 times higher than with hysterosalpingography.[71] More recent studies have suggested that radiation exposure to the ovaries between the 2 investigations is equivalent or even reduced with this study.[72] Because of anatomical variability, it can prove impossible to determine if there is unilateral or bilateral tubal patency. It is difficult to differentiate between patency and migration of the microspheres into a distended hydrosalpinx.[73]

Comparison with other techniques
A significant number of patients who do not have evidence of tubal patency are found to have tubal pathology at laparoscopy, even if chromotubation reveals patency.[73] Because of the disadvantages mentioned above, even advocates of this technique suggest that it should in general be used in conjunction with some other technique of tubal patency testing.[73]

Other ascending tests dependent on the transport of particles

The detection of sperm by culdocentesis or endoscopy within the Pouch of Douglas confirms tubal patency. The test suffers from the same technical problems as the methylene blue test.

'Descending tests'

Various descending tests have been described. Decker and Decker described the use of starch.[74]

Technique
A sterile specimen of starch is deposited over the fimbrae by culdoscopy or needling of the Pouch of Douglas. After 24 h, the cervical mucus is sampled with pipelle. The material is stained with iodine. The presence of starch and, therefore, patency is confirmed by the detection of blue granules.

Advantages
A relative cheap, low-tech procedure. Gives evidence of tubal function as well as patency.

Disadvantages
It is impossible to differentiate between unilateral and bilateral patency.

Other descending tests dependent on transport

Other media that have been used in this fashion include gold given as a suspension of microparticles by injection into the peritoneal cavity through the abdominal walls. Detection of the particles on a cotton plug left occluding the cervix for several hours indicated tubal patency.[75]

CONCLUSIONS

There is no ideal test to determine tubal patency. Many authorities use 2 complimentary investigations.[2,73] Laparoscopic chromotubation is the only method that gives a definitive diagnosis of peritubal adhesions. However, the high concordance levels of HSG and HyCoSy with laparoscopy suggests that they could be used as screening tests. The minority of patients with borderline test results or failing to conceive within a set time after initial investigation would then progress to laparoscopic chromotubation with sufficient time allotted to perform laparoscopic tubal surgery or adhesiolysis as deemed necessary.

REFERENCES

1 Hull M G R, Glazener C M A, Kelly N J et al. Population study of causes, treatment, and outcome of infertility. BMJ 1985; 291: 1693–1697

2 Campbell S, Bourne T H, Tan S L, Collins W P. Hysterosalpingo contrast sonography HyCoSy and its future role within the investigation of infertility in Europe. Ultrasound Obstet Gynecol 1994; 4: 245–253

3 Steck T, Wurfel W, Becker W, Albert P J. Serial scintigraphic imaging for visualization of passive transport processes in the human fallopian tube. Hum Reprod 1991; 6: 1186–1189

4 Hayashi N, Kimoto T, Sakai T et al. Fallopian tube disease: limited value of treatment with fallopian catheterisation. Radiology 1994; 190: 141–143

5 Karande V C, Pratt D E, Rabin D S, Gleicher N. The limited value of hysterosalpingography in assessing tubal status and fertility potential. Fertil Steril 1995; 63: 1167–1171

6 Watson A, Vandekerckhove P, Lilford R, Vail A, Brosens I, Hughes E. A meta-analysis of the therapeutic role of oil soluble contrast media at hysterosalpingography: a surprising result? Fertil Steril 1994; 61: 470–477

7 Rasmussen F, Larsen C, Justesen P. Fallopian tube patency demonstrated at ultrasonography. Acta Radiol 1986; 27: 61–63

8. Owens O M, Schiff I, Kaul A F, Cramer D C, Burt R A P. Reduction of pain following hysterosalpingogram by prior analgesic administration. Fertil Steril 1985; 43: 146–148

9 Ansari A H. Foley catheter for salpingography, Tubal insufflation and hydrotubation. Obstet Gynecol 1977; 50: 108–112

10 Balen F G, Allen C M, Siddle N C, Lees W R. Ultrasound contrast hysterosalpingo-graphy – evaluation as an outpatient procedure Br J Radiol 1993; 66: 592–599.

11 Forsey J P, Caul E O, Paul I D, Hull M G R. *Chlamydia trachomatis*, tubal disease and the incidence of symptomatic and asymptomatic infection following hysterosalpingography. Hum Reprod 1990; 5: 444–447

12 Pittaway D E, Winfield A C, Maxson W, Daniell J, Herbert C, Colston Wentz A. Prevention of acute pelvic inflammatory disease after hysterosalpingography: efficacy of doxycycline prophylaxis. Am J Obstet Gynecol 1983; 147: 623–626

13 Page E P. Use of isoxuprine in hysterosalpingography and uterotubal insufflation. Am J Obstet Gynecol 1968; 101: 358–364

14 World Health Organization. A new hysterographic approach to the evaluation of tubal spasm and spasmolytic agents. Fertil Steril 1983; 39: 105–107

15 Thurmond A S, Novy M, Uchida B T. Terbutaline in diagnosis of interstitial fallopian tube obstruction. Invest Radiol 1988; 23: 209–213

16 Grant A. Infertility surgery of the oviduct. Fertil Steril 1971; 22: 496–503

17 Sulak P J, Letterie G S, Hayslip C C, Coddington C C, Klein T A. Hysteroscopic cannu-lation and lavage in the treatment of proximal tubal occlusion. Fertil Steril 1987; 48: 493–49

18 Kerin J, Surrey E, Williams D, Daykhovsky L, Grundfest W. Falloscopic observations of endotubal isthmic plugs as a cause of reversible obstruction and their histological characterisation. J Laparoendosc Surg 1991; 1: 103–110

19 Duignan N M, Jordan J A, Coughlan B M. One thousand cases of diagnostic laparoscopy. J Obstet Gynaecol Br Commonw 1972; 79: 1016–1024

20 Fergusson I L C. Laparoscopic investigation of tubal infertility. In: Chamberlain G, Winston R. (eds) Tubal infertility diagnosis and treatment. Oxford: Blackwell, 1992; 30–46

21 Cary W H. Note on determination of patency of fallopian tubes by the use of collargol and x-ray shadow. Am J Obstet Dis Women Child 1914; 69: 462–466

22 Nunley W C, Bateman B G, Kitchen J D, Pope T L. Intravasation during hysterosalpingography using oil base contrast media, a second look. Obstet Gynecol 1987; 70: 309–312

23 Soules, M R. Spadoni L R. Oil versus aqueous media for hysterosalpingography: a continuing debate based on many opinions and few facts. Fertil Steril 1982; 38: 1–11

24 Bateman B G, Nunley W C, Kitchin J D, Kaiser D L. Utility of the 24 hour delay hysterosalpingogram film. Fertil Steril 1987; 47: 613–617

25 Eisenberg A D, Winfield A C, Page D L, Holburn G E, Schiffer T, Segars J H. Peritoneal reaction resulting from iodinated contrast material: comparative study. Radiology 1989; 172: 149–151

26 Byeth Y, Navot D, Lax E. A simple improvement in the technique of hysterosalpingography achieving optimal imaging and avoiding possible complications. Fertil Steril 1985; 44: 543–545

27 Lindequist S, Justesen P, Larsen C, Rasmussen F. Diagnostic quality and complications of hysterosalpingography: oil versus water soluble media. A randomized prospective study. Radiology 1991; 179: 69–74

28 Moore D E. Pain associated with hysterosalpingography: ethiodol versus salpix media. Fertil Steril 1982; 38: 629–631

29 Brokensha C, Whitehouse G. A comparison between iotrolan, a non-ionic dimer, and a hyperosmolar contrast medium, urograffin, in hysterosalpingography. Br J Radiol 1991; 64: 587–590

30 Snowden E U, Jarrett J C, Dawood M Y. Comparison of diagnostic accuracy of laparoscopy, hysteroscopy, and hysterosalpingography in the evaluation of female infertility. Fertil Steril 1984; 41: 709–713

31 Maguiness S D, Djahanbakhch O, Grudzinskas J G. Assessment of the fallopian tube. Obstet Gynecol Surv 1992; 47: 587–603

32 Watson A J S, Lilford R J. Is there still a place for open access tubal surgery in infertility – the case against. Adv Obstet Gynaecol 1995; 109: 12–15

33 Rutherford R N. The therapeutic value of repetitive lipiodol tubal insufflations. West J Surg Obstet Gynaecol 1948; 56: 145–154

34 Arronet G H, Eduljee S Y, O'Brien J R. A nine year survey of fallopian tube dysfunction in human infertility. Fertil Steril 1969; 20: 903–918

35 Vandekerckhove P, Watson A, Lilford R, Harada T, Hughes E. Therapeutic effect of oil-soluble and water-soluble media used for tubal patency testing (hysterosalpingography or laparoscopy). In: Farquhar C, Barlow D, Cooke et al (eds). Menstrual disorders and subfertility module of the Cochrane Database of Sytematic Reviews [updated 01 December 1997]. Available in the Cochrane Library [datbase on disk and CD-ROM]. The Cochrane Collaboration; Issue 1. Oxford: Update Software; 1998. Updated Quarterly

36 Weir W C, Weir D R. Therapeutic value of salpingograms in infertility. Fertil Steril 1951; 2: 514–522

37 Rasmusssen F, Lindequist S, Larsen C, Justesen P. Therapeutic effect of hysterosalpingography: oil-versus water- soluble contrast media – a randomized prospective study. Radiology 1991; 179: 75–78

38 Sawatari Y, Horii T, Hoshiai H. Oily contrast medium as a therapeutic agent for infertility because of mild endometriosis. Fertil Steril 1993; 59: 907–911

39 Johnson J V, Montoya I A, Olive D L. Ethiodol oil contrast medium inhibits macrophage phagocytosis and adherence by altering membrane electronegativity and microviscosity. Fertil Steril 1992; 58: 511–517

40 Goodman S B, Rein M S, Hill J A. Hysterosalpingography contrast media and chromotubation dye inhibit peritoneal lymphocyte and macrophage function in vitro: a potential mechanism for fertility enhancement. Fertil Steril 1993; 59: 1022–1027

41 Ansari A H. Tubal patency evaluation by the methylene blue test. Am J Obstet Gynecol 1969; 103: 1170–1175

42 Rubin I C. The non operative determination of patency of fallopian tubes: preliminary report. JAMA 1920; 74: 1017

43 Furniss H D. The Rubin test simplified. Surg Gynecol Obstet 1921; 33: 567–568

44 Sweeney W J. Pitfalls in present day methods of evaluating tubal function. 1: Tubal insufflation. Fertil Steril 1962; 48: 113–117

45 Sobrero A J, Silberman C J, Post A, Cimer L. Tubal insufflation and hysterosalpingography. A comparative study in 500 infertile couples. Obstet Gynecol 1961; 18: 91–93

46 World Health Organization. Comparative trial of tubal insufflation, hysterosalpingography and laparoscopy with dye hydrotubation for assessment of tubal patency. Fertil Steril 1986; 46: 1101–1107

47 Speck G. Phenolsulfonaphthalein as a test for the determination of tubal patency. Am J Obstet Gynecol 1948; 55: 1048–1052

48 Gromadzki W, Lukasik J, Papierowski Z. A comparative evaluation of the phenolsulphonaphthalein test and the Rubin test for tubal patency. Am J Obstet Gynecol 1963; 92: 1094–1101

49 Speck G. The revised PSP Speck test for tubal patency. South Med J 1967; 60: 1187–1190

50 Randolf J R, Ying Y K, Maier D B, Schmidt C L, Riddick D H. Comparison of real time ultrasonography, hysterosalpingography, and laparoscopy/hysteroscopy in the evaluation of uterine abnormalities and tubal patency. Fertil Steril 1986; 46: 828–832

51 Tufekci E C, Girit S, Bayirli E, Durmusoglu F, Yalti S. Evaluation of tubal patency by transvaginal sonosalpigography. Fertil Steril 1992; 57: 336–340

52 Shapiro B S, DeCherney A H. Ultrasound and infertility. J Reprod Med 1989; 34: 151–155

53 Deichert U, Schlief R, van de Sandt M, Daume E. Transvaginal hysterosalpingo-contrast sonography for the assessment of tubal patency with gray scale imaging and the additional use of pulsed wave Doppler. Fertil Steril 1992; 57: 62–67

54 Allahbadia G N. Fallopian tubes and ultrasonography: the Sion experience. Fertil Steril 1992; 58: 901–907

55 Deichert U, Schlief R, van de Sandt M, Juhnke I. Transvaginal hysterosalpingo-contrast-sonography Hy-Co-Sy compared with conventional tubal diagnostics. Hum Reprod 1989; 4: 418–424

56 Peters A J, Coulam C B. Hysterosalpingography with color Doppler ultrasonography. Am J Obstet Gynecol 1991; 164: 1530–1534

57 Mitri F F, Andronikow A D, Perpinyal S, Hofmeyr G R, Sonnendecker E W W. A clinical comparison of sonographic hydrotubation and hysterosalpingography. Br J Obstet Gynaecol 1991; 98: 1031–1036

58 Schurmann R J, Schlief R. Transvaginale Hysterosalpingo-Kontrastsonographie mit Echovist: ein nues Verfahren zur Diagnostik von Tubendurchgangigkeit und Uterusanomalien. In: Ertan A K, Schmidt W. (eds) Jahrbuch der Gynakologie und Geburtschlife. Zulpich: Biermann, 1993; 211–216

59 Pertynski T, Jakubowski W, Stelmachow J, Grabon W, Zurowski S. A scintographic method of examining the patency of oviducts using ^{133}Xe. Eur J Nucl. Med 1977; 2: 159–164

60 Maroulis G B, Yeko T R. Treatment of cornual obstruction by transvaginal cannulation without hysteroscopy or fluoroscopy. Fertil Steril 1992; 57: 1136–1138

61 Novy M J, Thurmond A S, Patton P, Uchida B T, Rosch J. Diagnosis of cornual obstruction by transcervical fallopian tube cannulation. Fertil Steril 1988; 50: 434–440

62 Deaton J L, Gibson M, Riddick D H, Brumsted J R. Diagnosis and treatment of cornual obstruction using a flexible tip guidewire. Fertil Steril 1990; 53: 232–236

63 Confino E, Friberg J, Gleicher N. Transcervical balloon tuboplasty. Fertil Steril 1986; 46: 963–965

64 Martensson O, Nilsson B, Ekelund L, Johansson J, Wickman G. Selective salpingography and fluoroscopic transcervical salpingoplasty for diagnosis and treatment of proximal fallopian tube occlusions. Acta Obstet Gynecol Scand 1993; 72: 458–464

65 Lisse K, Sydow P. Fallopian tube catheterization and recanalization under ultrasonic observation: a simplified technique to evaluate tubal patency and open proximally obstructed tubes. Fertil Steril 1991; 56: , 198–201

66 Hovsepian D M, Bonn J, Eschelman D J, Shapiro M J, Sullivan K L, Gardiner G A. Fallopian tube recanalization in an unrestricted patient population. Radiology 1994; 190: 137–140

67 Thurmond A S, Burry K A, Novy M J. Salpingitis isthmica nodosua: results of transcevical fluoroscopic catheter recannalization. Fertil Steril 1995; 63: 715–722

68 Gleicher N, Parrilli M, Pratt D E. Hysterosalpingography and selective salpingography in the differential diagnosis of chemical intrauterine versus tubal pregnancy. Fertil Steril 1992; 57: 553–558

69 McCalley M G, Braunstein P, Stone S, Henderson P, Egbert R. Radionuclide hysterosalpingography for evaluation of tube patency. J Nucl Med 1985; 26: 868–874

70 Arduini D, Valenza V, Pietrangeli D et al. A new radioisotopic method in the study of female reproductive apparatus. Nucl Compact 1985; 16: 66–70

71 Van der Weiden R M F, van Zijl J. Radiation exposure of the ovaries during hsterosalpingography. Is radionuclide hysterosalpingography justified? Br J Obstet Gynaecol 1989; 96: 471–472

72 Becker W, Steck T, Albert P, Borner W. Hysterosalpingography: a simple and accurate method of evaluating fallopian tube patency. Nucl Med 1988; 27: 252–257

73 McQueen D, McKillop J H, Gray H W, Bessent R G, Black W P. Investigation of tubal infertility by radionuclide migration. Hum Reprod 1991; 6: 529–532

74 Decker A, Decker W H. A tubal function test. Obstet Gynecol 1954; 4: 35–38

75 Caballero A, Hurtado E, Perez-Modrego S, Lasa E. Studies of the patency and function of apprehension and transportation of the fallopian tube with Au198. Am J Obstet Gynecol 1964; 90: 437–442

U. B. Knudsen J. Aagaard

Acute pelvic pain

The definition of acute pelvic pain (APP) is arbitrary. Often duration is only a few hours, but it can be days. It usually presents with a sudden onset, but may be insidious and the pain just increasing with time.

EPIDEMIOLOGY

The incidence of the different aetiologies of acute pelvic pain during a certain period is difficult to estimate. It is influenced by several factors, e.g. different medical practice, the distance to medical care and the age profile of the population in a certain area. In a 10 week period, 425 patients attended the gynaecological/obstetric department in Aarhus, Denmark, with acute pelvic problems. Of these women, 56% were pregnant with symptoms of imminent abortion. Of the 188 patients with gynaecological problems, 26% were seen at the hospital because extra-uterine pregnancy was suspected: 14% (7/49) of these women had a laparoscopy performed on the day of admittance. A further 24% attended the ward because of sequelae following an operation, more than

Table 21.1 Keypoints in the woman's history for assessing acute pelvic pain

Location
Mode of onset
Constant versus colic pain
Radiation
Relation to menstrual cycle

Dr U. B. Knudsen, Department of Obstetrics and Gynecology, Skejby Sygehus, Aarhus University Hospital, DK 8200 Aarhus N, Denmark

Dr J. Aagaard, Department of Obstetrics and Gynecology, Skejby Sygehus, Aarhus University Hospital, DK 8200 Aarhus N, Denmark

Correspondence to Dr U.B. Knudsen, Casper Mollers vej 5, DK-8240 Risskov, Denmark

half of them (53%) following termination of pregnancy (TOP). Six women had a suspected torsion of the adnexa (only one actually had this condition) and were operated on immediately; 8.5% had symptoms of PID; and 12% had abdominal pain without obvious cause (U.B. Knudsen, personal observation).

HISTORY

The history is extremely important when seeing a patient with acute pelvic pain. The description of the pain is also very important and the specific points summarised in Table 21.1 should always be covered. For women of reproductive age it is important to ask the following questions: the date of her last menstrual period (LMP), the regularity of the periods, contraception, any vaginal discharge, pyrexia, previous operations, current medication, other family members with similar symptoms, and recent journeys abroad. Furthermore, it is important to ask about gastrointestinal and urological symptoms, such as heartburn, nausea, vomiting, diarrhoea, frequency, dysuria or haematuria.

PHYSICAL EXAMINATION

The patient's behaviour must be observed. Is the patient able to move easily in the bed, or is she lying crouched up in the bed hardly moving. Abdominal exam-ination is mandatory: the location of the pain? Right side only (appendicitis?). Left side (diverticulitis?, constipation?), both sides (salpingitis?). A diagnosis of unilateral salpingitis can not be made until the pelvic organs have been visualised either by laparoscopy or laparotomy. Is there direct or rebound tenderness. Is there tenderness in the region of the kidneys? Look for a hernia, and auscultate for bowel sounds? Women, who have had their sexual début, always have to have a gynaecological examination. Vaginal discharge should be looked for, the smell noted and swabs (high vaginal or endocervical) obtained for examination by microscopy and inoculations for micro-organisms are obtained. Bleeding, products of conception in the cervical canal or cervical pathology (e.g. ectopion) should be excluded.

To assess the size of the uterus and the location of pain in relation to the uterus, bimanual palpation is performed together with palpation of the adnexae for

Table 21.2   Primary investigations of a patient with acute pelvic pain

Mid-stream urine specimen Swabs (high vaginal and endocervical) for micro-organisms Blood samples: haemoglobin, white blood cell count, CRP Pregnancy test (βhCG): urinary or serum βhCG

Table 21.3   Secondary investigations of a patient with pelvic pain

Ultrasound scan: vaginal/abdominal Operation: laparoscopy, laparotomy

enlarged ovaries, cysts, tubal pregnancy, or pyo-ovarial abscesses. Furthermore, a rectal examination must be performed to gain all relevant information and to exclude fresh blood (rectal tumour).

INVESTIGATIONS

The primary investigations of a patient with acute pelvic pain that should be performed routinely are summarised in Table 21.2. Depending on the results obtained, further investigations may be required (Table 21.3).

DISEASES

Diseases will be discussed in relation to: (i) premenarche; (ii) fertile status (gynaecological and obstetric); (iii) postmenopause; and finally (iv) non gynaecological diseases.

Premenarche

In the premenarche, APP most often is related to non-gynaecological diseases. Torsion of an ovarian cyst is rare, but Meyers et al[1] reviewed their recent experience with 12 children with 13 episodes of ovarian torsion. Of these 12 patients, three presented as neonates, six were premenarchal, and three were postmenarchal. Torsion of an ovarian cyst usually starts with a sudden onset of colicky pelvic pain, often located to one or other of the fossae. Later, the pain may become more constant, or after several hours even disappear. Usually the cysts are benign tumours (dermoids), but malignant tumours occasionally occur. Usually there are no gastrointestinal symptoms, although sometimes vomiting occurs. Furthermore, in the first hours the patient is usually apyrexic, but if the torsion is not operated on within these first few hours, necrosis can occur, resulting in pyrexia. Detorsion of the ischaemic adnexa appears to be successful.[2]

Persistent hymen can result in APP. Abdominal ultrasound reveals a solid mass in the vagina and, if a vaginal examination is attempted, the hymen will be visualised with a blue background due to altered blood. A small operation making an incision in the hymen, relieves the pain. Diseases in the premenarche are summarised in Table 21.4.

Table 21.4 Diseases in the premenarche

Torsion (cysts, adnexa)
Rupture of cysts
Persistent hymen (haematocolpos)

Fertile women

After the menarche, the origin of APP in fertile women can be due to gynaecological, pregnancy related (Table 21.5) or non-gynaecological causes (discussed later).

Table 21.5 Diseases in fertile women divided into gynaecological and obstetric causes

GYNAECOLOGICAL	OBSTETRIC
Pelvic inflammatory disease (PID)	
Sexual transmitted disease (STD)	I. Trimester
Iatrogenic PID	Sub-chorionic haematoma
termination of pregnancy (TOP)	
intra-uterine contraceptive device (IUCD)	II. Trimester
hystero-salpingo-graphy (HSG)	Abruption
hysteroscopy	Fibroids (necrosis)
Tubo-ovarian abscess	
pyo-ovary	III. Trimester
Ectopic pregnancy	Partial abruption
Miscarriage	Abruption
Cysts: rupture, torsion	Braxton-Hicks contractions
Complications to assisted reproduction:	Contractions
PID	
Hyperstimulation syndrome	**Postpartum**
Torsion of adnexa	Paravaginal haematoma
Mittelschmerz	Contractions
Hematometra (cervical stenosis)	Urinary retention
Fibroids (necrosis)	
Urinary retention	
Abscesses (external genital)	

Gynaecological diseases in fertile women

Pelvic inflammatory disease (PID) indicates an upper genital tract infection. Current estimates from industrialized countries indicate an annual incidence of PID of 9.5–14 cases per 1000 women in their fertile years.[3] PID is the most common cause of hospitalization among reproductive-age women based on the average annual discharge summaries in the US.[4] The infection may involve the endometrium, tubes and the ovaries.

Salpingitis can either be due to sexually transmitted disease (STD) or iatrogenic, e.g. by hystero-salpingo-graphy, or instrumentation of the uterine cavity, i.e. termination of pregnancy (TOP), hysteroscopy or after insertion of IUCD. The most common cause of STD is *Chlamydia trachomatis*, accounting for around 50% of the cases, whereas *Neisseria gonorrhoea* now is rare in the Scandinavian countries.[3] The spectrum of symptoms of salpingitis is wide ranging, from no symptoms at all to a clinical picture presenting with some or all of the symptoms seen in Table 21.6.

No single clinical or laboratory finding is pathognomonic for salpingitis. In addition, pain located in the right hypogastric area (Fitz-Hugh-Curtis syndrome) due to *Chlamydia trachomatis* infection can occur. The diagnosis is often made without sufficient investigation. This is accepted practice because hesitation can cause significant morbidity in women of the childbearing age and more intensive investigations, i.e. laparoscopy, seldom change the management. The consequences of the PID depend on the severity. The earlier antibiotic treatment is introduced, the better.

Approximately 75% of women with salpingitis have never been pregnant, and infection of the salpinx has the most important prognostic consequences

Table 21.6 Frequency of signs and symptoms of salpingitis (modified with permission from Mårdh et al[3])

	% (n = 623)
Low abdominal pain	100.0
Metrorrhagia	35.5
Urethritis symptoms	18.6
Lower genital tract infection (LGTI)	
Purulent vaginal content on microscopy	100.0
Symptoms of discharge	54.6
Vomiting or nausea	10.3
Proctitis symptoms	6.9
Fever (> 38°C) at admission	32.9
Palpable adnexal swelling	49.4

for fertility (see Fig. 21.1, Weström et al[5]). Following PID, the rate of ectopic pregnancy is 10-fold higher than that in women who never had the disease.

Termination of pregnancy (TOP) results in around 0.5–3.2% of PID.[6] The experience of the staff performing the operation and the accuracy of the documentation of complications influence the number recorded. Screening for *Chlamydia* infection prior to TOP is now recommended in most Western countries. Retained products in the uterine cavity are usually the main cause of infection following TOP, and re-evacuation under antibiotic cover is necessary.

PID after hysteroscopy is rare. In a follow-up study including more than 500 out-patient hysteroscopies, no PID were reported (S. Duffy MD, St James's University Hospital, Leeds, UK, personal communication). Postoperative infection after transcervical resection of the endometrium (TCRE) was seen in 24 (6%) of 412 patients.[7]

The role of IUCDs in the spread of PID is controversial. By the mid-1980s, several studies had reported an increased risk of PID among IUCD-users as compared with non-users, whereas recent re-analysis show that IUCDs per se, especially the medicated ones, are not associated with increased risk of PID,

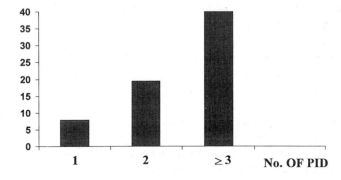

% OF TUBAL OCCLUSION

Fig. 21.1 The diagram shows the rate of tubal factor infertility in relation to episodes of PID. Modified with permission from Weström et al.[5]

nor are they associated with an increased risk of ectopic pregnancy or subsequent infertility.[8]

The most frequent complication of PID is the development of a tubo-ovarian abscess, occurring in up to 30% of hospitalized patients.[9]

Vaginal bleeding and APP are common signs of spontaneous abortion. The overall risk for spontaneous abortion was 11% in a unselected Danish population including approximately 300 500 pregnancies.[10] In an ultrasound screening study at 10–13 weeks of gestation, the prevalence of early pregnancy failure was 2.8% (501 cases out of 17 870 women). The prevalence was higher in women with a history of vaginal bleeding.[11] In a study of 347 patients with confirmed viable intra-uterine pregnancy between 6 and 14 weeks of gestation, women with vaginal bleeding had a significant higher risk of miscarriage (12.7%) than women without vaginal bleeding (4.2%).[12]

Ectopic pregnancy is the fourth most common cause of maternal death during pregnancy ,and accounts for about 10% of total maternal death in the UK.[13] The clinical diagnosis of ectopic pregnancy still remains a challenge for the gynaecologist and the diagnosis is only correct in less than 50% of cases.[14] Abdominal pain is the commonest symptom, often associated with rebound tenderness, and is frequently present before rupture. The pain can be ipsilateral, bilateral or even contralateral to the site of the ectopic. Amenorrhoea is reported in 75–95% of patients. The last menstrual period is often described as lighter than normal and may occur earlier or later than expected.

The development of high resolution ultrasound scan and sensitive human chorionic gonadotropin (β-hCG) assays has made early detection of tubal pregnancy easier. Transvaginal ultrasound scan allows identification of intra-uterine pregnancies at a β-hCG level of 1000 IU/l and can, therefore, confirm or exclude an intra-uterine pregnancy in suspected cases of ectopic pregnancy. If the pregnancy has been found to be intra-uterine, ectopic pregnancy is unlikely, because the combination of intra-uterine and ectopic pregnancy is rare (1:4000–15 000 in spontaneous conception[15,16]) and (1:100 after assisted reproductive technology[17,18]).

Torsion of adnexa, cysts or fibroids are also seen in the APP clinic. Often only an operation (laparoscopy/tomy) can differentiate. Traditionally salpingo-oophorectomy has been carried out. Detorsion of twisted ischemic adnexa can be carried out either laparoscopically, or at laparotomy and seems to be safe and 'adnexal-sparing'. Long-term follow-up of the twisted ischemic adnexa managed by detorsion in 40 patients has shown that this approach has a high success rate as measured by subsequent follicular development, which was demonstrated in 35 of 37 patients (3 were lost to follow-up).[2] Of the removed cysts at detorsion, 9 out of 15 were functional, whereas 2 were dermoids, 2 simple neoplastic cysts, and one serous and one mucinous cystadenomas. The postoperative course was uneventful, except for a transient temperature elevation in five patients. Some authors report success from Doppler ultrasound examination to differentiate between healthy, viable ovaries and ovaries that need to be removed,[19,20] whereas others describe the usefulness of colour Doppler ultrasonography to be limited due to the non-specificity.[21]

Dermoid cysts/teratomas often present with pain, an abdominal tumour, and metromenorrhagia. Of 286 cases of teratomas, only 7.7% appeared with torsion. Bilaterality was found in around 15%.[22,23] The rate of malignant transformation of dermoid cysts was 0.9% overall, but 4.3% in patients over 40 years.[23]

Rupture of a cyst is often an 'exclusion diagnosis'. At times, endometriosis can appear as APP, often due to bleeding from an endometriosis cyst.

Ovulation pain (Mittelschmerz) occurs at mid cycle with sudden onset and sharp lower abdominal pain followed by several hours of dull aching in the pelvis. The onset of pain most frequently corresponds to the peak LH level 24 h prior to ovulation, suggesting that the pain is caused by the rapid expansion of the dominant follicle, rather than because of rupture of the ovarian follicle at ovulation.[24] This is supported by ultrasound studies of ovulation.[25]

Hematometra can presents it self as APP, but most frequently it develops over some weeks after surgical procedures on the cervix (large loop excision of the transformation zone, LLETZ) or isthmus (trans cervical endometrial resection, TCER) have been carried out. The treatment is drainage by dilatation.

Adenomyosis mainly appear as chronic pelvic pain encountered in later life. Adenomyosis seldom causes APP, but can be seen.[26] Ultrasound may unveil adenomyosis, but often the diagnosis is made by the pathologist after hysterectomy.

Necrosis in fibroids can appear as constant, or colicky APP, sometimes accompanied with pyrexia. Often the patient is at least 40 years old as fibroids increase in frequency and size with age in the fertile period, and the fibroids usually get smaller after the menopause. The peak incidence for myomas requiring surgery occurs around age 45 years and declines thereafter.[27]

Women undergoing assisted conception can develop PID due to contamination in connection with aspiration of the oocytes. Pyo-ovarion may occur, and the infection can be long lasting. Women with severe sepsis require surgical intervention either aspiration of abscesses or more radical surgery.

Hyperstimulation-syndrome characterized by enlargement of the ovaries, intra-abdominal ascites, and sometimes pleural and pericardial-exudate is another complication of assisted conception. The incidence of symptoms giving ovarian hyperstimulation syndrome is between 1–10% and more severe hyperstimulation occurs in 0.5% of all induced cycles.[28,29] The clinical picture is one of APP occurring at 5 or 10 days after HCG has been administered to induce ovulation, depending on whether the syndrome is caused by exogenous or endogenously produced HCG. The diagnosis of APP is obvious, but the syndrome is important as the frequency of women attending for assisted reproduction are rising. The symptoms are nausea, vomiting and diarrhoea and, in severe cases, haemodynamic and electrolyte imbalance. If pregnancy has been achieved, especially in multiple, the syndrome is more severe and longer lasting. Gynaecological examination should not be attempted to avoid rupturing the enlarged ovaries. The most important parameters to monitor are the patient's weight, urinary output, haemoglobin concentration, haematocrit and white blood cell count. If haematocrit rises to > 55% and white blood cell count > 25×10^9/l, the risk of secondary complications is high, and the patient may require intensive care. Otherwise, the treatment is symptomatic.

Adnexal torsion in pregnancies after gonadotropin therapy is seen in 0.6% of cases and is found in up to 16% of pregnancies complicated by hyperstimulated ovaries.[30] Around 1/3 (13/40) of the adnexal torsions Oelsner et al.[2] operated on were due to hyperstimulated ovaries.

Abscesses, giving APP located in the vulva, bartholinitis, perirectal, are usually obvious during the physical examination.

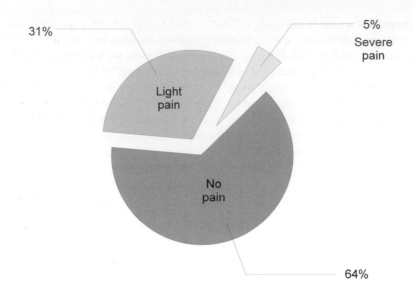

Fig. 21.2 Haemorrhage-associated abdominal pain among women with vaginal bleeding in the first and second trimester. Modified with permission of *Elsevier Science* from Axelsen et al.[31]

Obstetric diseases

Pregnancy related events are the most common reason for attending the hospital during the reproductive years. In fertile woman, a urine pregnancy test is mandatory, even though pregnancy may be unlikely based on the patient's history. APP and bleeding in early pregnancy can be due to miscarriage, ectopic pregnancy or sub-chorionic haematoma, but even in pregnancies terminated by childbirth, bleeding is common. A descriptive study based on information obtained by questionnaires administered during pregnancy has reported a frequency of 1 in 5 women, who had experienced bleeding in the first and second trimester. However, most women did not experience any pain (see Fig. 21.2).[31]

Intra-uterine haematoma in women can cause pain and vaginal bleeding. The underlying mechanism is thought to be placental separation with blood appearing as a space between the membranes and the uterine wall. The incidence of subchorionic hemorrhage in women with viable pregnancies was 1.3%.[32] Some reports indicate intra-uterine haematoma to increase the risk of miscarriage, stillbirth, abruptio placentae, and preterm birth,[32] whereas others find no correlation of large intra-uterine haematomata to pregnancy outcome.[33]

The prevalence of fibroids in pregnancy is around 0.5–1%. Myomas can increase rapidly in size in early pregnancy, whereafter only few continue to increase in size. APP can be due to necrosis or torsion, and abdominal pain occur in 10% of pregnant women with fibroids.[34]

Abruption of the placenta is usually associated with vaginal bleeding, but, in cases of pain and tenderness of the uterus without bleeding (20–35% of cases with abruptio[35]), this diagnosis has to be kept in mind, as delivery may well be required. Differential diagnosis will be placenta praevia and rupture of the uterus. The incidence of abruption of the placenta is approximately 1%, with a recurrency rate of 5–15%.[35] Predisposition to abruptio is smoking, poly-hydramnios, twin pregnancies, pre-existing intra-uterine growth retardation and high alcohol consumption, whereas correlation to hypertension is controversial.[35]

Braxton-Hicks contractions are non-regular intermittent uterine contractions, which can be detected by the month 4 of pregnancy.[36] Labour contractions can, at times, appear as APP, and several case reports describe the surprise to both the mother and her relatives, in cases where they are not aware of the pregnancy.

Postmenopausal

In the menopause, torsion of cysts (cysts/malignant tumours) or adnexa can occur. Pyometra is also a rare cause of APP, usually due to stenosis of the cervical canal, and most often seen in cases of endometrial cancer[37] or as mentioned previous secondary to, for example, earlier TCER.[38] Urinary retention due to cystocele or prolapse of the uterus can also cause APP (Table 21.7).

Table 21.7 Diseases in postmenopausal women

Torsion of cysts
Pyometra
Urinary retention

Non gynaecological diseases

Urinary tract infection (UTI) can occur in all age groups (babies, 'honeymoon-cystitis', pregnancy, the elderly) and may present with pelvic pain without any obvious symptoms such as dysuria and frequency. Therefore, it must be excluded by an urinary dipstick test before other diagnoses are considered.

Calculi in the urinary tract can also present as APP

Appendicitis

Although appendicitis has the highest incidence in children and young adults from 3–30 years of age, it can occur in all age groups, and with different clinical presentations. Usually there are three stages:

Stage I: lasting from 6–18 h where the symptoms are weak, diffuse abdominal pain, often located periumbilically, or in the epigastrium. Furthermore, nausea, anorexia and vomiting are often present. Objectively, there may only be mild tenderness in the right fossa.

Stage II: lasting several hours, but usually less than 48 h. The pain is localised to the right iliac fossa, with maximal tenderness at McBurney's point. The pain can either be constant or colicky in nature. The temperature is seldom more than 38°C, and the pulse is increased adequately. Generally, the patient will have passed no flatus nor defaecated for several hours, although children may have diarrhoea. The patient should be operated on at this stage. Otherwise one

Table 21.8 Diseases causing acute pelvic pain which can occur in all age groups

> Urinary tract infection (UTI)
> Appendicitis
> Mechels diverticulitis
> Viral mesenterial adenitis
> Invagination
> Diverticulitis
> Ileus
> Hernia
> Ischaemic abdominal pain
> Aneurism
> Skeletal causes?

of two things occur: either the pain disappears and the patient will be well within the next day or two, or the third stage appears.

Stage III: the pain increases, the patient's condition deteriorates, and the temperature and pulse increase. This leads to diffuse peritonitis, or a peri-appendicular abscess. Laparoscopy should be undertaken on liberal indication in young fertile women to exclude appendicitis.

Meckels diverticulitis
Meckels diverticulitis has a prevalence of approximately 2% in the population, and 90% are clinically not apparent.[39] Meckels diverticulitis and viral mesenteric adenitis can mimic appendicitis.

Invagination
Invagination of the bowel in children often presents as APP.

Diverticulitis
Diverticulitis occurs mainly among the elderly, usually with more diffuse abdominal pain, but can appear as left sided APP.

Ileus
More rarely ileus, especially seen in previously operated patients, appears as APP. Furthermore, ischaemic abdominal pain or ruptured aneurysm of the aorta can appear as APP and, because of the serious consequences these illnesses can cause, they always have to be kept in mind.

Hernia
A hernia can occur in all age groups. It is most often located in the inguinal region, being either a direct or indirect hernia, or in the femoral region. Furthermore, umbilical hernia and divarication of the recti abdominis can occur. All cicatrices even small ones after laparoscopy have to be examined carefully. With increasing numbers of laparoscopies in gynaecological surgery, hernias in trocar ports will increase in numbers. The average incidence is around 1%, but rising with increasing size of trocars.[40] The localization is approximately 27% umbilical and 73% extra-umbilical. This implies that the

risk of trocar hernia is present regardless of the position of the fascial defect. The diagnosis is typically based on the presence of vomiting or nausea with an extended and painful abdomen, usually within 2 weeks of surgery. However, the course can be prolonged and ileus can occur up to one year following laparoscopy. In most cases, the hernial content was small intestines or omentum.[40]

Psychosomatic APP

In rare cases, no somatic pathological cause for APP can be found and psychosomatic APP appears to be the diagnosis.

KEY POINTS FOR CLINICAL PRACTICE

- In any patient suffering from acute pelvic pain a systematic history is mandatory

- A careful physical examination, including precise description of pain location, exploration of scar tissue, and gynaecological examination is required. Biochemical tests are secondary

- All fertile women with acute pelvic pain must be considered pregnant until a pregnancy test has shown otherwise

- The diagnosis of ectopic pregnancy still remains a challenge for the gynaecologist, and it remains the fourth most common cause of maternal death during pregnancy

- Consider the diagnosis of PID even if the patient is apyrexial. Early treatment with antibiotics will greatly reduce the morbidity in women of childbearing age

- UTI can occur among the pregnant, non pregnant and in all age groups of women. Urinary dipstick tests should always be performed.

REFERENCES

1   Meyer J S, Harmon C M, Harty M P, Markowitz R I, Hubbard A M, Bellah R D. Ovarian torsion: clinical and imaging presentation in children. J Pediatr Surg 1995; 30: 1433–1436
2   Oelsner G, Bider D, Goldenberg M, Admon D, Mashiach S. Long-term follow-up of the twisted ischemic adnexa managed by detorsion. Fertil Steril 1993; 60: 976–979
3   Mårdh P A, Möller B, Paavonen J, Weström L. Pelvic inflammatory disease.In: Mandell L G, Rein M F. (eds) Atlas of infectious diseases, Vol. V, ch 5. Philadelphia: Churchill Livingstone, 1996
4   Velebil P, Wingo P A, Xia Z, Wilcox L S, Peterson H B. Rate of hospitalization for gynecologic disorders among reproductive-age women in the United States. Obstet Gynecol 1995; 86: 764–769
5   Weström L, Joesoef R, Reynolds G, Hagdu A, Thompson S E. Pelvic inflammatory disease and fertility. A cohort study of 1,844 women with laparoscopically verified disease and 657 control women with normal laparoscopic results. Sex Transm Dis 1992; July-August: 185–192
6   Heisterberg L, Kringelbach M. Early complications after induced first-trimester abortion. Acta Obstet Gynecol Scand 1987; 66: 201–204
7   Istre O. Transcervical resection of endometrium and fibroids: the outcome of 412 operations performed over 5 years. Acta Obstet Gynecol Scand 1996; 75(6): 567–574

8 Chi I. What we have learned from recent IUD studies: a researcher's perspective. Contraception 1993; 48: 81–108

9 Landers D V, Sweet R L. Current trends in the diagnosis and treatment of tuboovarian abscess. Am J Obstet Gynecol 1985; 151: 1098–1110

10 Knudsen U B, Hansen V, Juul S, Secher N J. Prognosis of a new pregnancy following previous spontaneous abortions. Eur J Obstet Gynecol Reprod Biol 1991; 39: 31–36

11 Pandya P P, Snijders R J, Psara N, Hilbert L, Nicolaides K H. The prevalence of non-viable pregnancy at 10–13 weeks of gestation. Ultrasound Obstet Gynecol 1996; 7: 170–173

12 Hill L M, Guzick D, Fries J, Hixson J. Fetal loss rate after ultrasonically documented cardiac activity between 6 and 14 weeks, menstrual age. J Clin Ultrasound 1991; 19: 221–223

13 HMSO. Report on confidential inquiries into maternal deaths in the UK. London: HMSO, 1994

14 Tuomivaara L, Kauppila A, Puolakka J. Ectopic pregnancy – an analysis of the etiology, diagnosis and treatment in 552 cases. Arch Gynecol Obstet 1986; 237: 135–147

15 Kitchin J D, Wein R M, Nunley Jr W C, Thiagarajah S, Thornton Jr W N. Ectopic pregnancy: current clinical trends. Am J Obstet Gynecol 1979; 134: 870–876

16 Bello G V, Schonotz D, Moshirpur J, Jeng D Y, Berkowitz R L. Combined pregnancy: the Mount Sinai experience. Obstet Gynecol Surv 1986; 41: 603–613

17 Molloy D, Deambrosis W, Keeping D, Hynes J, Harrison K, Hennessey J. Multiple-sited (heterotopic) pregnancy after in vitro fertilization and gamete intrafallopian transfer. Fertil Steril 1990; 53: 1068–1071

18 Dor J, Seidman D S, Levran D, Ben-Rafael Z, Ben-Shlomo I, Mashiach S. The incidence of combined intrauterine and extrauterine pregnancy after in vitro fertilization and embryo transfer. Fertil Steril 1991; 55: 833–834

19 Tepper R, Lerner Geva L, Zalel Y, Shilon M, Cohen I, Beyth Y. Adnexal torsion: the contribution of color Doppler sonography to diagnosis and post-operative follow-up. Eur J Obstet Gynecol Reprod Biol 1995; 62: 121–123

20 Fleischer A C, Stein S M, Cullinan J A, Warner M A. Color Doppler sonography of adnexal torsion. J Ultrasound Med 1995; 14: 523–528

21 Quilling S P, Siegel M J, Transabdominal color Doppler ultrasonography of the painful adolescent ovary. J Ultrasound Med 1994; 13: 549–555

22 Ayhan A, Aksu T, Develioglu O, Tuncer Z S, Ayhan A. Complications and bilaterality of mature ovarian teratomas (clinicopathological evaluation of 286 cases). Aust N Z J Obstet Gynaecol 1991; 31: 83–85

23 Shiromiizu K, Kawana T, Sugase M, Izumi R, Mizuno M. Clinicostatistical study of ovarian tumors of germ cell origin. Asia Oceania J Obstet Genaecol 1991; 17: 207–215

24 Speroff L, Glass R H, Kase N G. Clinical gynecologic endocrinology and infertility, 5th edn. London: Williams & Wilkins, 1994

25 de Crespigny L Ch, O'Herlihy C, Robinson H P. Ultrasonic observation of the mechanism of human ovulation. Am J Obstet Gynecol 1981; 139(6): 636–639

26 Fujino T, Watanabe T, Shinmura R, Hahn L, Nagata Y, Hasui K. Acute abdomen due to adenomyosis of the uterus: a case report. Asian Oceania J Obstet Gynaecol 1992; 18: 333–337

27 Cramer D W. Epidemiology of myomas. Semin Reprod Endocrinol 1992; 10: 320–324

28 Golan A, Ron-el R, Herman A, Soffer Y, Weinraub Z, Caspi E. Ovarian hyperstimulation syndrome: an updated review. Obstet Gynecol Surv 1989; 44: 430–440

29 Smitz J, Camus M, Devroey P, Erard P, Wisanto A, Steirteghem A C. Incidence of severe ovarian hyperstimulation syndrome after GnRH agonist/HMG superovulation for in vitro fertilization. Hum Reprod 1990; 5: 933–937

30 Maschiach S, Bider D, Moran O, Goldenberg M, Ben-Rafael Z. Adnexal torsion of hyperstimulated ovaries in pregnancies after gonadotropin therapy. Fertil Steril 1990; 53: 76–80

31 Axelsen S M, Henriksen T B, Hedegaard M, Secher N J. Characteristics of vaginal bleeding during pregnancy. Eur J Obstet Gynecol Reprod Biol 1995; 63: 131–134

32 Ball R H, Ade C M, Schoenborn J A, Crane J P. The clinical significance of ultrasonograph-ically detected subchorionic hemorrhages. Am J Obstet Gynecol 1996; 174: 996–1002

33 Pedersen J F, Mantoni M. Large intrauterine haematomata in threatened miscarriage. Frequency and clinical consequences. Br J Obstet Gynaecol 1990; 97: 552–553

34 Rice J P, Kay H H, Mahony B S. The clinical significance of uterine leiomyomas in pregnancy. Am J Obstet Gynecol 1989; 160: 1212–1216

35 Fraser R, Watson R. Bleeding during the latter half of pregnancy. In: Chalmers I, Enkin M, Keirse M. (eds) Effective care in pregnancy and childbirth. Oxford: Oxford University Press, 1989

36 Brody S. Obstetrik Gynekologi. Liber, 9th edn 1993

37 Goodman A, Zukerberg L R, Rice L W, Fuller A F, Young R H, Scully R E. Squamous cell carcinoma of the endometrium: a report of eight cases and a review of the literature. Gynecol Oncol 1996; 61: 54–60

38 Amin-Hanjani S, Good J M. Pyometra after endometrial resection and ablation. Obstet Gynecol 1995; 85 (Suppl 5 pt 2): 893–894

39 Phillips F, Maiterth T. Akutes Abdomen durch Entzundung eines konkrementhaltigen Meckel-Divertikels. Aktuelle Radiol 1992; 2: 243–245

40 Lajer H, Widecrantz S, Heisterberg L. Hernias in trocar ports following abdominal laparoscopy. A review. Acta Obstet Gynecol Scand 1997; 76: 389–393

22

Ezzat L. Kozman   Malcolm I. Frazer   Nigel Holland

Use of mechanical devices in the management of stress incontinence

Incontinence can have a devastating effect on the life of sufferers and their families and is of enormous cost to the nation.[1] Genuine stress incontinence is the commonest cause of urinary incontinence in women. It is widely accepted that the most effective treatment of severe or persistent genuine stress incontinence is surgery.[2] Nevertheless, some form of non-surgical conservative therapy is usually the first approach in the majority of women. Conservative therapies are relatively inexpensive, have fewer complications and do not compromise future surgical treatment. Conservative management of genuine stress incontinence includes physiotherapy techniques to improve the tone in the pelvic floor musculature, oral medications such as alpha-adrenergic agonists in association with oestrogen preparations and mechanical devices worn either within the vagina or within the urethra. This review addresses the role of mechanical devices in the management of stress incontinence. We have excluded weighted vaginal cones and electrical devices since these are essentially modalities that have as their final common pathway the pelvic floor musculature and its functional improvement. We have also excluded catheters, pads and other collecting devices in order to concentrate on an area of treatment that is poorly represented in the literature.

ANATOMICAL CONSIDERATIONS

Efficient urinary control depends on proximal urethral support, bladder neck closure and the intrinsic urethral mechanism.[3] The bladder neck and proximal

Mr E.L. Kozman, Department of Urogynaecology, Women's Health Directorate, Warrington Hospital NHS Trust, Lovely Lane, Warrington, Cheshire WA5 1QG, UK

Mr Malcolm I. Frazer, Department of Urogynaecology, Women's Health Directorate, Warrington Hospital NHS Trust, Lovely Lane, Warrington, Cheshire WA5 1QG, UK

Mr Nigel Holland, Department of Urogynaecology, Women's Health Directorate, Warrington Hospital NHS Trust, Lovely Lane, Warrington, Cheshire WA5 1QG, UK

urethra are normally situated in an intra-abdominal position above the pelvic floor and are supported by the pubo-urethral ligaments. Another component thought to play an important role in the suspension of the bladder neck is the pubo-vesical ligament complex attached between the symphysis pubis and the intrinsic striated muscles of the urethra which is believed to maintain the spatial relationships of the urethra and bladder within the pelvis. During rises in intra-abdominal pressure, the contraction of these muscles stretches the urethral functional length and increases its closure pressure. They also pull the vagina against the urethra compressing the latter posteriorly.[4] Increases in the intra-abdominal pressure are also transmitted to the proximal urethra. Patients suffering from genuine stress incontinence have excessive mobility of the urethrovesical junction and proximal urethra. During increases in intra-abdominal pressure, normal spatial relationships between the urethra, bladder and pelvis are disrupted resulting in deficient transmission of the pressure rise to the proximal urethra. Attempted restoration of these spatial relationships is the aim of many intravaginal devices.

MECHANICAL DEVICES

Somewhat predictably, the ancient Egyptians are reported to have had a device for the treatment of incontinence. It probably took the form of a golden phallus which was inserted in the vagina and is believed to have been used to treat post-partum stress incontinence.[5]

Despite this long tradition, mechanical devices are not often used in the management of incontinence today. They are also seldom mentioned as a serious treatment option in established textbooks and monographs. The aim of this review is to investigate whether this silence is justified from available objective clinical trials. We have divided mechanical devices into two main categories: vaginal devices and urethral devices.

VAGINAL DEVICES

Historical perspectives

In the late 1960s and early 1970s, Habib, Edwards and Bonnar suggested the use of three occlusive vaginal devices.

Habib intravaginal device

The Habib intravaginal device was carved from a solid piece of silicone plastic to fit each patient.[6] It was composed of three parts, the first part fitted over the mons pubis, the second between the labia, and the third was sited inside the vagina supporting the anterior vaginal wall and compressing the bladder neck (Fig. 22.1A,B). Habib's preliminary report remains to this day the only information on this device in the literature. He detailed seven 'representative' cases in whom he had used the device and indicated that it had been used successfully in more than 15 incontinent patients. Details on the exact diagnoses are limited and outcomes are apparently entirely subjective.

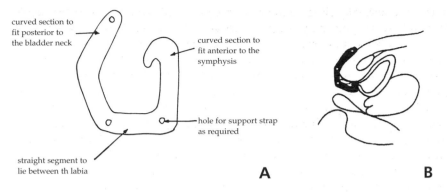

curved section to
fit posterior to
the bladder neck

curved section to
fit anterior to the
symphysis

hole for support strap
as required

straight segment to
lie between th labia

A

B

Fig. 22.1 (**A**) Habib's device (by permission of W B Saunders). (**B**) Habib's device in situ (by permission of W B Saunders).

Edward's pubo-vaginal spring device

Edward's pubo-vaginal spring device also consisted of three parts.[7] The first part was a triangular shaped fenestrated pressure pad that fitted anterior to the symphysis pubis. This pad was attached by a pair of spring wires covered by plastic tubes to a vertical pressure pad that was positioned inside the vagina and supported the bladder neck region from behind. This latter pad also compressed the urethra (Fig. 22.2). After Edward's initial description of the device in 1970 and detailing its experimental development in 1971,[8] Edwards and Malvern reported its use in 36 patients with urodynamically diagnosed sphincter weakness.[9] Of these patients, 25 (69.5%) were said to have had a 'successful outcome'. Success, however, was not defined. The highest success rates were reported in the 61–70 year-old age group. Nevertheless, closer study of the results indicate that 12 of the 25 'successful patients' underwent a repair operation subsequently.

Bonnar's device

Bonnar's device consisted of a triangular piece of silicone plastic with a bifid base. It carried an inflatable pad that when inserted in the vagina with the bifid

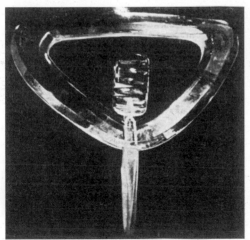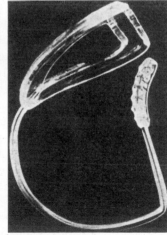

Fig. 22.2 Edwards device (by permission, BMJ Publishing Group).

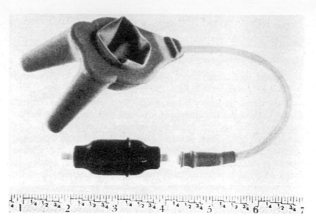

Fig. 22.3 Bonnar's device (by permission of *Lancet* from Bonnar J: Silicone vaginal appliance for control of stress incontinence 1977, 1161).

base at the posterior fornices and the balloon inflated, would compress the urethra and support the bladder neck (Fig. 22.3). Bonnar reported trying this device on 60 women with urinary incontinence with a success rate of 60%. Failures were attributed to difficulty with insertion or retention of the device. Unfortunately, Bonnar's account lacked a specific urodynamic diagnosis and the success reported was not objectively described. He also stated that his device was also tried in women with unstable bladder and proved beneficial in restoring normal function by inhibiting both urgency and frequency during the period of bladder re-education.[10]

The Edwards and Habib devices had to be removed to allow the patient to void, while the Bonnar's device only had to be deflated and then re-inflated. None of these devices were comfortable to use and needed considerable dexterity. Their main mode of action was by urethral compression. They do not appear to have withstood the test of time.

Tampons

Tampons are often suggested in the management of mild or intermittent stress incontinence. A small, prospective, randomised, single blind controlled study was undertaken by Nygaard of the effectiveness of a Tampax Super tampon in controlling incontinence during aerobic exercise sessions.[11] Data from 14 women were available for analysis. Mean urine loss decreased from 45.3 g without a tampon to 31.0 g wearing the super tampon. Eight participants whose urine loss was greater than 4 g in the control session (range 4.1–82 g) had less than 4 g loss with the tampon in situ. Nygaard's data hint at mostly modest decreases with, nevertheless, a number of spectacular successes. The use of tampons remains largely anecdotal.

Vaginal pessaries

The earliest vaginal pessaries were made of cork, ivory or ebony and were ring-shaped. They were primarily used for the correction of prolapse. Control of incontinence was an incidental feature in some patients.

Bhatia et al studied the urodynamic effects of a Smith-Hodge pessary in 12 women with genuine stress incontinence diagnosed on urodynamics.[12] They demonstrated a consistent and significant increase in urethral functional length and urethral closure pressure under varying stressful conditions, when compared with pre-pessary studies. Uroflowmetry post-pessary showed absence of obstruction and 10 of the 12 patients studied became continent. They concluded that the vaginal pessary restored continence by stabilising the urethra and urethrovesical junction allowing normal physiological pressure transmission.

Bergman and Bhatia used the pessary during the pre-operative evaluation of women with genuine stress incontinence and found a similarity in the resting and stress urethral closure pressure profiles of pessary users and those patients who had undergone successful continence surgery.[13] Based on these findings, the authors suggested the 'pessary test' to replace 'Bonney's test' which restores continence by obstructing the urethra and urethrovesical junction.

Bhatia and Bergman showed that the Smith-Hodge pessary not only can be used as a conservative management for genuine stress incontinence but also as a prognostic tool aiding in the selection of incontinent patients suitable for continence surgery.[14] The study by Bhatia and Bergman concentrated on assessing the effects of the vaginal pessary on various urodynamic parameters, such as functional urethral length, urethral closure pressures, both static and under stress, and uroflowmetry. Unfortunately, they did not comment on the long term efficiency of the pessary, or on the patient's acceptability. They also omitted reporting on the side effects associated with the use of vaginal pessaries. It is not even clear from the text the length of the study period. A major defect of the paper, as indeed of many papers of that era, is that there was no objective assessment of incontinence.

Standard contraceptive diaphragm

Suarez et al reported achieving complete resolution of genuine stress incontinence in 11 of 12 patients (91%) by using a standard contraceptive diaphragm.[15] Two of the 11 patients who achieved continence withdrew from the study because of discomfort associated with wearing the diaphragm. Urodynamic reassessment of the 9 continent patients with the diaphragm in situ showed an increase in urethral closure pressures and a decrease in urine flow rates; however, there was neither a change in time to peak flow nor significant residual urine. Their results were comparable to Bhatia and Bergman,[12] except that Suarez found it difficult to interpret the changes in the urethral functional length. Suarez et al concluded that a vaginal diaphragm of appropriate size presented a viable alternative to surgery in selected patients.[15] They felt it could be used as a temporising measure in patients awaiting surgery as well as an alternative diagnostic and prognostic test predicting successful outcome of continence surgery, a concept previously reviewed by Bhatia and Bergman.[14]

Bladder neck support prosthesis

Biswas first reported the use of a silastic device of his own design for the treatment of genuine stress incontinence in 1988.[16] It has undergone an increasing amount of clinical assessment and is now available for use in its

A

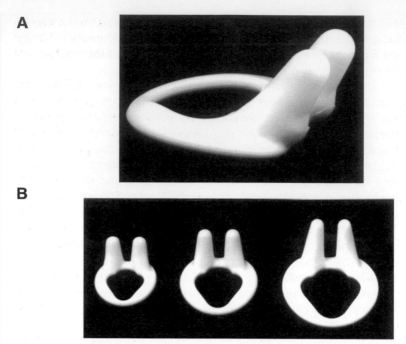

B

Fig. 22.4 Bladder neck support prosthesis. **(A)** lateral view; **(B)** top view of three sizes of device. (Photographs kindly provided by Dr K H Moore, St George's Hospital, Sydney, Australia).

native Australia and the US (Johnson and Johnson Medical, Inc., Arlington, TX, USA). The device is a flexible ring made of medical grade silicone rubber. It has two blunt prongs located at one end (Fig. 22.4A,B) and, when placed in the vagina, the prongs are said to elevate the urethrovesical angle in a manner similar to a Burch colposuspension. Although, as originally described, the device was transparent and came in only one standard size, more recently barium has been added to the silicone to colour it white and a variety of four prong lengths and six ring diameters are now offered. Biswas reported his initial experience with 44 women using the bladder neck support prosthesis in 1988.[16] The patients were assessed before fitting the device and after wearing it continuously for 3 months. The details of assessment are not clear from the published report, but 38 patients (85%) achieved continence which was 'objectively demonstrated'. The device was quite successful in both patients who had had previous surgery and those who were unsuitable for surgery. The expulsion rate was 11% and only 4 patients found the device unacceptable.

A further, better documented, study was reported by Biswas et al in 1993.[17] Thirty patients with proven genuine stress incontinence were enrolled in this study intending to use the device for a 3 month trial. Five-day urinary diaries and pad tests were used to assess urinary leakage. At the time of this publication, the bladder neck support prosthesis was made in 24 sizes, but five patients were still excluded because they needed a larger size than was available. The study reported on 25 patients, in 20 of which the bladder neck support prosthesis was deemed to be clinically successful although the specific criteria of success were not described. In 12 out of the 20 patients, the pad test was dry (less than 2 g) with the device still in situ. Overall, in the 20 successful patients, mean pad values fell from 56 g without the device to 4 g with the device in situ. Clearly, these patients were becoming drier and the results were encouraging.

Davila and Ostermann[18] reported on the short term use of the bladder neck support prosthesis in 30 women with urodynamically proven genuine stress incontinence. Incontinence was graded mild, moderate and severe depending upon the results of three provocative tests performed with 250 ml bladder volume. The patients were asked to cough, heel bounce and jump. A grade of 'severe' was given to those who lost urine with all three activities, 'moderate' with two, and 'mild' if loss occurred with only one. At initial testing, 9 subjects had severe, 13 had moderate, and 7 had mild incontinence. At study termination, 25 (83.3%) subjects were dry and 5 (16.6%) were improved but had mild incontinence. The opportunity for bias in this semi-objective assessment is obvious. Patients also reported the number of incontinence episodes per week and despite the statement above that 25 patients were 'dry', no patient reported zero incontinence episodes in any week when wearing the device. The mean number of incontinence episodes did fall, however, from nearly 10 episodes without the device to just over 3 episodes per week with the device. On the basis of repeat urodynamics, including urethral pressure profilometry, both static and stress, and urethral Q tip angles, the authors concluded that in the 'successful' group of women, the device mimicked the action of the Burch colposuspension with a similar success rate.

Foote et al presented the results of a prospective study on the long term use of the bladder neck support prosthesis assessing both efficacy in achieving continence and complications.[19] Fifteen women out of a total of 26 continued wearing the device for one year. Subjectively, 87.5% of patients gave the device greater than 85% rating for comfort and success. The objective success rate at 12 months was 87.5%. Success was defined as either complete dryness or greater than 50% reduction in urine leakage on both pad test and frequency/volume chart, and with comfortable fit of the device. The mean pad weighing test fell significantly over the 12 months from 57 g to 9 g. Over the same period, the number of leaks per week fell from 4.0 to 0.4 and the adverse impact on QOL (quality of life) assessment fell from a baseline of 8.1/10 to 1.5/10. The reported side effects were bacterial cystitis in 4 (15.4%), and increased vaginal loss in 14 (54%). This increased loss was attributed to the oestrogen cream which was used to reduce vaginal abrasions. Two patients had superficial abrasions and two developed vaginal granulation tissue related to pressure areas of the ring in the posterior fornix. They concluded that although the bladder neck support prosthesis was associated with a reduction of urinary leakage in 87.5% of women who could tolerate the device, it needed appropriate surveillance for urinary tract infections and vaginal abrasions. The latter should be reduced with the use of a more loosely fitting device. Women with a history of previous vaginal surgery were not considered suitable for the device because of fitting difficulties and reduced long lasting benefits. The authors of this study also noted that after removal of the device, there was an ongoing reduction of urinary leakage. This residual effect was attributed to remoulding of the connective tissue around the prongs thus improving the support of the bladder neck.[19]

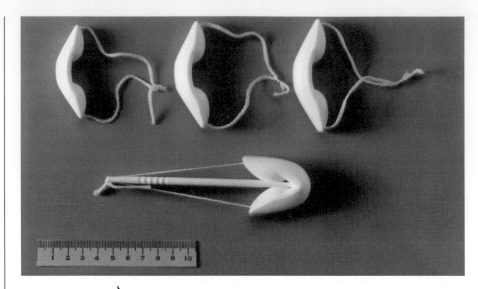

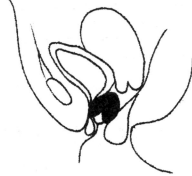

Fig. 22.5 **(A)** Continence guard device (three sizes with applicator); photograph kindly supplied by Dr Hans Thyssen. **(B)** Continence guard device in situ.

Continence guard

The continence guard is an intravaginal device made of polyurethane foam (Fig. 22.5A,B). It is soft, smooth and hydrophilic. When saturated with water it increases in size by 30%. Different shapes were tested by Thyssen and Lose[20] as to their bladder neck stabilising effect assessed by ultrasound. The prototype was produced in three sizes. Women were instructed on how to insert the device using an applicator. They were advised to use the largest device that gave minimum discomfort and to change the device daily in order to minimise the risk of toxic shock syndrome, as *Staphylococcus aureus* was able to grow on the surface of the device in vitro. They assessed the device in 26 women with the symptom of stress incontinence. Their initial assessment was for one month. A 24 h home pad weighing test, uroflowmetry, post-void residual urine and a 3 day voiding diary were made, but they did not attempt to make a urodynamic diagnosis. Four of the 26 women discontinued the treatment, two because of discomfort and two because of difficulties in placing the vaginal device. The preliminary study showed that of the remaining 22 women, 9 (41%) were subjectively cured and 10 (45%) improved whilst 3 (14%) claimed unchanged incontinence. They reported that all women with device in situ had unchanged voiding characteristics and all had a significantly decreased urinary loss on a repeat 24 h pad weighing test ($P < 0.0005$). Despite this report, many women were still 'wet' on pad testing. There were no vaginal or urinary infections. All 22 women found the device acceptable and wanted to continue to use it. They followed up 19 of these patients for one year.[21] They used the same methods for assessment but the 24 h home pad test and the 3 day voiding diary were done with and without the device in place. Thirteen of the 19 patients (68%) were subjectively cured, 5 (26%) were improved whilst one (5%) reported unchanged incontinence. Eighteen patients (95%) showed decreased leakage at the 24 h pad weighing test. Patients whose average leak before treatment was 69 g (range 10–194 g) had a decrease in loss to 18 g (range 0–75 g) after one year with the device in situ and 45 gm (range 11–125 g) without the device. The overlapping of the ranges and mean values of the pad-test results illustrate the inappropriateness of using parametric descriptive statistics in non-normally distributed data. There was no evidence of urinary or vaginal infection. Vaginal examination failed to show any evidence of irritation or erosion.

While Thyssen and Lose concluded that the device was relevant for younger patients with mild stress incontinence, Hahn and Milsolm[22] in a larger multicentre study on 90 women showed that even patients with severe leakage and women up to 65 years of age were also improved or became dry. However, the length of the study period was very short at only 4 weeks.

URETHRAL DEVICES

Where vaginal devices are designed to restore the normal anatomical relationship between the urethra and bladder, urethral devices primarily obstruct the outflow of urine.

Urethral plug

Nielsen et al used a urethral 'plug' made of thermoplastic elastomere on 31 patients with genuine stress incontinence.[23] The urethral plug consists of a meatal plate, a soft stalk and either one or two spheres along the stalk (Fig. 22.6). The spheres were located according to the results of the urethral pressure profile. The mid-point of the proximal sphere was placed at the bladder neck in order to reduce the amount of urine pushed into the proximal urethra during increased intra-abdominal pressure. The distal sphere was placed just at the maximum urethral pressure point aiming at increasing the maximal urethral closure pressure during stress. The plug was removed at voiding and replaced by a new plug. They planned to test the plug with two spheres in week one and the plug with only the distal sphere in week two of the study.

Patients were evaluated by symptom analysis, pad weighing test, uroflowmetry, cystometry, urethral closure pressure profile, voiding cystourethrography, gynaecological examination and urine culture. Of the 31 women, 4 (13%) could not learn to insert the plug, and 5 (16%) considered the incontinence to be a minor problem and were satisfied simply with the

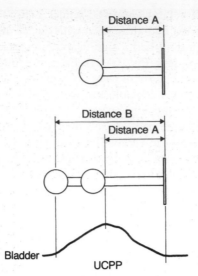

Fig. 22.6 The urethral plug (kindly supplied by Kurt Nielsen and by permission of Williams and Wilkins Publishing).

examination! Thus 22 women completed period one. Only 14 completed period two because 3 patients repeatedly lost the plug with one sphere and 5 patients refused to participate in period two due to unchanged incontinence in period one. A median of four plugs were used daily (range 1–9). Subjectively, 8 of the 14 patients (57%) preferred the plug with two spheres due to easier insertion and less tendency to dislocation. Objectively, Nielsen et al showed a statistically significant decrease in urinary leakage after both periods of use. A mean pad test result of 29.5 g before the study was reduced to an impressive 0.5 g after both periods one and two. However, we would make the point again that pad test data are not normally distributed and, therefore, the presentation of data as means is misleading. The authors reported an overall subjective and objective success rate of 73%. The urethral plug was very soft and insertion was difficult. The fact that the plug had to be individually fashioned according to the results of the urethral closure pressure profile also made it inconvenient and expensive. An improved design, the urethral plug II was developed and evaluated by Nielsen et al.[24] The new plug still consisted of an oval meatal plate, a soft stalk and either one sphere (2.0 cm from the metal plate) or two spheres (1.8 and 3.0 cm from the metal plate) along the stalk. Inside the stalk was a removable semi-rigid guide pin to ease insertion. They recruited 40 women with genuine stress incontinence who were randomly allocated to treatment with either the two spheres or the one sphere plug during period one (2 weeks). In period two (2 weeks) they used the other plug. They then continued using the 'preferred plug' for a further 2 months (period three). Of the 40 recruited women, only 18 completed period three. Of these 18 women, 14 preferred the plug with two spheres, 17 were subjectively and objectively continent or improved, but only 9 preferred to continue using the device after completion of the study. This amounts to only 22.4% of the original recruited group. The reported complications were urinary tract infections and loss of the plug into the bladder which occurred in two patients. Further evaluation of the

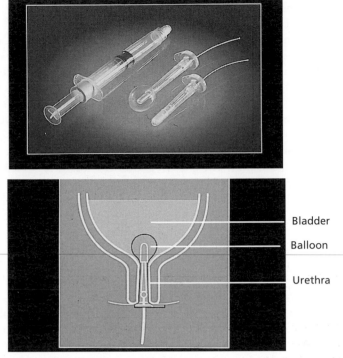

Bladder

Balloon

Urethra

Fig. 22.7 (A) Reliance insert and introducer. (B) Reliance insert in situ (both photographs supplied by Astra Tech, Berkshire, UK).

long-term effects on incontinence, urethral tolerance and possible complications may be worthwhile.

Reliance™ urinary control insert (Astra Tech)

The device is catheter-like, 14F gauge and made of thermoplastic elastomere (Fig. 22.7A,B). A meatal tab on the proximal end ensures correct positioning and prevents its migration into the urethra. Once inserted into the urethra, it is held in place by a small balloon at the distal end of the shaft. The shaft of the insert has a lumen that allows air into the balloon via a removable applicator. A tiny ball valve seals the air inside. The balloon is deflated by pulling a release string It is intended for single-use and hence a new device is inserted each time. The device is available in five sizes, increasing in length in 5 mm increments from 3 cm to 5 cm. It comes with a sizing device, a single use calibrating catheter with applicator, which is used to measure the urethral length.

Staskin et al initially enrolled 215 patients in a multicentre study.[25] Patient's evaluation was by detailed history, clinical examination, urine analysis and culture, cystometrography and cystourethroscopy. Assessment of effectiveness was by pad weighing tests, 7 day urinary diaries, patient's perception of ease and comfort using a five-point rating scale and finally an evaluation of quality of life improvements via a standard SF-36 health status survey. Before completion of a preliminary 4 month period, 80 patients (37%) withdrew from the study mainly because of discomfort and inability/unwillingness to use the device. Other reasons for withdrawal were urinary urgency and infection, haematuria, bladder irritation, leakage with device use, loss to follow-up and non-compliance with the protocol. The remaining 135 patients used a total of 16 200 devices (average daily use 2–3; range 1–6) for an average of 2–3 h (range 1–6 h) per usage. A further 21 patients declined to participate in the 4 month pad weighing test. Results were available on 51 patients who completed 12 months' product use.[26] The authors showed that 80% of the 114 patients who used the device for 4 months reported complete dryness, and 95% achieved greater than 80% improvement in their urine loss. The pad weighing test measuring urine loss in grams showed a statistically significant reduction from 44.0 g to 2.5 g after 4 months of use and from 41.1 g to 3.7 g after 12 months ($P < 0.0001$) Only one of the 114 patients failed to improve when the device was inserted. They also showed no significant changes in either bladder capacity or urodynamic results after 4 months of device use. One hundred of 135 patients completed their urinary diaries for the fourth month, of which 89% showed improvement in their incontinence and 72% remained completely dry. Of the patients who completed a urinary diary for 12 months, 65% reported complete dryness. Comfort of the device improved significantly during the study. Only 13% of the 135 patients reported device discomfort by the end of the study.

The SF-36 quality of life data showed a statistically significant improvement from 78.80 to 84.70 at 4 months ($P = 0.004$) and 81.60 to 88.95 at 12 months ($P < 0.01$). In 17% of users there was symptomatic bacteriuria which was successfully treated by a short course of antibiotics. They related this rate of infection, which later settled, to a learning curve in the use of the device. They also reported microscopic haematuria but on cystourethroscopy there was no anatomical damage apparent. Five patients experienced migration of the device into the urethra but were able to remove the device themselves. Two other patients had to have their device removed cystoscopically from the bladder. The invasive nature of urethral devices per se, and the expense of the Reliance™ insert in particular, may work to reduce its overall applicability to the majority of women with urethral sphincter incompetence.

Autocath 100

This device is a cylinder constructed of surgical steel coated with silver. Proximal and distal retention elements secure the device in situ in the urethra. A spring loaded plunger within the cylinder regulates the flow of urine. The opening pressure of the device can be adjusted by the spring tension selected so that a range of pressures can be utilised. The insertion is under local anaesthetic and can be performed as an out-patient procedure. Once the device is inserted, the patient activates it by contracting the lower abdominal muscles for about 4 s. The device remains open until the bladder is empty and then closes automatically. The valve device remains closed during momentary rises in intra-abdominal pressure, such as coughing or sneezing, only opening on sustained contraction of the lower abdominal muscles.

Wright et al assessed the Autocath 100 on 24 patients with urodynamically diagnosed genuine stress incontinence for an average of 43.4 days (range 0–93 days) with an average pressure setting of 54 cm/H_2O.[27] They also tried the device in another group of women with urinary retention. In the genuine stress incontinence group, the mean number of daily incontinence episodes was 5.53 without the device and 0.44 ($P < 0.001$) after insertion; pad testing was not performed. There was no change in maximal urethral closure pressure and no reported cystoscopic changes post-device. The complaints reported were lower urinary tract infection (23%), mild discomfort and migration of the device proximally into the bladder (5%) which was later resolved by modifying the design of the device. Patients with mild symptoms found that the initial discomfort far outweighed the inconvenience of their incontinence. The patients who accepted the device best were those who suffered from significant incontinence.

Continence control pad

The continence control pad (CCP) is a hydrogel-coated contoured foam pad. It is claimed that the adhesive hydrogel can stick to the wet skin for a period of up to 5 h. The pad has a tapered end that is oriented towards the front of the patient and a blunt end that is oriented towards the vagina. Eckford et al recruited 24 women with the symptom of stress incontinence of urine.[28] They argued that a urodynamic diagnosis was not necessary because the CCP was primarily designed for use in the primary care setting. They assessed their patients during the week before, and again after using the CCP for 2 weeks, by urinary diaries, pad-tests and a review of their symptoms. Although 24 women initially responded to an invitation to take part in the study, only 19 (79.2%) completed it. It was not clear from the published article why 5 (20.8%) women failed to complete the study. The authors reported a significant decrease in the number of incontinent episodes per week ($P = 0.002$). Three women were rendered completely continent, 14 had fewer episodes of leakage, one was the same and one had an increased number of incontinent episodes. From the pad-test results, they were able to show a statistically significant reduction in the urinary leakage with the CCP in situ ($P < 0.001$). As expected, they noted that women with minor degrees of leakage found the pads to be more efficacious. Of the 19 women who completed the study, 4 reported poor adherence of the CCP to the skin, 2 complained of introital discomfort on removing it, and one of introital discomfort on placing the device. Only one woman developed urinary infection and two complained of urinary urgency and frequency.

It is generally accepted that women with occasional, milder degree of incontinence, while waiting for, or unwilling to have, an operation or who have not completed child-bearing can benefit from a continence device. Nevertheless, the authors' hint, that the CCP was primarily designed for use in the primary care setting, is slightly worrying in that it might delay referring these women for a definitive diagnosis and an appropriate specialist treatment. It would have also been more informative to know why 20.8% of the recruited women did not continue with the study. From the report it was not clear how often the CCP needed to be changed or how it should be cleaned.

Femassist™ device

The Femassist™ device attaches like a suction cup with the help of a mild sealing ointment, to the flat area about 2–3 cm in diameter around the urethra.

The mild vacuum action supports surrounding tissue as it gently squeezes the urethra. The exact mode of action of the device remains a little obscure, since occlusion of the urethra distal to the point of maximal urethral pressure would not necessarily result in decreased incontinence. Once in place, the device folds against the body and is generally concealed within the labia. When a patient wishes to urinate, she pulls the device by the edge to remove it. The device can then be washed with hand soap and water and reapplied. A single device can be used for up to 1 week before disposal.

Versi et al recruited women with an average age of 54 years (range 29–81 years) for their study.[29] Their patients were fitted with one of two sized devices and were assessed before and after 1 month's use. The subjective assessment consisted of incontinence impact questionnaires, urogenital distress inventories and visual analogue scales assessing the symptoms of stress and urge incontinence, urgency and urethral irritation. The objective assessments consisted of 1 h standardised ICS pad tests, 48 h home pad tests and pre and post treatment mid-stream urine tests: 91 patients completed the study. It is not clear from the paper how many women were originally recruited. Of the 91 women, 44 had mixed incontinence, 38 had stress incontinence and 9 had urge incontinence. Urodynamics do not seem to have been performed and so these categories are derived from the patient's symptoms. They claimed that the use of the device was associated with a dramatic improvement in the quality of life. Of the 91 women who completed the study, 68% had an objective improvement in their 1 h pad test results without a significant increase in bacteruria, irritation or urinary tract infections rates. These results were reproduced by Prashar et al, particularly in regard to the improvement in the quality of life scores.[30]

In a further multicentre clinical trial reported by the company but which does not appear to have been published, it was concluded that only patients with genuine stress incontinence benefited from the device.[31] Of these patients, 55% were 100% dry, 22% had 90% reduction of their urine loss, and 22% had a reduction of 50%. The incidence of irritation was only 2% and was satisfactorily treated with topical oestrogen cream. They concluded that the Femassist™ device was effective, safe and comfortable to use. Nevertheless, of the 52 women who withdrew from the study, 9 had difficulty with placing the device, 6 found the device not effective and 10 found the device either uncomfortable or inconvenient.

CONCLUSIONS

There are now a number of devices available for the treatment of genuine stress incontinence. In only a small minority, most notably the bladder neck support prosthesis, Reliance™ insert and more recently the Femassist™ device, has there been any substantial objective data on their efficacy. Early indications suggest that these three devices may deserve to be more widely available and used, particularly in those patients where a surgical solution is not being contemplated. Of some concern, however, is the invasive nature of the Reliance™ insert and other intra-urethral devices which may eventually lessen their overall usefulness.

Perhaps for obvious reasons, there are no data comparing devices with dummy or placebo interventions. Most trials have tended to be small scale and 'explanatory'. Rather than asking 'can this intervention improve incontinence when tested in an ideal setting?', it is more important to address the pragmatic question, 'is this treatment policy better than alternative policies for managing people with incontinence in an everyday care setting?' With this in mind, many studies tend to report results using the number of patients finishing the trial as the denominator rather than the total number of patients initially recruited. If results are converted to 'intention to treat', then the overall success rates are generally much less impressive but the information much more useful and meaningful. We would counsel against the widespread and uncritical adoption of mechanical devices in the management options of women with incontinence until their exact usefulness and cost-effectiveness has been proven. The Cochrane Urinary and Faecal Incontinence Group (the CURE project) of the Cochrane database has set up a team to evaluate the effectiveness of mechanical devices for incontinence of which one of the authors (MIF) is a member. Hopefully, some of the deficiencies in the data will be corrected as this project gathers momentum. As yet there is no one entirely satisfactory mechanical device for the treatment of incontinence. The search for one will no doubt continue to tax the imagination of enthusiasts and device manufacturers for the foreseeable future.

KEY POINTS FOR CLINICAL PRACTICE

- Mechanical devices currently available work either by altering the spatial relationships of the bladder neck and pelvic floor or by urethral occlusion

- No device is wholly without complications but the intra-urethral devices have the potential to give rise to more serious problems

- Mechanical devices may prove to be an important adjunct to more conventional methods of managing incontinence in women but there is simply not enough good quality data to be enthusiastic

- Reported success rates are always falsely elevated by investigators' reluctance to present their data using 'intention to treat' criteria

- No clinical trials exist that compare one device with another, therefore, it is not clear which is the most effective device, if any

- Much of the data on these devices are incomplete and poorly represented in the mainstream peer-review literature.

- Until the exact role of these devices (some of which are very expensive) becomes clear, we would caution against their indiscriminate use in the primary care setting prior to full specialist assessment.

- Ideally women who are using these devices should be part of ongoing clinical research trials

1 Report of the Royal College of Physicians. Incontinence causes, management and provision of services. London: Royal College of Physicians, 1995; 4–5

2 Klarskov P, Belving D, Bischoff N et al. Pelvic floor exercises versus surgery for female urinary stress incontinence. Urol Int 1986; 41: 129–132

3 Bourcier A, Juras J. Nonsurgical therapy for stress incontinence. Urol Clin North Am 1995; 22: 613–627

4 DeLancey J O. Structural aspects of the extrinsic continence mechanism. Obstet Gynecol 1988; 72: 296–301

5 Edwards S L. Mechanical and other devices. In: Caldwell K P S, ed. Urinary incontinence. London: Academic Press, 1970; 115–127

6 Habib H. Non operative treatment of recurrent stress incontinence in female subjects: preliminary report of a new device. J Urol 1969; 101: 854–856

7 Edwards L. Device for control of incontinence of urine in women. BMJ 1970; 3: 104

8 Edwards L. The control of incontinence of urine in women with a pubovaginal spring device: objective and subjective results. Br J Urol 1971; 43: 211–225

9 Edwards L, Malvern J. Long term follow up results with the pubovaginal spring device in incontinence of urine in women; comparison with electronic methods of control. Br J Urol 1973; 45: 103–108

10 Bonnar J. Silicone vaginal appliance for control of stress incontinence. Lancet 1977: 1161

11 Nygaard I. Treatment of exercise incontinence with mechanical devices. Neurourol Urodyn 1992; 11: 367–368

12 Bhatia N N, Bergman A, Gunning J E. Urodynamic effects of a vaginal pessary in women with stress urinary incontinence. Am J Obstet Gynecol 1983; 147: 876–884

13 Bergman A, Bhatia N N. Pessary test: simple prognostic test in women with stress urinary incontinence. Urology 1984; 24: 109–110

14 Bhatia N N, Bergman A. Pessary test in women with urinary incontinence. Obstet Gynecol 1985; 65: 220–226

15 Suarez G M, Baum N H, Jacobs J. Use of standard contraceptive diaphragm in management of stress urinary incontinence. Urology 1991; 37: 119–122

16 Biswas N C. A silastic vaginal device for the treatment of stress urinary incontinence [abstract]. Neurourol Urodyn 1988; 7: 271–272

17 Biswas N C, Spencer P, King J. Conservative management of stress incontinence with a bladder neck support prosthesis (BSP). Neurourol Urodyn 1993; 12: 311–313

18 Davila G N, Ostermann K V. The bladder neck support prosthesis: a non-surgical approach to stress incontinence in adult women. Am J Obstet Gynecol 1994; 171: 206–211

19 Foote A J, Moore K H, King J. A prospective study of the long term use of the bladder neck support prosthesis [abstract]. Neurourol Urodyn 1996; 15: 404–406

20 Thyssen H, Lose G. New disposable vaginal device (continence guard) in the treatment of female stress incontinence. Acta Obstet Gynecol Scand 1996; 75: 170–173

21 Thyssen H, Lose G. Long term efficacy and safety of a vaginal device in the treatment of stress incontinence [abstract]. Neurourol Urodyn 1996; 15: 394–395

22 Hahn I, Milsom I. Treatment of female stress urinary incontinence with a new anatomically shaped vaginal device (Conveen continence guard). Br J Urol 1996; 77: 711–715

23 Nielsen K K, Kromann-Andersen B, Jacobsen H et al. The urethral plug: a new treatment modality for genuine urinary stress incontinence in women. J Urol 1990; 144: 1199–1202

24 Nielsen K K, Walter S, Maegaard E et al. The urethral plug II: an alternative treatment in women with genuine stress incontinence. Br J Urol 1996; 72: 428–432

25 Staskin D, Bavendam T, Miller J et al. Effectiveness of urinary control insert in the management of stress urinary incontinence: early results of a multicenter study. Urology 1996; 47: 629–636

26 Staskin D, Bavendam T, Davila G W et al. Multicenter experience using an expandable urethral insert for management of urinary stress incontinence. Data presented at the International Continence Society meeting in Sydney, Australia, October 17, 1995

27 Wright M, Bladou F, Bordowski A et al. Restoring continence with the Autocath 100 in women [abstract]. Neurourol Urodyn 1996; 15: 401-402

28 Eckford S, Jackson S, Lewis P, Abrams P. The continence control pad – a new external urethral occlusion device in the management of stress incontinence. Br J Urol 1996; 77: 538–540

29 Versi E, Griffiths D, Giovannini D. Improvement in 'quality of life' and urinary incontinence using the Femassist™ device [abstract S66]. Int Urogynecol J 1997; 8: 78

30 Prashar S, Moore K, Bryant C et al. The urethral occlusive device for the treatment of urinary incontinence: changes in quality of life [abstract S130]. Int Urogynecol J 1997; 8: 159

31 Femassist™ multicentre clinical trial, unpublished data on file. Insight Medical Devices Ltd, Asmec Centre, Eagle House, The Ring, Bracknell, Berkshire RG12 1HB, UK

Janice M. Rymer   Edward P. Morris   Ignac Fogelman

Gonadotrophin-releasing hormone analogues and addback therapy in current gynaecological practice

The use of GnRH analogues in clinical gynaecological practice is expanding. The hypo-oestrogenic state that they produce is associated with side effects such as hot flushes and dry vagina. In addition, many studies report bone loss with GnRH analogue use.[1,2] The extent of this loss appears to be equivalent to that found after a surgical menopause. However, as the state of hypo-oestrogenism is limited (usually) to 6 months, the stimulus to bone loss is withdrawn and most studies report that the loss is partially reversible, although few studies have had adequate follow-up to assess accurately long-term bone loss. GnRH analogue use for periods longer than 6 months would make this effect on bone mass more concerning. West et al in 1987[3] assessed women over 12 months of GnRH analogue therapy and noted an 8% spinal bone loss. Accepting that studies report differing bone loss depending on whether it is measured by quantitative computed tomography (QCT) or dual X-ray absorptiometry, if this degree of bone loss were to be permanent it would significantly increase an individual's risk of developing osteoporosis. In this situation, bone density measurements would be required to monitor the patient's bone mass which may not be practical or available.

In the modern days of women's choice, many are opting for long-term medical treatment of their gynaecological conditions, rather than resorting to radical surgery.

The concept of addback therapy aims to counteract the hypo-oestrogenic side-effects, including bone loss, without stimulating the condition for which the GnRH analogue was originally given. This introduces the possibility of

Dr Janice M. Rymer, Senior Lecturer/Consultant in Obstetrics and Gynaecology, UMDS, Guy's Hospital, Guy's and St Thomas' Hospital Trust, St Thomas Street, London SE1 9RT, UK

Mr Edward P. Morris, Research Fellow, HRT Research Unit, Guy's Hospital, Guy's and St Thomas' Hospital Trust, St Thomas Street, London SE1 9RT, UK

Professor Ignac Fogelman, Consultant in Nuclear Medicine, Guy's Hospital, Guy's and St Thomas' Hospital Trust, St Thomas Street, London SE1 9RT, UK

Table 23.1 Amino acid substitutions in GnRH agonists used in current clinical practice compared to endogenous GnRH

	Position 6	Positions 9–10
GnRH	Gly	Pro–Gly–NH$_2$
Goserelin	D-Ser(Bu^t)	Pro–Az-Gly
Nafarelin	(D-Nal)^2	Pro–Gly–NH$_2$
Leuprolide	D-Leu	Pro–NH–CH$_2$–CH$_3$
Buserelin	D-Ser(Bu^t)	Pro–NH–CH$_2$–CH$_3$

longer courses of treatment. Gynaecological conditions for which long-term treatment would be useful include diseases such as endometriosis, fibroids and dysfunctional uterine bleeding (DUB) that tend to recur after short treatment periods. A variety of agents have been considered as addback therapy to combat the effects of the hypo-oestrogenic state, these include progestogens, oestrogens, oestrogens and progestogens combined, tibolone, bisphosphonates, parathyroid hormone and calcitonin.

GnRH RELEASE

GnRH is synthesised by neurones within the medial basal and preoptic area of the hypothalamus after cleavage of a larger 92 amino acid precursor and released in a pulsatile fashion into the hypothalamic-hypophyseal portal system to the anterior pituitary where it stimulates production of luteinizing hormone (LH) and follicle-stimulating hormone (FSH) from the gonadotroph cells.

The pulsatile release of GnRH is essential for normal reproductive function. Feedback from gonadal steroids acting on the hypothalamus influences both amplitude and frequency of GnRH release during the normal menstrual cycle, contributing to cyclical variation in circulating levels of LH and FSH.[4,5] Other known modulators of gonadotrophin secretion include catecholamines, endogenous opioids, prolactin, inhibin, progesterone and testosterone.[6]

GnRH RECEPTORS

GnRH binds to receptors located in the phospholipid plasma membrane of the gonadotroph cell. After GnRH binding, there is a rise in intracellular calcium which leads to activation of protein kinase C which, in turn, both releases preformed gonadotrophins and increases cellular synthesis of gonadotrophins.[7]

An important feature of gonadotroph cells is their ability to regulate the number of GnRH receptors. Receptor numbers increase to amplify the synthesis and release of gonadotrophins during pulsatile GnRH secretion or following use of short-acting GnRH agonists.[7] However, long term stimulation of the GnRH receptor with analogues of GnRH leads to an overall downregulation of receptor function, or desensitisation. Downregulation is partially explained by a marked reduction in GnRH receptor numbers during tonic stimulation, possibly partly as a result of internalisation of the ligand–receptor complex. Reduction in receptor numbers does not, however, fully account for the degree of desensitisation encountered with GnRH agonists, as inhibition of receptor internalisation does not appear to reduce the effects of GnRH analogues.[8] Other mechanisms thought to be involved in GnRH-induced receptor downregulation result from prolonged presence of GnRH analogue on the receptor preventing further stimulation and post-receptor events, such as reduced calcium flux following inactivation of calcium channels during desensitisation.[9]

PROTEIN CHEMISTRY AND DEVELOPMENT OF GnRH ANALOGUES

Endogenous GnRH is a decapeptide with a plasma half-life of about 15 min, which is inactivated by enzymatic cleavage.

GnRH agonists are generally formed following modifications to the GnRH molecule at position 6 and at position 9–10 (Table 23.1). Amino acid substitutions at these points improve both metabolic stability and potency.

Extensive changes in the GnRH molecule are required to produce a GnRH analogue with antagonistic effects. GnRH antagonists have increased receptor affinity and reduced metabolism at the receptor which is achieved by producing molecules with high hydrophobicity.[10]

There are also data to suggest that in rats, using photoaffinity labels, GnRH antagonists bind to a different region of the gonadotroph receptor than agonists.[11] This information suggests that the design strategy of molecules with antagonistic activity should differ from that of agonists. In practice, most antagonist molecules barely resemble the initial GnRH decapeptide, retaining few original amino acids.

ADMINISTRATION AND FORMULATION OF GnRH ANALOGUES

Due to complete inactivation of GnRH analogues within the gut,[12] parenteral routes remain the sole means of administration at present.

Agonists

Half-lives of GnRH agonists vary considerably – from 35 min for Buserelin[13] to 4.5 h for Goserelin.[14] The unacceptability of daily subcutaneous injections for prolonged periods to achieve steady-state plasma levels of these compounds has resulted in the development and clinical use of various modes of administration. Currently available routes are intranasal, intramuscular or subcutaneous injection of a suspension of microcapsules and subcutaneous injection of a biodegradable implant that releases GnRH analogue over a 28 day period (Table 23.2).

Nasally administered GnRH agonist preparations are of variable efficacy which may vary according to the potency of the agonist used, the absorption of the drug and compliance with therapy.[15–17] Nafarelin (Synarel®, Roche) has

Table 23.2 Doses and preparations of currently available GnRH agonists

Compound	Proprietary name	Manufacturer	Route	Dose
Buserelin	Suprecur®	Hoechst Marion Roussel	Nasal	One 150 µg spray per nostril, 3–4 times daily
Nafarelin	Synarel®	Searle	Nasal	One 200 µg spray twice daily (alternate nostrils)
Leuprorelin	Prostap SR®	Lederle	Subcut. or i.m.	One injection of microcapsules containing 3.75 mg of drug every 4 weeks
Goserelin	Zoladex®	Zeneca	Subcut.	One injection of biodegradable depot containing 3.6 mg of drug every 4 weeks

Subcut. = suncutaneous
i.m. = intramuscular

been identified as a good GnRH agonist for nasal administration as it has a mean plasma half-life of 4.4 h with high biological potency of between 200 and 300 times greater than endogenous GnRH.[17,18] Buserelin has a high biological potency (100 times that of native GnRH),[19] but has a shorter half-life which necessitates more frequent administration than nafarelin. Frequent dose regimens may lead to poor compliance with therapy, especially over periods as long as 6 months. Nasal rhinitis or use of long-acting nasal decongestants were thought to interfere significantly with absorption and subsequent bio-availability of these drugs when taken nasally. A recent study has shown that no difference in plasma levels of nafarelin over 8 h was noted in women with perennial rhinitis against controls without rhinitis when 400 µg of the drug was administered intranasally.[17] The same study also noted that use of long-acting decongestants did not significantly affect the absorption of nafarelin provided that the decongestant is administered at least 30 min after the drug is given.

Microcapsules of a biodegradable co-polymer of lactic and glycolic acids (PLGA) containing leuprorelin (Prostap SR®, Lederle) are on average 20 µm in diameter and are small enough to pass through a conventional needle (23 gauge) for subcutaneous or intramuscular injection.[20] This form of depot results in a sudden release of drug on the first day of administration, followed by a steady serum level for the remainder of the 28 day period as the PLGA breaks down, releasing leuprorelin. The sudden high initial release of drug is thought to be due to release of free drug or drug that has only a weak association with the PLGA and not as a consequence of rapid degradation of the PLGA. As leuprorelin has relatively few adverse effects, an elevated serum level for the first 24 h is not thought to be clinically relevant.[20]

For several years the GnRH analogue goserelin (Zoladex®, Zeneca) has been widely available. It is administered as a rod 1 mm in diameter and 1 cm in length, containing 3.6 mg of goserelin dispersed within a biodegradable polymer – poly D,L-lactide-co-glycolide. Once injected subcutaneously, goserelin is released over a 28 day period from the polymer by diffusion of the drug from aqueous channels and by release of the drug as the polymer degrades, achieving effective pituitary desensitisation.[21]

More recent developments in the technology of depot forms of GnRH analogue administration include a 10.8 mg goserelin depot which has been shown in men to be pharmacologically equivalent to the 3.6 mg depot, but delivering the drug over a longer period of 12 weeks.[22] Early animal studies with subcutaneous injection of buserelin (Suprecur®, Hoechst Marion Roussel) microparticles has shown that oestradiol and testosterone secretion is reversibly suppressed with a dose interval of 4 weeks.[23] A recently produced subcutaneous implant containing 6.6 mg of buserelin has been shown to be effective in maintaining ovarian suppression over a period of more than 90 days in women.[24]

It is hoped that future developments will include carrier protein technology that will allow the production of drugs that contain GnRH analogues in such a way as to render these fragile peptides immune to the damaging effects of the gut.

Antagonists

Due to the unwanted histaminic side-effects and relatively low biological potency of early GnRH antagonists, the introduction of a potent and safe preparation into clinical practice has been significantly delayed. Two recent preparations still in development, ganirelix and cetrorelix, appear to have promise. Both these drugs require regular subcutaneous administration. More recently, however, a report of six cases of perimenopausal women with uterine leiomyomata given depot injections of cetrorelix for at least 7 weeks prior to hysterectomy has shown encouraging results.[25] In this study, the depot was composed of 30 or 60 mg of cetrorelix in a pamoate microparticle formulation, which lasted between 21 and 28 days. This was the first report of such a preparation, but the future production of a clinically available GnRH antagonist is an exciting prospect.

CLINICAL APPLICATIONS OF GnRH ANALOGUES

Agonists

GnRH agonists are widely used in current gynaecological practice. Short courses are administered as part of pituitary down regulation prior to superovulation techniques. Slightly longer courses of GnRH analogues may be administered for pre-operative endometrial thinning prior to endometrial ablation. Three month courses for shrinkage of uterine fibroids are now frequently used. Six month treatment schedules for the treatment of endometriosis represent the longest currently accepted regimes of GnRH agonist administration.

GnRH agonists are also used in the management of menorrhagia, hirsuitism, premenstrual syndrome, true precocious puberty and breast cancer.

Antagonists

As this group of drugs has still to be evaluated fully in clinical research, and acceptable dose regimens developed, there are as yet no recognised clinical indications for antagonists that are not adequately treated by GnRH agonists. GnRH antagonists are, however, widely used as neuroendocrine probes, contributing to greater understanding of the physiology and pathology of the reproductive system.

One of the main potential advantages of antagonists over agonists is the rapid suppression of pituitary function. Plasma oestradiol levels fall over a period of 3 days to trough levels and return to normal within 4 days of cessation of therapy following GnRH antagonist administration.[26] Agonists may take up to 3 weeks to reduce oestradiol levels to effective levels at commencement of therapy, and up to 4 weeks for normal oestradiol levels to be achieved on stopping the drug.[27] As the aim of GnRH agonist administration during superovulation is to prevent unwanted LH surges, the almost immediate actions of GnRH antagonists have considerable benefits in accurately and predictably regulating ovarian stimulation while reducing the risks of ovarian hyperstimulation.[28]

When safe and effective GnRH antagonists are licensed for use in indications similar to those currently used for agonistic analogues, antagonists may well become the drugs of choice in the treatment of many gynaecological disorders.

UNWANTED EFFECTS OF GnRH ANALOGUES

Agonists

Adverse effects related to GnRH agonist administration are due to the relatively rapid suppression of oestrogen administration in an otherwise healthy premenopausal woman. A well-known unwanted effect of GnRH analogues is the oestrogen 'flare'. This follows the initial stimulation of the gonadotroph cells, releasing LH and FSH, with subsequent increase in sex steroid production. This may result in a transient increase in symptoms from the disease that is being treated. The effects of the flare and its duration can be minimised by commencing GnRH agonist therapy from the midluteal phase (after day 21) to the early follicular phase (day 1). Thereafter, oestrogen levels fall to effective therapeutic concentrations.

Whilst receiving long term parenteral GnRH agonists, most women experience vasomotor symptoms.[3,29] Other less frequent but widely recognised symptoms include vaginal dryness, reduction in libido, headaches and psychological symptoms associated with hypo-oestrogenism such as lack of concentration, mood changes and forgetfulness.

Doubts about the endometrial safety of GnRH agonists have been raised[27,30] following reports of irregular bleeding whilst on intranasal therapy.[31] This may be due to inadequate circulating levels of agonist, as a result of poor absorption of nasal dose or poor compliance, leading to breakthrough ovarian activity with consequent endometrial stimulation. There are no known reports questioning the endometrial safety of regularly administered depot preparations on GnRH agonists. Women with large fibroids, particularly those within the uterine cavity or those with submucous fibroids, may experience episodes of bleeding, possibly as a result of local atrophic changes leading to mucosal fragility over the surface of the fibroid, or by degeneration and resultant necrosis of the tumour.[32]

There is little doubt as to the importance of oestrogen in the maintenance of the female skeleton.[33] In young women treated with GnRH agonists, oestrogenic protection of the skeleton is lost during the treatment course. This has been shown to result in bone loss in the region of 3–5% following a 6 month course of GnRH agonists, the reversibility of which is the subject of considerable debate.[1,2] This easily demonstrable unwanted effect of GnRH agonists on the female skeleton, though of doubtful clinical significance when short term courses are administered, remains the main reason that the maximum duration of GnRH therapy has been limited to 6 months. If there is an element of irreversible bone loss following a course of GnRH therapy, then the most serious potential adverse effect of GnRH therapy would be a reduction in bone density that would lead to patients entering the menopause with lower bone mass. In young women this may be even more important if, in addition, therapy prevents attainment of peak bone mass. At present this does not adversely affect use of GnRH agonists for courses of 3 months or less in ovulation induction, pre-operative endometrial preparation or fibroid shrinkage. However, long term non-surgical relief of symptoms from endometriosis and fibroids from prolonged courses of GnRH agonists is prevented due to theoretical possibility of development of osteoporosis during therapy.

Antagonists

These drugs, as previously discussed, achieve 'medical castration' by occupancy and competitive blockade of the gonadotroph receptors. Unlike agonistic analogues, their effect is dose-related and they do not stimulate any receptor or post-receptor events, thus producing no initial release of gonadotrophins or 'flare'.[34] It is important to realise that as antagonists have the same effect as agonists in reducing serum oestrogen concentrations to minimal levels, any treatment course is likely to result in the unwanted effects of hypo-oestrogenism such as menopausal symptoms and bone loss that accompany GnRH agonist therapy.

Due to the extensive changes that occur to the molecule to produce a compound with antagonistic effects, this group of peptides is considerably more antigenic than agonists. These molecular differences, combined with the fact that higher concentrations of antagonists are needed to exert an effect have been shown to produce local and systemic histamine release.[35] This then may produce local redness, induration and pruritis at injection sites and occasionally evidence of systemic reaction such as bronchoconstriction. These unwanted effects, combined with the need for administration by regular injection have prevented these drugs from being successfully used in clinical practice. The development of newer compounds such as Ganirelix (Organon) and Cetrorelix (ASTA), which appear to have few histaminic side-effects,[26,36] is an encouraging development which may allow long term use of antagonists in the future.

Tissue oestrogen sensitivity

In oestrogen dependent conditions, such as endometriosis and uterine fibroids, the effective reduction of oestradiol to negligible levels is the key to treatment of both conditions. More specifically, it has been shown by Dickey et al in 1984[37] that treatment of extensive endometriosis (AFS original classification) required oestradiol levels of < 15 pg/ml for ≥ 75 days, and AFS severe and moderate class endometriosis required serum oestrogen levels of < 22 pg/ml and < 41 pg/ml, respectively, before complete remission could be achieved. Uterine fibroids appear to be more oestrogen sensitive than endometriosis, in that there is measurable shrinkage when oestradiol levels of 15–25 pg/ml are attained.[38,39]

By replacing oestrogen transdermally to achieve differing oestrogen levels in postmenopausal women, Chetowski et al[40] showed that bone is the most oestrogen sensitive tissue, requiring a level of between 25 and 30 pg/ml to reduce bone loss. At these low levels, there was little measurable oestrogen response in the vaginal epithelium and blood lipids.

The oestrogen threshold hypothesis

The above data suggest that were it possible to find the specific level at which a particular tissue responds to oestrogen, it may be possible to treat safely an oestrogen dependent condition with GnRH analogues whilst preserving bone and minimizing other unwanted hypo-oestrogenic effects.[41,42]

Knowing in advance the oestrogen level needed to treat safely a gynaecological disease such as endometriosis potentially has significant benefits to patients, but as the theory depends on very accurate measurement of circulating oestradiol levels, it would be extremely hard to attain in practice, as there may be considerable variations between laboratory 'normal' ranges and assay senstivities from unit to unit. However, as assays improve in quality generally, and for units with high quality facilities for oestradiol measurement, the oestrogen threshold hypothesis may be used in the future.

Titration of the oestrogen level to reach a specified target may be achieved by either altering the dose of analogue administered or by maximally blocking oestrogen production with full dose GnRH analogue therapy and administering replacement oestrogen or other therapies to prevent unwanted effects, a concept widely known as 'addback therapy'.

STRATEGIES FOR MINIMISING THE CONSEQUENCES OF GnRH ANALOGUE INDUCED HYPO-OESTROGENISM

Modifying GnRH analogue doses

Alteration of doses of GnRH analogues, though an attractive option, may lead to problems with compliance, breakthrough gonadotrophin secretion and consequent treatment failure.

The ability to alter doses of GnRH agonists is limited as most drug development data for the treatment of oestrogen dependent disorders are from continuous doses of agonist – enough to ensure complete pituitary gonadotroph downregulation – with the express intent of avoiding breakthrough secretion of gonadotrophins. This has lead to the production of several slow release compounds which are unsuitable for such dosage manipulation. Nasal administration would, therefore, seem to be the only reliable route for such an activity. As mentioned above, though this is an effective way of administering GnRH agonists, it is vulnerable to difficulties with compliance. A proposed protocol for this treatment in a very compliant woman would be to start therapy at a high dose, then reducing the dose to attain a pre-determined oestrogen level.

Such patients would need to be counselled on the importance of continuing therapy and advised on the need for continued non-hormonal means of contraception. Though this protocol may be effective when strictly adhered to in individual cases in the short term, the two main oestrogen dependent conditions that are indications for GnRH agonist therapy – endometriosis and uterine fibroids – would benefit from the ability to administer safely GnRH agonists for much longer periods. Long-term nasal drug administration may well prove unacceptable for this and, therefore, GnRH agonist dose manipulation may not be possible until varying dose slow-release preparations become available.

GnRH antagonists, through their dose-dependent competitive blockade of the gonadotroph cell, may be the future way in which oestradiol levels can be reduced with a degree of accuracy and reliability to a pre-determined target. Unfortunately, antagonists will have to be more widely understood before such studies can be commenced to investigate this interesting possibility.

Addback therapy

This strategy entails 'adding' another therapeutic agent or combination of agents to be administered in conjunction with GnRH analogue. When evaluating an 'addback therapy' the following need to be considered: (i) the effect on the GnRH's therapeutic effect on the original disease process; (ii) the effect on hypo-estrogenic symptoms; (iii) the effect on bone; and (iv) the effect on lipid profile.

Progestogens

Progestogens alone, in the absence of oestrogens, have been shown to inhibit bone loss and alleviate menopausal symptoms.[43-46] It has been suggested that the 19-nortestosterone derivatives (e.g. norethisterone) may produce more significant anti-oestrogenic effects on the endometrium than drugs such as medroxyprogesterone acetate (MPA). The two compounds that have been studied in conjunction with GnRH analogues are norethisterone and MPA. Progestogens are known to promote endometrial atrophy – sometimes referred to as a 'pseudopregnancy effect'. The published studies regarding GnRH analogues and progestogens are difficult to evaluate as the numbers are small; different GnRH analogues have been used in conjunction with different progestogens and varying doses.

Norethisterone in doses of 10 mg daily has been shown to reduce bone loss in postmenopausal women,[47] although smaller doses of norethisterone (up to 3.5 mg) did not appear to prevent bone loss. In combination with GnRH analogues in premenopausal women using 10 mg of norethisterone daily, Surrey and Judd[48] demonstrated a beneficial effect on bone density and full recovery after 24 weeks of cessation of therapy. Riis et al[49] found bone sparing effects with 1.2 mg of NET but the numbers were small and the control group was historical. Eldred et al[50] used doses from 0.7 mg up to 2.5 mg of NET and, although significant bone loss still occurred, this was less with increasing doses of NET. With regard to biochemical markers of bone metabolism, the increase in hydroxyproline and calcium/creatinine ratios was abolished in the 2.5 NET group. MPA at a dose of 15 mg daily did not appear to be bone protective, although it eliminated hypo-oestrogenic symptoms.[51] It appears that norethisterone is superior to MPA in protection of bone loss.

The dose of norethisterone as addback therapy has yet to be determined and is probably in the order of 5–10 mg daily. When contemplating long-term use of progestogens in this context, the effect on lipid parameters gains increasing importance. NET decreases HDL and the lipid changes with MPA have not been reported. No data are available on the effects of progestins as addback therapy and their direct effect on vessel wall and blood flow. This is of obvious importance when assessing the long-term cardiovascular risk. Higher doses of progestogens require investigation as well as the use of alternative progestogens such as dydrogesterone.

Oestrogen and progestogen combined therapy

It is unacceptable to give unopposed oestrogen replacement therapy. In the conditions mentioned above, oestrogen may stimulate the original disease and, even if this is not the case, there is the risk of producing unwanted endometrial histological changes.

The combined oestrogen and progestogen regimens show promise with respect to alleviation of hypo-oestrogenic symptoms and protection of the skeleton, although the published studies are difficult to evaluate as the protocols are so varied, the controls poor and the numbers small. Many different combinations of oestrogens and progestogens have been used and all appear to be beneficial for relief of menopausal symptoms. Conjugated oestrogens should be used in a dose of at least 0.625 mg to prevent bone loss. Transdermal oestrogens in a dose of 25 μg do not appear to be completely effective for prevention of bone loss[52] and should be evaluated in a higher dose such as 50 μg. It would seem unwise to give cyclical hormone replacement therapy, especially treating endometriosis or premenstrual syndrome (PMS). With endometriosis the endometriotic tissue may be stimulated, leading to pain and, with PMS, the added progestogen may well stimulate the progestogenic side-effects perceived in the normal menstrual cycle. Therefore, the ideal HRT addback therapy should be continuous combined therapy of which none have been published to date.

With the oestrogen and progestogen therapies studied there are many ranges in dosages used and, as mentioned previously, the important features of an addback therapy are the effect on the skeleton, plasma lipids, the original disease, and additional side-effects. The majority of the oestrogen and progestogen therapies studied have used bone sparing doses and appear to be effective.[53-55] If continuous combined therapies are used, then a lower dose of progestogen can be used and, theoretically, this should be beneficial for the lipid profile.

Tibolone

Tibolone is a synthetic steroid with weak oestrogenic, progestogenic and androgenic properties which has been used as HRT in postmenopausal women. Tibolone is metabolised to 3 isomers of which the progestogenic delta 4 isomer predominates at the level of the endometrium, inducing endometrial atrophy. Tibolone relieves hypo-oestrogenic symptoms, is bone protective and yet does not stimulate endometrium.[56] Shaw and Lindsay studied 33 women who had endometriosis or fibroids and they were randomised to tryptorelin 3.75 mg every 4 weeks with placebo or tryptorelin and tibolone 2.5 mg daily for 24 weeks.[6] The group receiving tibolone had significantly less flushes and yet improvements in endometriosis were similar in each group with regard to bone loss. The placebo group lost 5.1% in the lumbar vertebrae (assessed by dual energy X-ray absorptiometry, DXA) compared with 1.1% in the tibolone group. The effect on lipids was not reported. Previous authors have shown a decrease in total cholesterol, triglycerides and HDL cholesterol and decrease in lipoprotein (a).[57,56] Tibolone appears to have potential as an effective addback therapy as it appears to act on bone in a way comparable to oestrogen,[56] is more potent than pure progestogens yet without the stimulatory effect of oestrogen on the endometrium.

Bisphosphonates

Bisphosphonates are synthetic analogues of pyrophosphate characterised by 2 C–P bonds on the same carbon atom resulting in a PCP structure. The chemical structure allows a great number of possible variations by changing the 2 lateral chains on the carbon atom. The main pharmacological effect of the bisphosphonates is the ability to inhibit bone resorption and this is exerted through the strong affinity of bisphosphonates with the bone surface. The mode of action is not well understood and the activity of bisphosphonates on bone resorption varies greatly from one compound to another.

Etidronate, a first generation bisphosphonate, is given for 14 consecutive days (400 mg/day) followed by calcium carbonate 500 mg/day for 76 days. The cycle is then repeated. Cyclical etidronate has been shown to reduce fractures when given to postmenopausal women with osteoporosis. Etidronate should be taken on an empty stomach, as food and fluids can significantly reduce absorption. Side-effects are rare, but some patients may have nausea and diarrhoea. To date, bisphosphonates have not been evaluated alone as addback therapy. Sodium etidronate has been studied in conjunction with norethindrone and compared directly to high doses of norethindrone with GnRH agonists.[58] The aim of the study was to assess bone mineral density, vasomotor symptoms, circulating oestrogens and lipids. The rationale behind this combination of low dose norethindrone with etidronate was to see whether it was more lipid friendly than the higher doses of progestogen needed to protect the skeleton when progestogen is given alone as addback. There were no significant changes in lumbar spine bone mineral density over 48 weeks which were no different to those of matched controls. With regard to vasomotor symptoms, the subjects receiving either 10 mg of norethindrone compared to 2.5 mg of norethindrone and sodium etidronate experienced minimal symptoms during the agonist therapy. The group receiving GnRH analogue alone experienced significant hot flushes and these persisted throughout the therapy. Bone density in the lumbar spine (DXA) significantly declined only in the groups receiving GnRH analogue alone –4.8 % ($P < 0.05$). It is of interest that bone density increased slightly in the patients receiving GnRH analogues with low dose norethindrone and cyclic sodium etidronate. The women who received both doses of norethindrone had decreased HDL levels, the extent of which was greater for patients receiving the higher 10 mg daily dosage.

The conclusion from the study was that sodium etidronate, in conjunction with low dose norethindrone, was as good as high dose norethindrone for vasomotor symptoms and prevention of bone loss and was not as detrimental to the lipoprotein profile. It appears that either of the 2 addback regimens could safely be used for prolonged therapy of endometriosis, as they did not negate the effect of GnRH analogue on the original disease process. The main difference between the 2 regimens was the greater abnormal lipoprotein changes (and weight gain) associated with administration of higher norethindrone doses.

There are several newer and more potent bisphosphonates which have not, as yet, been evaluated in this context. It is probable that these drugs will also prevent bone loss alone but will not prevent hypo-oestrogenic symptoms.

Calcitonin

Calcitonin is a natural polypeptide hormone that is a weak antiresorptive that can reduce pain associated with vertebral fractures. Calcitonin can either be given by injection or nasal preparation. Roux et al investigated 40 patients who had endometriosis and were given 3.75 mg monthly of triptorelin and 1 mg of calcium daily for 6 months and, in addition, they were randomised to receive placebo, nasal salmon calcitonin (SCT) 100 IU daily or SCT 200 IU daily.[59] Biochemical markers of bone metabolism and bone density measurements were performed at baseline and after 6 months. There was no difference in bone loss at the lumbar spine (DXA) between the three groups and biochemical markers of bone metabolism reflected post menopausal status, again with no difference between the 3 groups. Therefore, it appears that these doses of calcitonin are insufficient to prevent GnRH analogue induced bone loss.

Parathyroid hormone

Continuous administration of parathyroid hormone (PTH) decreases bone mass but intermittent administration of low dose PTH stimulates bone formation leading to increased bone mass. There is only one study that has looked at parathyroid hormone in conjunction with GnRH analogues. Finkelstein et al studied 50 women who had symptomatic laparoscopically proven endometriosis.[60] They were randomised to receive nafarelin at a dose of 200 µg intranasally twice daily for 6 months or nafarelin and PTH at a dose of 40 mg (500 units) subcutaneously, daily for 6 months. The women were also asked to maintain a daily calcium intake of approximately 120 mg. The aim of the study was to assess the effect of this regimen on the skeleton. The women in the nafarelin only group lost significant bone in the lateral lumbar spine (3.5% - P <0.001) whereas in the group receiving additional PTH the spinal bone mineral density increased (3.4%, P = 0.01). With regards to the femoral neck, both groups showed significant decreases (1.8%, P = 0.01) for the nafarelin group, (1.7%, P = 0.02) for the nafarelin and PTH group. The authors concluded that the addition of PTH prevented spinal bone loss in women receiving GnRH analogues and this increased bone density was accompanied by increases in biochemical markers of bone formation and resorption. Because bone density at all sites in the women who had received nafarelin and parathyroid hormone equalled or exceeded that in the women who received nafarelin alone, it appeared that increased bone formation offset the increase in bone absorption. Although LDL increased in the nafarelin and parathyroid hormone groups, the rates of change in serum LDL did not differ significantly between the groups. HDL did not change. Therefore, PTH appeared to prevent spinal bone loss but bone loss occurred in the femur. PTH did not appear to be detrimental to the lipid profile. However, even if satisfactory, its use may be significantly limited due to its expense and clinical availability.

SUMMARY

In the context of GnRH analogue use, for addback therapy to be most beneficial it should be instituted as early as possible. Progestogens are potentially able to inhibit bone loss and have some effect on alleviating menopausal symptoms and do not stimulate the endometrium. Due to its superior prevention of bone loss, norethisterone is preferred to MPA and, although the ideal dose has not been ascertained, this is probably 5 or 10 mg daily. The disadvantage of progestogens are their effects on the lipid profile, the relevance of which is unclear if they are administered as addback therapy for a few years.

Tibolone relieves hypo-oestrogenic symptoms, does not stimulate the endometrium and prevents bone loss but at present its effect on lipoproteins is unclear. This agent shows promise as an ideal addback agent.

Similarly, continuous combined oestrogen/progestogen regimens would be beneficial as bone mass would be maintained, the original disease should not be stimulated, and menopausal symptoms would be relieved. Again, the long-term effect on the cardiovascular system has yet to be assessed.

To date, cyclical etidronate alone has not been investigated, but one would assume it would prevent bone loss without eliminating the vasomotor symptoms. The newer bisphosphonates would undoubtedly prevent bone loss, but continued menopausal symptoms would be a major drawback. Progestogens and bisphosphonates show promise as there is relief of vasomotor symptoms, prevention of bone loss and the effect on lipoproteins is not as detrimental as with progestogens alone. This combination merits further investigation, although etidronate with low dose oestrogen/progestrogen combinations may also prove to be effective. There is one report on the use of parathyroid hormone in conjunction with GnRH analogue which primarily looks at the effect on bone loss. PTH appeared to prevent spinal bone loss but bone loss occurred in the femur. PTH did not appear to be detrimental to the lipid profile. However, even if satisfactory its use may be significantly limited due to its expense and clinical availability.

Other approaches to addback therapy are at present experimental with no practical alternatives to the above at the present time.

CONCLUSION

GnRH agonists are widely available and, with increasing indications for GnRH therapy, their use is becoming widespread. Advances such as the development of new methods of administration, especially for those who need long term administration, continue to be made. Development of GnRH antagonists may produce ideal drugs in the future, but these are undergoing further evaluation.

Use of strategies to limit the long-term effects of this group of drugs, such as modifying the dose of GnRH analogue and concomitant administration of addback therapy, appear to be effective, but need further development.

Addback therapy would enable GnRH analogues to be used long-term. The studies to date are relatively short-term (mostly 6 months). The ideal addback therapy would relieve hypo-oestrogenic symptoms, prevent the GnRH analogue induced bone loss, not alter the efficacy of GnRH analogues and not be detrimental to the lipid profile (though long-term importance of this is currently unknown).

At the present time, it would appear that tibolone or oestrogen/progestogen continuous combined preparations should be considered as first line addback agents. Bisphosphonates and progestogens show promise as second line treatments. However, the optimal regimen/dosage for the treatment of endometriosis and fibroids has yet to be established.

REFERENCES

1 Johansen J S, Riis B J, Hassager C, Moen M, Jacobson J. The effect of a gonadotropin-releasing hormone agonist analog (nafarelin) on bone metabolism. J Clin Endocrinol Metab 1988; 67: 701–706

2 Dawood M Y, Lewis V, Ramos J. Cortical and trabecular bone mineral content in women with endometriosis: effect of gonadotrophin-releasing hormone agonist and danazol. Fertil Steril 1989; 52: 21–26

3 West C P, Lumsden M A, Lawson S, Williamson J, Baird D T. Shrinkage of uterine fibroids during therapy with goserelin (Zoladex): a luteinizing hormone-releasing hormone agonist administered as a monthly subcutaneous depot. Fertil Steril 1987; 48: 45–51

4 Crowley W F, Filicori M, Spratt D I, Santoro N F. The physiology of gonadotrophin-releasing hormone (GnRH) in men and women. Recent Prog Hormone Res 1985; 41: 473–525

5 Conn P M, Crowley J R. Gonadotrophin-releasing hormone and its analogues. N Engl J Med 1991; 324: 93–103

6 Shaw R W. Mechanisms controlling gonadotrophin secretion. Adv Reprod Endocrinol 1994; 6: 1–15

7 Clayton R N. Gonadotrophin-releasing hormone: its actions and receptors. J Endocrinol 1989; 120: 11–19

8 Gorospe W C, Conn M. Agents that decrease gonadotrophin-releasing hormone (GnRH) receptor internalization do not inhibit GnRH mediated gonadotrope desensitisation. Endocrinology, 1987; 120: 222–229

9 Stojilkovic S S, Rojas E, Stutzin A, Izumi S, Catt K J. Desensitization of pituitary gonadotrophin secretion by agonist-induced inactivation of voltage-sensitive calcium channels. J Biol Chem 1989; 264: 10939–10942

10 Vickery B H, Nestor J J J. Luteinizing hormone-releasing hormone analogs: development and mechanism of action. Semin Reprod Endocrinol 1987; 5: 353–369

11 Janovick J A, Haviv F, Fitzpatrick T D, Conn P M. Differential orientation of a GnRH agonist and antagonist in the pituitary GnRH receptor. Endocrinology, 1993; 133: 942–945

12 Sandow J, Fraser H M, Geisthovel F. Pharmacology and experimental basis of therapy with LHRH agonists in women. Prog Clin Biol Res 1986; 225: 1–5

13 Holland F J, Fishman L, Costigan D C et al. Pharmacokinetic characteristics of the gonadotrophin-releasing hormone analogue D-Ser(TBU)-6EA-10-luteinising hormone-releasing hormone (buserelin) after subcutaneous and intranasal administration in children with central precocious puberty. J Clin Endocrinol Metab 1986; 63: 1065–1070

14 Swaisland A J, Adam H K, Barker Y, Holmes B, Hutchinson F G. Tailored release profiles for Zoladex using biodegradable polymers. Pharm Weekblad Sci Ed 1988; 10: 57

15 Rajfer J, Handelsman D J, Crum A, Steiner B, Peterson M, Swerdlof R S. Comparisons of the efficacy of subcutaneous and nasal spray buserelin treatment in suppression of testicular steroidogenesis in men with prostate cancer. Fertil Steril 1986; 46 :104–110

16 Henzl M R, Kwei L. Efficacy and safety of nafarelin in the treatment of endometriosis. Am J Obstet Gynecol 1990; 162: 570–574

17 Henzl M R. Gonadotropin-releasing hormone analogs: update on new findings. Am J Obstet Gynecol 1992; 166: 757–761.

18 Chaplin M D. Bioavailability of nafarelin in healthy volunteers. Am J Obstet Gynecol 1992; 166: 762–765

19 Erickson L D, Ory S J. GnRH analogues in the treatment of endometriosis. Obstet Gynecol Clin North Am 1989; 16: 123–145

20 Ogawa Y. Small-size microcapsules for long-term GnRH agonist administration. In: Filicori M, Flamigni C (eds) Treatment with GnRH analogs: controversies and perspectives. New York: Parthenon, 1996; 47–52

21 Dutta A S, Furr B J A, Hutchinson F G. The discovery and development of Goserelin (Zoladex⁰). Pharm Med 1993; 7: 9–28

22 Debruyne F M, Dijkman G A, Lee D C et al. A new long acting formulation of the luteinizing hormone-releasing analogue goserelin: results of studies in prostate cancer J Urol 1996; 155: 1352–1354

23 Sandow J, von Rechenberg W, Jerabek-Sandow G, Krauss B, Fenner-Nau D, Lill N. Pharmacokinetics of buserelin microparticles in three animal species. Gynaecol Endocrinol 1996; 10: 9

24 von Rechenberg W, Sandow J, Seidel R, Trabant H. Biopharmaceutical studies with buserelin implants. Gynaecol Endocrinol 1996; 10: 8

25 Felberbaum R, Riethmüller-Winzen H, Germer U et al. First clinical experiences with a slow release formulation of the GnRH antagonist cetrorelix (SB-75) in patients with uterine fibroma to undergo surgery. Gynaecol Endocrinol 1996; 10: 52

26 Nelson L R, Fujimoto V Y, Jaffe R B, Monroe S E. Suppression of follicular phase pituitary-gonadal function by a potent new gonadotropin-releasing hormone antagonist with reduced histamine-releasing properties (ganirelix). Fertil Steril 1995; 63: 963–969

27 West C P. LHRH analogues in the management of uterine fibroids, premenstrual syndrome and breast malignancies. In: Healy D. (ed) Baillière's Clinical Obstetrics and Gynaecology. London: Baillière Tindall, 1988; 689–709

28 Frydman R, Cornel C, de Ziegler D, Taieb J, Spitz I M, Bouchard P. Prevention of premature luteinizing hormone and progesterone rise with a gonadotropin-releasing hormone antagonist, Nal-Glu, in controlled ovarian hyperstimulation. Fertil Steril 1991; 29: 257–266

29 Maheux R, Guilloteau C, Lemay A, Bastide A, Fazekas A. Luteinizing hormone-releasing hormone agonist and uterine leiomyoma: a pilot study. Am J Obstet Gynecol 1985; 152: 1034–1039

30 Schmidt-Gollwitzer M, Hardt W, Schmidt-Gollwitzer K, von der Ohe M, Nevinney-Stickel J. Influence of the LH-RH analogue buserelin on cyclic ovarian function and on endometrium. A new approach to fertility control? Contraception 1981; 23: 187–195

31 Brenner P F, Shoupe D, Mishell D R. Ovulation inhibition with naferelin acetate nasal administration for 6 months. Contraception 1985; 32: 531–551

32 Friedman A J. Vaginal haemorrhage associated with degenerating submucous leiomyomata during leuprolide acetate treatment. Fertil Steril 1989; 52: 152–154

33 Fogelman I. The effects of oestrogen deficiency on the skeleton and its prevention. Br J Obstet Gynaecol 1996; 103: 1–4

34 Pavlou S N, Sharp S C. Clinical applications of GnRH antagonists in men. In: Bouchard P, Caraty A, Coelingh Bennink H J T, Pavlou S N. (eds) GnRH, GnRH analogs, gonadotropins and gonadal peptides. New York: Parthenon, 1993; 285–292

35 Hall J E, Whitcomb R W, Rivier J E, Vale W W, Crowley W F J. Differential regulation of luteinizing hormone, follicle stimulating hormone, and free α-subunit secretion from the gonadotrope by gonadotropin-releasing hormone(GnRH): evidence from the use of two GnRH antagonists. J Clin Endocrinol Metab 1990; 70: 328–335

36 Reissmann T, Felberbaum R, Diedrich K, Engel J, Comaru-Schally A M, Schally A V. Development and applications of luteinizing hormone-releasing hormone antagonists in the treatment of infertility: an overview. Hum Reprod 1995; 10: 1974–1981

37 Dickey R P, Taylor S N, Curole D N. Serum estradiol and danazol. I. Endometriosis response, side effects, administration interval, concurrent spironolactone and dexamethasone. Fertil Steril 1984; 42: 709–716

38 Friedman A J, Barbieri R L, Doubilet P M, Fine C, Schiff I. A randomized double-blind trial of a gonadotropin releasing hormone agonist with or without medroxyprogesterone acetate in the treatment of leiomyomata uteri. Fertil Steril 1988; 49: 404–409

39 Friedman A J, Harrison-Atlas D, Barbieri R L, Benacerraf B, Gleason R, Schiff I. Medical management of uterine leiomyomata: treatment with depot leuprolide: a gonadotropin releasing hormone agonist. Fertil Steril 1989; 51: 241–256

40 Chetowski R J, Meldrum D R, Steingold K A et al. Biological effects of transdermal oestradiol. J Clin Endocrinol Metab 1986; 314: 1615–1620

41 Barbieri R L, Gordon A C. Hormonal therapy of endometriosis: the estradiol target. Fertil Steril 1991; 56: 820–822

42 Barbieri R L. Hormone treatment of endometriosis: the estrogen threshold hypothesis. Am J Obstet Gynecol 1992; 106: 740–745

43 Paterson M E L. A randomised double-blinded cross-over trial into the effects of norethisterone on climacteric symptoms and biochemical profiles. Br J Obstetr Gynaecol 1982; 89: 464–472

44 Erlik Y, Medrum D R, Lagasse L D, Judd H L. Effect of megestrol acetate on flushing and bone metabolism in post-menopausal women. Maturitas 1981; A3: 167–172

45 Mandel F P, Davidson B J, Erlik Y, Judd H L, Meldrum D R. Effects of progestins on bone metabolism in post-menopausal women. J Reprod Med 1982; 13: 511–514

46 Abdalla H I, Hart D M, Lindsay R, Leggate I, Hooke A. Prevention of bone mineral loss in postmenopausal women by norethisterone. Obstet Gynecol 1985; 66: 789–792

47 Horowitz M, Wishart J, Need A G, Morris H, Philcox J, Nordin B E. Treatment of post-menopausal hyperparathyroidism with norethindrone. Arch Intern Med 1987; 147: 681

48 Surrey E S. Reduction of vasomotor symptoms and bone mineral density with combined norethindrone and long acting gonadotrophin-releasing hormone agonist therapy of symptomatic endometriosis: a prospective randomised trial. J Clin Endocrinol Metab 1992; 75: 558–563

49 Riis B J, Christiansen C, Johansen J S, Jacobson J. Is it possible to prevent bone loss in young women treated with luteinizing hormone-releasing hormone agonists? J Clin Endocrinol Metab 1990; 7: 920–924

50 Eldred J M, Haynes P J, Thomas E J. A randomised double-blind placebo controlled trial of the effects on bone metabolism of the combination of nafarelin acetate and norethisterone. Clin Endocrinol 1992; 37: 354–359

51 West C P, Hillier H. Long term treatment of uterine fibroids with 'Zoladex' (goserelin). 'Zoladex' (goserelin) and Gynaecology: Reinforcing the Partnership, 1994; Abstract: Satellite Symposium 14th FIGO World Congress

52 Howell R, Edmonds D K, Lees B, Stevenson J, Dowsett M. A randomized controlled trial of goserelin with addback (HRT) for endometriosis – effect on bone density. Fertil Steril 1993; 143 (Suppl): 137

53 Tiitinen A, Simberg N, Stenman U H, Ylikorkala O. Estrogen replacement does not potentiate gonadotrophin-releasing hormone agonist induced androgen suppression in treatment of hirsuitism. J Clin Endocrinol Metab 1989; 79: 447–451

54 Leather A T, Studd J W W, Watson N R, Holland E F N. The prevention of bone loss in young women treated with GnRH analogues with 'addback' estrogen therapy. Obstet Gynecol 1993; 81: 104–107

55 Thomas E J, Okuda K J, Thomas N M. The combination of depot gonadotrophin-releasing hormone agonist and cyclical hormone replacement therapy for dysfunctional uterine bleeding. Br J Obstet Gynaecol 1991; 98: 1155–1159

56 Rymer J, Chapman M G, Fogelman I. Effect of tibolone on postmenopausal bone loss. Osteoporos Int 1994; 4: 314–319

57 Farish E, Barnes J F, Rolton H A, Spowart K, Fletcher D C, Hart D M. Effect of tibolone on lipoprotein (a) and HDL subfractions. Maturitas 1994; 20: 215–219

58 Surrey E S, Voight B, Fournet N, Judd H L. Prolonged gonadotrophin-releasing hormone agonist treatment of symptomatic endometriosis: the role of cyclic sodium etidronate and low-dose norethindrone 'add-back' therapy. Fertil Steril 1995; 63: 747–755

59 Roux C, Pelissier C, Listrat V et al. Bone loss during gonadotrophin-releasing hormone agonist treatment and use of nasal calcitonin. Osteoporos Int 1995; 5: 185–190

60 Finkelstein J S, Klibanski A, Schaefer E H, Hornstein M D, Schiff I, Neer R M. Parathyroid hormone for the prevention of bone loss induced by estrogen deficiency. N Engl J Med 1994; 331: 1618–1623

Thomas Ind

Management of post-menopausal bleeding

Abnormal post-menopausal vaginal bleeding (PMB) accounts for a significant proportion of gynaecological referrals. Excluding endometrial carcinoma is the primary aim of initial investigations. Traditionally, this was achieved by performing uterine curettage under general anaesthetic. However, new methods of examining the endometrium have been introduced into clinical practice, many without proper clinical assessment. Current reports have led to more questions than answers and the best method of investigating women with PMB is still disputed.

This chapter highlights the important issues concerning the management of women with PMB. In particular, the chapter concentrates on the clinical aspects that may lead to suspicion of an endometrial malignancy or other important pathological causes. In addition, the arguments for and against different methods of investigating uterine bleeding in post-menopausal women are discussed.

INCIDENCE, AGE AND GEOGRAPHICAL DISTRIBUTION

Post-menopausal bleeding is a phenomenon of the Western world and is most common in Caucasian women of high socio-economic class.[1] The incidence increases with migration from developing to Western countries[1] and implicates environmental reasons as the main cause. This is of particular interest as it does not take into account the proportion of hysterectomised women in the developed world. The disparity is probably due to the increased use of exogenous oestrogens; the higher degree of obesity and, therefore, peripheral conversion of plasma androstenedione to estrone;[2] and a higher accessibility to medical services and, therefore, increase in reporting.

Mr Thomas Ind, Senior Registrar, O&G Professorial Suite, Prince William Wing, St George Public Hospital, Gray Street, Kogarah, Sydney, New South Wales 2217, Australia

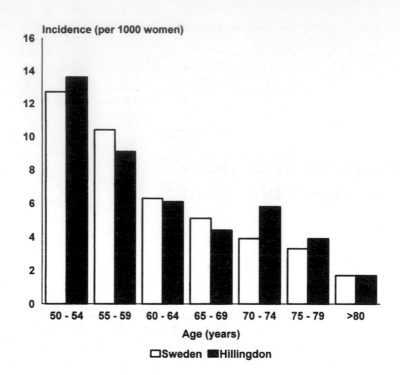

Fig. 24.1 Incidence of postmenopausal bleeding in Sweden and in Hillingdon.

In Sweden, the incidence of PMB varies between 13 per 1000 post-menopausal women at the age of 50 years to 2 per 1000 post-menopausal women at the age of 80 years (Fig. 24.1).[3] In contrast, the risk of endometrial carcinoma in women with PMB rises with age from about 1% at the age of 50 years to about 25% at the age of 80 years.[3]

The incidence of PMB in the UK is unknown. However, at Hillingdon Hospital between the years of 1995 and 1996 PMB accounted for 4.6% (316/6929) of new gynaecological referrals and 23.6% (316/1337) of new gynaecological referrals for women of menopausal age. Based on the population served by the hospital, the local incidence of PMB has been estimated to be 7.0/1000 post-menopausal women. This varies between 13.6/1000 women at the age of 50 years to 1.7/1000 women at the age of 80 years (Fig. 24.1).

PATHOLOGY

The causes of PMB are summarised in Table 24.1. Early studies reported the risk of endometrial cancer associated with PMB as 53–58%.[4,5] However, more recent reports suggest the incidence to be 1.5–28% with an average of 11% (Table 24.2).[3,6–22] This may reflect increasing awareness of the importance of PMB with all women referred for investigation rather than just those at high risk.

Other causes of PMB include endometrial hyperplasia or polyps (Table 24.2). However, a significant proportion of women with PMB have atrophic endometria (Table 24.2). Payne et al[23] found benign or non-neoplastic causes

Table 24.1 Causes of vaginal bleeding in post-menopausal women

Systemic	Bleeding disorders	
	Exogenous oestrogens	Hormone replacement
		Ginseng
	Endogenous oestrogens	Peripheral conversion of androstenedione
		Oestrogen producing tumours
Local	Benign	Endometrial polyps
		Endometritis
		Cervical polyps
		Cervicitis
		Cervical trauma
		Senile atrophic vaginitis
		Vaginal trauma
		Vaginal inflammation
		Vaginal polyps
		Vulval dystrophies
		Vulval dermatitis
		Vulval trauma
	Malignant/premalignant	Fallopian tube carcinoma
		Leiomyosarcoma of uterus
		Endometrial carcinoma
		Endometrial hyperplasia
		Cervical carcinoma
		Vaginal carcinoma
		Vulval carcinoma
		Secondary tumours

Women with lesions of the bladder, urethra, rectum and anus may also describe their bleeding as being per vagina.

for PMB in 66% of women (Table 24.3): these included a significant proportion of women with cervicitis, cervical polyps and atrophic vaginitis. Other sites of origin include the bladder, urethra, rectum and anus which are often described by patients to be per vagina in origin.[7,11,23]

Table 24.2 Histopathological findings of the endometrium in women with postmenopausal bleeding. A meta-analysis

Histopathology	Percent (n/total)	References
Normal endometrium	57.0 (2464/4322)	3,6,7,10–22
Atrophic/insufficient sample	44.7 (1809/4050)	3,6,7,10–17,19–22
Proliferative	8.8 (227/2574)	3,6,7,10,12,18,20–22
Secretory	1.0 (25/2574)	3,6,7,10,12,18,20–22
Benign polyps	13.1 (535/4081)	3,6,7,10–15,17–22
Hyperplasia	10.3 (442/4278)	3,7,9,10–15,17–22
Simple	8.6 (90/1042)	3,7,9,12,17,22
Complex	1.9 (20/1042)	3,7,9,12,17,22
Cancer	11.0 (507/4592)	3,6–22
Other pathology	8.4 (321/3815)	3,6,7,10–15,17–22

Table 24.3 Benign causes of postmenopausal bleeding arising from the female reproductive tract (from Payne et al[23])

	Total	Infective (%)	Neoplastic (%)	Trauma (%)	Exogenous (%)
Vulvo/vaginal	73	58	27	15	0
Cervix	184	0	51	49	0
Corpus	150	7	56	0	37
Adnexa	0	0	0	0	0

Table 24.4 Non-endometrial malignancies associated with postmenopausal bleeding. A meta-analysis

Site	Percent (n/total)	References
Ovary	1.2 (18/1522)	3,7,11,23
Cervix	5.7 (222/3885)	3,7,11,13,18,23
Vulva/vagina	1.4 (27/1945)	6,18,23
Other	0.8 (9/1065)	6,11,23

Post-menopausal bleeding is also associated with other non-endometrial cancers.[3,7,11,18,23] The most common of these is carcinoma of the cervix with a reported incidence in women with PMB of 0.8–13% (Table 24.4).[3,7,11,13,18,23] Other associated tumour sites of the female reproductive tract include the fallopian tubes, vagina and vulva (Table 24.4).[7,11,23] In addition, post-menopausal women who complain of vaginal bleeding have a small but significant risk of having ovarian, breast or colorectal carcinomas (Table 24.4).[3,7,11,23]

HISTORY, EXAMINATION AND CERVICAL CYTOLOGY

A thorough history and examination is the most important step in assessing women with PMB. It is an integral part of diagnosis and results of investigations should only be interpreted in conjunction with the whole clinical picture.

Table 24.5 Probability of having endometrial cancer associated with postmenopausal bleeding in women with different risk factors. A meta-analysis

Risk factor	Percent (n/total)	References
Early menarche (< 10 years)	80.0 (4/5)	7
Late menopause (> 55 years)	45.5 (5/11)	7
Nulliparity	41.8 (28/67)	7,24
Unopposed oestrogen therapy	40.0 (10/25)	19,24
Bleeding moderate or severe*	33.5 (77/230)	7,19,24
Obesity	33.0 (30/91)	7,24
Diabetes	31.0 (13/42)	7,24
Hypertension	30.7 (42/137)	7,24
Liver disease	30.0 (9/30)	7
Persistent/recurrent bleeding	27.0 (38/141)	24

*Mild bleeding was defined as spotting.

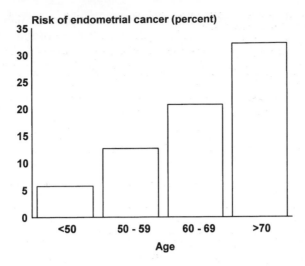

Fig. 24.2 Probability of having endometrial cancer associated with postmenopausal bleeding in women of different age groups. A meta-analysis of 881 women from three different studies.[3,7,24]

A history should elicit the exact nature of the bleeding. This may assist in diagnosis as the exact nature of the bleeding may lead the clinician to suspect an endometrial neoplasm (Table 24.5).[7,19,24] Furthermore, a thorough history may alert the clinician to factors that are associated with an increased risk of endometrial cancer and hyperplasia, such as diabetes, nulliparity and use of unopposed oestrogens (Table 24.5).[7,19,24,25] The incidence of complex endometrial hyperplasia or carcinoma varies greatly with these risk factors in women with PMB (Table 24.5). The risk of endometrial cancer increases with age and the number of risk factors present (Figs 24.2 & 24.3).[3,7,25] In one study,[24]

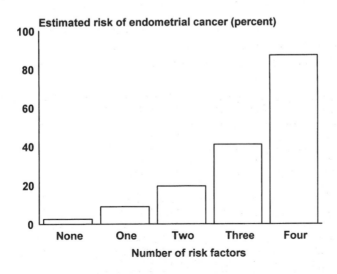

Fig. 24.3 Probability of having endometrial cancer associated with postmenopausal bleeding in women with different numbers of risk factors. Modified from Feldman et al.[24]

the risk was calculated to be as high as 87% in nulliparous, diabetic women over the age of 70 years compared to only 2.6% if none of these risk factors were present. In that study,[24] the odds ratio for endometrial malignancy was 9.1 for women over 70 years, 3.7 for women with diabetes, and 2.7 for nulliparous women.

A thorough examination may help in the diagnosis of vulval, vaginal, cervical or pelvic pathology. Vaginal and cervical pathology such as cervical polyps, senile atrophic vaginitis or ulceration from a ring pessary may be directly visualised. Furthermore, an indication of the patient's general health can be obtained which is important before considering a general anaesthetic.

Some argue that abnormal uterine bleeding in a menopausal woman is a clinical indication for cervical cytology irrespective of when last performed. Endometrial carcinoma may be detected by cervical cytology in up to 30% of cases.[26] Furthermore, there is a significant risk of carcinoma of the cervix (Table 24.3). In a recent survey of 457 women with PMB, 6 cases of cervical carcinoma were diagnosed.[3] As cervical cytology will miss a significant proportion of cases of cervical neoplasia, any further suspicion of cancer of the cervix, such as a history of post-coital bleeding, should result in a thorough colposcopic examination.

INVESTIGATIONS

The aim of investigations is to exclude both endometrial cancer and atypical hyperplasia. Previously this has been performed using fractional curettage under general anaesthesia. More recently hysteroscopy has enabled visualisation of the uterine cavity and directed biopsy. However, many women with PMB are overweight, diabetic and hypertensive. The risks of general anaesthesia are substantial in such women. This has led to the development of outpatient investigations such as endometrial sampling. A list of common methods for excluding endometrial carcinoma in women with PMB is detailed in Table 24.6.

Dilatation and curettage

Until recently, fractional endometrial curettage under general anaesthetic has been advocated as the investigation of choice for women with PMB.[27,28] By

Table 24.6 Methods for excluding endometrial cancer or hyp[erplasia in women with menopausal bleeding

Outpatient procedures	Endometrial sampling Hysteroscopy and directed endometrial biopsy Trans-vaginal ultrasound (endometrial thickness) Sonohysteroscopy
Inpatient procedures	Dilatation and curettage Dilatation and fractional curettage Hysteroscopy and curettage Hysteroscopy and directed endometrial biopsy

sampling tissue from the endocervical canal separately, an assessment of spread to the cervix can be made when the woman has endometrial cancer. The technique is well accepted and used as the gold standard in many studies of alternative methods for endometrial sampling. However, uterine curettage itself seems to have escaped careful scientific assessment. The sensitivity for detecting endometrial cancer is unknown. Less than half of the endometrium is sampled in 60% of patients[29] and, as the uterine cavity is not visualised, areas of neoplasia may be missed. When compared to a simple outpatient device for endometrial sampling (the Pipelle) in women with PMB, Ben-Baruch et al[30] reported that curettage only provided adequate tissue for histological analysis in 45.8% of cases compared to 84.1%. Furthermore, worrying data were reported by Feldman et al,[31] who found that 6 (2%) of 263 women who had a benign or inadequate specimens at initial curettage for PMB had endometrial carcinoma 2 years following the procedure. A further 17 (6%) of the women had complex hyperplasia.[31]

When dilatation and curettage has successfully made a diagnosis of endometrial cancer, the pathology may be incorrect. In a study of 577 women who subsequently had hysterectomies for endometrial cancer,[32] the specimen at curettage correctly diagnosed only 91.6% of adenocarcinomas, 30.7% of adenoacanthomas and 37.5% of adenosquamous carcinomas.

The complications of curettage include perforation, haemorrhage and infection. The risks of these are significant. The incidence of perforation following uterine curettage is 6–13 per 1000;[33–36] the risk of infection is 3–5 per 1000;[35,36] and the risk of haemorrhage is 4 per 1000 procedures.[36] The consequences of these complications is not to be understated. Perforation may result in damage to the bowel, bladder or ureters and any of these three complications could result in an unplanned laparotomy and even hysterectomy.[37–42] In a meta-analysis of 12 598 patients who underwent dilatation and curettage, Grimes[43] reported the incidence of unanticipated major operations as being 1.4 per 1000 procedures (range 0.3–5 per 1000). In that series of 12 598 women,[43] 8 patients had hysterectomies and 10 patients had laparotomies which did not lead to hysterectomy.

In 1982, Grimes[43] estimated that the annual cost of dilatation and curettage in the US to be US$ 703 million. Dilatation and curettage is: (i) expensive; (ii) associated with a significant complication rate; (iii) ineffective at yielding a diagnosis; and (iv) may miss a significant proportion of endometrial neoplasms. With modern techniques of assessing the endometrium, there is no longer a place for uterine curettage in the management of post-menopausal women with uterine bleeding.

Outpatient endometrial sampling

There are now many devices for performing endometrial biopsies in the outpatient setting (Fig. 24.3). Grimes[43] reported a 20 year experience with Vabra aspiration techniques in which the complication rate was lower, and the detection rate for endometrial abnormalities higher, when compared with curettage. However, Vabra aspiration only samples an average of 41.6% of the endometrial surface[44] and is less tolerated than other forms of office endometrial sampling.[45]

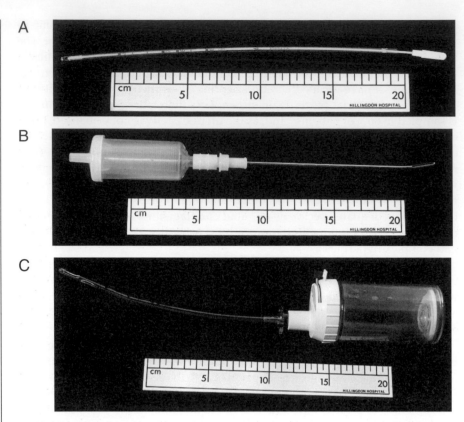

Fig. 24.4 Devices for office endometrial sampling. **(A)** Pipelle de Cournier, **(B)** Vabra aspirator, **(C)** Vaukutage.

The Pipelle de Cournier[46] is tolerated better than most other forms of office endometrial biopsy device[45,47,48] but only samples an average of 4.2% of the endometrial surface.[47] The sensitivities reported for detecting endometrial carcinoma by the Pipelle range between 98% (39/40)[49] and 68% (25/37)[50] with two other authors reporting the detection rates as 83% (54/65)[51] and 92% (24/26).[52] The figures are similar to the detection rates for endometrial cancer reported for the Novak curette (85% and 93%),[53,54] Z-sampler (83%),[53] Permacurette (73%),[54] Mi-Mark Helix (93%)[55] and Endopap (68.2%).[56]

The complication rates for out-patient endometrial sampling devices have not been widely reported. The incidence of both uterine perforation and infection with the Vabra aspirator is 0–4 per 1000.[7] In a meta-analysis of 5851 cases of endometrial sampling using the Vabra aspirator, Grimes[43] was unable to find a single case where an unanticipated major operation was necessitated by complications.

Many no longer consider endometrial sampling without visualisation of the uterine cavity as the gold-standard investigation for PMB. This is clearly illustrated by Stovall et al,[57] who performed pre-operative endometrial sampling using Vabra aspiration, the Novak curette or traditional curettage on 619 women having elective hysterectomies. In that study,[57] there were 30 instances in which endometrial sampling failed to identify either endometrial hyperplasia or carcinoma.

Hysteroscopy with endometrial sampling

Until recently, hysteroscopy was only available at specialist centres. However, the first successful hysteroscopy on a women with post-menopausal bleeding was reported as long ago as 1869.[58] Hysteroscopy allows a visual inspection of the uterine cavity and can help ensure that foci of abnormal appearing endometrium are sampled for histological analysis. Furthermore, the endocervix can be directly visualised. This allows spread of endometrial cancer to be seen thus influencing management.[59] More uterine abnormalities are diagnosed when hysteroscopy is performed prior to curettage.[60-62] However, hysteroscopy without biopsy is unreliable in differentiating between pre-malignant and malignant endometrium.[63-65]

There is evidence that endometrial carcinoma is less likely to be missed when hysteroscopy is performed prior to curettage.[66,67] Altaras et al[66] performed microhysteroscopy and endometrial sampling in 39 women with PMB in whom curettage had failed to obtain adequate tissue for analysis. Pathology results were obtained in 29 (74.3%) of the women, three of whom had endometrial adenocarcinoma. In a further study of 202 patients with PMB in whom curettage failed, hysteroscopically directed endometrial sampling found 19 cases of endometrial hyperplasia and 7 cases of carcinoma.[67] In that study,[67] 70% of lesions were focal, thus accounting for them being missed at curettage.

The first hysteroscopes to gain use in routine clinical practice were rigid instruments (Fig. 24.5A). However, with improved fibreoptics came the introduction of flexible endoscopes (Fig. 24.5B) which allowed hysteroscopies to be performed in an out-patient setting. The procedure has a high degree of patient acceptability.[68-70] In one study following office hysteroscopy, only 3%

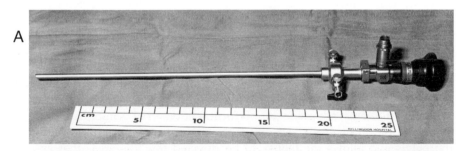

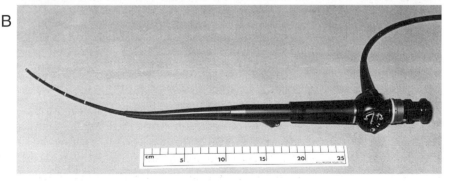

Fig. 24.5 Hysteroscopes. **(A)** 4.5 mm rigid hysteroscope, **(B)** 3 mm flexible hysteroscope.

(3/100) of women with PMB stated that they would have preferred the procedure to have been performed under general anaesthetic.[70] The efficiency of out-patient flexible hysteroscopy in detecting endometrial abnormalities is as good as that performed under general anaesthetic with one study demonstrating significantly better accuracy with a flexible hystero-fibrescope than with rigid hysteroscopy.[71] The impact of out-patient hysteroscopy is huge. One group calculated a potential saving to the Australian national health budget of A\$ 60 million (about £30 million) per annum with its routine use.[72]

The addition of hysteroscopy to endometrial sampling is associated with more possible operative complications. These include water intoxication, pulmonary oedema, air embolism and anaphylaxis due to distension fluid. The incidence of perforation at operative hysteroscopy has been reported as 13/1000 and other serious complications as 1/1000.[73] One would expect these complication rates to be significantly lower for diagnostic hysteroscopy and the procedure is generally considered to be safe.

There is presently concern about the possibility of neoplastic implantation into the pelvic cavity caused by hysteroscopy.[74,75] Sagawa et al[76] aspirated the pelvic peritoneum of 27 women with endometrial carcinoma before and after hysteroscopy. In that study, 3 (11.1%) women had tumour cells in the washings before hysteroscopy and a further 3 (12.5%) afterwards. Although the data are worrying, it is not known if the initial washings of the three cases were false negative results. Furthermore, one case was attributed to the endometrial biopsy, suggesting that curettage could also be associated with this phenomenon. Tanizawa et al[71] reported that the incidence of tumour cells in the pelvic cavity after hysteroscopy in 1115 patients with endometrial cancer was no different than in those patients who had not been hysteroscoped. In addition, Neis et al[77] performed careful histological examination of fallopian tubes in 118 women with endometrial carcinoma after hysteroscopy with carbon dioxide. In that study, only one tumour cell was found in a single fallopian tube. The risks of iatrogenic neoplastic implantation are overstated and are not a unique phenomenon of hysteroscopy. The rare occurrence of a tumour cell in the peritoneal cavity must be considered less dangerous to a patient than missing a case of endometrial cancer. To date, there is no information as to whether the risk alters with different distension media; however, it seems advisable to perform endometrial sampling after the hysteroscopy. This is likely to decrease the risk of tumour cell implantation in the pelvis and allows the biopsy to be directed towards areas that appear suspicious

Ultrasound

Measurements of endometrial thickness by transvaginal ultrasound (TVS) may play a role in screening for uterine malignancy in women with PMB. Many authors have reported the sensitivity for endometrial carcinoma as 100%.[9–13,78,79] However, the false positive rate is high (about 26% for atrophic endometrium).[13] Furthermore, about 55% of women require further investigations.[13] The specificity of TVS is even lower in women receiving oestrogen therapy[13] and small changes in the cut-off measurement may substantially lower the sensitivity.[13] One author reported a sensitivity for endometrial neoplasia as only 80% using a TVS measurement of endometrial thickness of 5 mm as a cut-off.[80] In that paper, 3 of 15 malignant tumours were missed. Although one of these included uterine spread from a lymphoma, there were two cases of stage 1 adenocarcinoma with endometrial thickness measurements of 2 mm and 3 mm, respectively.

There is clearly a discrepancy with different groups' results and a number of unanswered questions exist. Tsuda et al[8] found the sensitivity for endometrial carcinoma as only 86% using a cut-off of only 2 mm. However, that group used transabdominal sonography which produces less clear images of the endometrium than TVS due to the lower degree of proximity of the probe to the uterus.

Unanswered questions include the type of measurement which should be made and the cut-off level for which further investigations should be performed. Endometrial measurements can be of single thickness or can include both endometrial layers including the contents of the cavity. The latter has the advantage of being enlarged if the cavity is distended by fluid or a polyp. Although no direct comparison has been made, the larger measurement would be expected to increase the sensitivity for benign pathology at the expense of specificity. Numerous cut-off levels have been used, with 3, 4 or 5 mm being the most common.[9–13,78,79] However, there is a considerable ethnic variation in the normal thickness of the endometrium[81] and normal ranges from one unit cannot be used by another with a different racial population.

Inter-operator variability of endometrial thickness measurements has not been assessed. It is reasonable to suspect that the sensitivity of such measurements for endometrial carcinoma would be operator-dependent. Bockman reported that 40–50% of all endometrial neoplasms develop in a hormone-independent manner from atrophic endometrium and can be focal rather than diffuse.[82] It is, therefore, possible that areas of neoplastic endometrium could be missed when inexperienced sonographers fail to visualise the whole endometrium. This is more likely with a retroverted uterus. Furthermore, other pathology such as endometrial polyps are often missed.[13]

The failure of TVS to diagnose consistently benign pathology has led many groups to perform sonohysterography.[83–86] Cicinelli et al[83] reported the sensitivity for detecting benign polyps as only 33.3% for TVS compared to 75% for transabdominal sonohysterography. That same group found a sensitivity of 100% for hysteroscopy.[83] Furthermore, if intra-uterine instrumentation and fluid distension is being performed, visualisation of the uterine cavity with a hysteroscope adds little to the procedure. The sensitivity and specificity of TVS for endometrial cancer may be increased by combining sonographic measurements with endometrial sampling[16] or Doppler blood flow studies.[78,87] However, Sladkevicius et al[15] concluded that TVS measurements of endometrial thickness was a better discriminator between normal and pathological and between benign and malignant endometrium than any Doppler variable.

An advantage of ultrasound for investigating PMB is the opportunity for examining the whole pelvis. Gredmark et al[3] found that 8 of 457 women who presented with abnormal menopausal vaginal bleeding had ovarian tumours. As many ovarian cancers cannot be palpated on bimanual examination,[88,89] ultrasound is an important investigation. However, some ovarian neoplasms may be missed and ultrasound may increase the risk of unnecessary operative intervention for benign adnexal disease.[90]

Ultrasound measurements of endometrial thickness may play a role in screening for malignant disease in women with PMB. This has been suggested by the results of a large multicentre study,[13] but other reports are not in total agreement.[80] The best evidence presently available suggests that full double thickness measurements which include the contents of the cavity should be made using a transvaginal probe. As normal endometrial thickness varies with different ethnic groups,[81] it is reasonable for gynaecological ultrasound units to have their own cut-off levels for normality. The role of TVS in patients with persistent PMB has not been fully assessed and more detailed investigation of these women is, therefore, required.

Other specific investigations

Magnetic resonance imaging (MRI) has been advocated in the diagnosis of endometrial cancer.[91] Similar to ultrasound measurements of endometrial thickness, MRI measurements have a high degree of sensitivity for endometrial carcinoma but lack specificity.[91] MRI may also be used to predict myometrial invasion[91-95] in established cases of endometrial cancer and is more accurate at this than ultrasound.[92] However, the cost and time required for MRI imaging suggests that it is not a practical method for screening the large number of women with PMB that presently exist.

Many authors have studied the use of tumour markers for the diagnosis of endometrial cancer.[96-98] These include the cancer antigens 125, 19-9, 50 and 15-3 as well as carcino-embryonic antigen, alfa-fetoprotein, placental-type alkaline phosphatase, and the core fragment of urinary beta human chorionic gonadotrophin.[96-98] To date, these tumour markers have proved to be of little value in the screening of women with PMB for endometrial cancer.[96-98]

CONCLUSIONS

At present, there is little comparative data for each method of investigation. A simple power analysis shows that a study with a 90% power at a 5% significance level would require over 24 000 subjects with PMB to demonstrate a 10% difference in sensitivity for endometrial cancer between two forms of investigation. The only statistically sound method to compare all forms of investigation for PMB would be to examine the whole uterus histopathologically. The ethical nature of such a study would be dubious.

At present, the management of PMB should be tailored to suit an individual case's clinical merits. No clear evidence for the best method of investigation exists. The International Society for Gynecologic Endoscopy agreed that hysteroscopy could replace dilatation and curettage in the investigation of post-menopausal women with uterine bleeding.[99] The author of this review currently recommends hysteroscopy and endometrial sampling as the gold standard for diagnosis. This can be performed as an out-patient if suitable facilities are available. Vaginal ultrasound is a useful investigation which provides additional information. However, the sensitivity for detecting endometrial carcinoma may not be 100% and benign pathology is often missed.

Even hysteroscopically guided endometrial biopsy is not 100% sensitive at detecting endometrial carcinoma.[100] Furthermore, it is easy to miss premalignant endometrial hyperplasia with this technique.[63-65] Therefore, postmenopausal women with persistent or recurrent uterine bleeding should have repeat investigations and, in some rare cases, a hysterectomy should be considered if a diagnosis cannot be made.

ACKNOWLEDGEMENTS

The author would like to thank the library staff of the Royal College of Obstetricians and Gynaecologists and of the Royal Society of Medicine for their help. In addition, he would like to thank Jaqueline Hill of the information department at Hillingdon Hospital for providing data from the hospital.

REFERENCES

1 Gusberg S B. The individual at high risk for endometrial carcinoma. Am J Obstet Gynecol 1976; 126: 535–542
2 MacDonald P C, Edman C D, Hemsell D L, Porter J C, Siiteri P K. Effect of obesity on conversion of plasma androstenedione to estrone in post-menopausal women with and without endometrial cancer. Am J Obstet Gynecol 1978; 130: 448–455
3 Gredmark T, Kvint S, Havel G, Mattsson L A. Histopathological findings in women with postmenopausal bleeding. Br J Obstet Gynaecol 1995; 102: 133–136
4 Te Linde R W. Post-menopausal bleeding. Am J Surg 1940; 48: 289
5 Geist S H, Matus M. Causes of post-menopausal uterine bleeding. Am J Obstet Gynecol 1933; 25: 388
6 Choo Y C, Mak K C, Hsu C, Wong T S, Ma I I K. Postmenopausal uterine bleeding of non-organic cause. Obstet Gynecol 1985; 66: 225–228
7 Alberico S, Conoscenti G, Veglio P, Bogatti P, Di Bonito L, Mandruzzato G. A clinical and epidemiological study of 245 postmenopausal metrorrhagia patients. Clin Exp Obstet Gynecol 1989; 4: 113–121
8 Tsuda H, Kawabata M, Umesaki N, Kawabata K, Ogita S. Endometrial assessment by transabdominal ultrasound in postmenopausal women. Eur J Obstet Gynecol 1993; 52: 201–204
9 Smith P, Bakos O, Heimer G, Ulmsten U. Transvaginal ultrasound for identifying endometrial abnormality. Acta Obstet Gynecol Scand 1991; 70: 591–594
10 Goldstein S R, Nachtigall M, Snyder J R, Nachtigall L. Endometrial assessment by vaginal ultrasonography before endometrial sampling in patients with postmenopausal bleeding. Am J Obstet Gynecol 1990; 163: 119–123
11 Granberg S, Wikland M, Karlsson B, Norström A, Friberg L G. Endometrial thickness as measured by endovaginal ultrasonography for identifying endometrial abnormality. Am J Obstet Gynecol 1991; 164: 47–52
12 Nasri M N, Shepherd J H, Setchell M E, Lowe D G, Chard T. The role of vaginal scan in measurement of endometrial thickness in postmenopausal women. Br J Obstet Gynaecol 1991; 98: 470–475
13 Karlsson B, Granberg S, Wikland M et al. Transvaginal ultrasound of the endometrium in women with postmenopausal bleeding – a Nordic multicenter study. Am J Obstet Gynecol 1995; 172: 1488–1493
14 Osmers R, Völksen M, Schauer A. Vaginosonography for early detection of endometrial carcinoma? Lancet 1990; 335: 1569–1571
15 Sladkevicius P, Valentin L, Marsal K. Endometrial thickness and Doppler velocimetry of the uterine arteries as discriminators of endometrial status in women with post-menopausal bleeding: a comparative study. Am J Obstet Gynecol 1994; 171: 722–728

16 Van den Bosch T, Vandendael A, Van Schoubroeck D, Wranz P A, Lombard C J. Combining vaginal ultrasonography and office endometrial sampling in the diagnosis of endometrial disease in postmenopausal women. Obstet Gynecol 1995; 85: 349–352

17 Valle R F. Hysteroscopic evaluation of patients with abnormal uterine bleeding. Surg Gynecol Obstet 1981; 153: 521–526

18 Procopé B-J. Aetiology of postmenopausal bleeding. Acta Obstet Gynecol Scand 1971; 50: 311–313

19 Miyazawa K. Clinical significance of an enlarged uterus in patient with postmenopausal bleeding. Obstet Gynecol 1983; 61: 148–152

20 Lidor A, Ismajovich B, Confino E, David M P. Histopathological findings in 226 women with post-menopausal uterine bleeding. Acta Obstet Gynecol Scand 1986, 65: 41–43

21 Isaacs J H, Ross F H. Cytologic evaluation of the endometrium in women with postmenopausal bleeding. Am J Obstet Gynecol 1978, 131: 410–412

22 Nasri M N, Coast G J. Correlation of ultrasound findings and endometrial histopathology in post-menopausal women. Br J Obstet Gynaecol 1989; 96: 1333–1338

23 Payne F L, Wright R C, Fetterman H H. Postmenopausal bleeding. Am J Obstet Gynecol 1959; 77: 1216–1227

24 Feldman S, Cook E F, Harlow B L, Berkowitz R S. Predicting endometrial cancer among older women who present with abnormal vaginal bleeding. Gynecol Oncol 1995; 56: 376–381

25 Pace S, Grassi A, Ferrero S et al. Diagnostic methods of early detection of endometrial hyperplasia and cancer. Int J Gynecol Oncol 1995; 5: 373–381

26 Demirkiran F, Arvas M, Erkun E et al. The prognostic significance of cervico-vaginal cytology in endometrial cancer. Eur J Gynaecol Oncol 1995; 16: 403–409

27 Monaghan J M. Operations on the uterine cavity. In: Monaghan J M. (ed) Bonney's gynaecological surgery, 9th edn. East Sussex: Baillière Tindall, 1986; 40–43

28 Peel K R. Malignant disease of the uterine body. In: Whitfield C R. ed. Dewhurst's textbook of obstetrics and gynaecology for postgraduates, 5th edn. London: Blackwell Science, 1995; 747–758

29 Stock R J, Kanbour A. Pre-hysterectomy curettage. Obstet Gynecol 1975; 45: 537

30 Ben-Baruch G, Seidman D S, Schiff E, Moran O, Menczer J. Outpatient endometrial sampling with the Pipelle curette. Gynecol Obstet Invest 1994; 37: 260–262.

31 Feldman S, Shapter A, Welch W R, Berkowitz R S. Two year follow-up of 263 patients with post/perimenopausal vaginal bleeding and negative initial biopsy. Gynecol Oncol 1994; 55: 56–59

32 Romagnolo C, Zasso B, Maggino T, Blandamura S. Histopathological characterisation in carcinoma of the endometrium. Comparison between biopsy and pathological examination of specimens. Eur J Gynecol Oncol 1993; 14: 106–108

33 Word B, Gravlee L C, Wideman G L. The fallacy of simple uterine curettage. Obstet Gynecol 1958; 12: 642–645

34 Word B. Current concepts of uterine curettage. Postgrad Med 1960; 28: 450

35 McElkin T W, Bird C C, Reeves B D, Scott R C. Diagnostic dilation and curettage. A 20-year survey. Obstet Gynecol 1969; 33: 807

36 MacKenzie I Z, Bibby J G. Critical assessment of dilatation and curettage in 1029 women. Lancet 1978; 2: 566

37 Davies M F, Howat J M. Intestinal obstruction secondary to uterine perforation: an unusual cause of vaginal bleeding. Br J Clin Pract 1990; 44: 331–332

38 Miko T L, Lampe L G, Thomazy V A, Molnar P, Endes P. Eosinophilic endomyometritis associated with diagnostic curettage. Int J Gynaecol Pathol 1988; 7: 162–172

39 Sacks P C, Tchabo J G. Incidence of bacteremia at dilatation and curettage. J Reprod Med 1992; 37: 331–334

40 Kauff N D, Chelmow D, Kawada C Y. Intractable bleeding managed with Foley catheter tamponade after dilatation and evacuation. Am J Obstet Gynecol 1995; 173: 957–958

41 Tobias D H, Koenigsberg M, Kogan M, Edelman M, LevGur M. Pyomyoma after uterine instrumentation. A case report. J Reprod Med 1996; 41: 375–378

42 Lodh U, Kumar S, Arya M C, Tyagi A. Ureterouterine fistula as a complication of an elective abortion. Aust N Z J Obstet Gynaecol 1996; 36: 94–95

43 Grimes D A. Diagnostic dilation and curettage: a re-appraisal. Am J Obstet Gynecol 1982; 142: 1–6

44 Rodriguez G C, Yaqub N, King M E. A comparison of the Pipelle device and the Vabra aspirator as measured by endometrial denudation in hysterectomy specimens: the Pipelle device samples significantly less of the endometrial surface than the Vabra aspirator. Am J Obstet Gynecol 1993; 168: 55–59

45 Kaunitz A M, Masciello A, Ostrowski M, Rovira E Z. Comparison of endometrial biopsy with Pipelle and Vabra aspirator. J Reprod Med 1988; 33: 427–431

46 Cournier E. The Pipelle: a disposable device for endometrial biopsy. Am J Obstet Gynecol 1984; 148: 109–110

47 Stovall T G, Ling F W, Morgan P L. A prospective, randomized comparison of the Pipelle endometrial sampling device with the Novak curette. Am J Obstet Gynecol 1991; 165: 1287–1290

48 Silver M M, Miles P, Rosa C. Comparison of Novak and Pipelle endometrial biopsy instruments. Obstet Gynecol 1991; 78: 828–830

49 Stovall T G, Photopulos G J, Poston W M, Ling F W, Sandles L G. Pipelle endometrial sampling in patients with known endometrial carcinoma. Obstet Gynecol 1991; 77: 954–956

50 Ferry J, Farnsworth A, Webster M, Wren B. The efficacy of the Pipelle endometrial biopsy in detecting endometrial carcinoma. Aust N Z J Obstet Gynaecol 1993; 33: 76–78

51 Guido R S, Kanbour-Shakir A, Rulin M C, Christopherson W A. Pipelle endometrial sampling. Sensitivity in the detection of endometrial cancer. J Reprod Med 1995; 40: 553–555

52 Zorlu C G, Cobanoglu O, Isik A Z, Kutluay L, Kuscu E. Accuracy of Pipelle endometrial sampling in endometrial carcinoma. Gynecol Obstet Invest 1994; 38: 272–275

53 Larson D M, Krawisz B R, Johnson K K, Broste S K. Comparison of the Z-sampler and Novak endometrial biopsy instruments for in-office diagnosis of endometrial cancer. Gynecol Oncol 1994; 54: 64–67

54 Iossa A, Cianferoni L, Ciatto S, Cecchini S, Camptelli C, Lo Stumbo F. Hysteroscopy and endometrial cancer diagnosis: a review of 2007 consecutive examinations in self-referred patients. Tumori 1991; 77: 479–483

55 Buratti E, Cefis F, Masserini M, Goisis F, Vergadoro F, Bolis G. The value of endometrial cytology in a high risk population. Tumori 1985; 71: 25–28

56 Suprun H Z, Taendler-Stolero R, Schwartz J, Ettinger M. Experience with endopap endometrial sampling in the cytodiagnosis of endometrial carcinoma and its precursor lesions. I. A correlative cytologic- histologic-hysteroscopic diagnostic pilot study. Acta Cytol 1994; 38: 319–323

57 Stovall T G, Solomon S K, Ling F W. Endometrial sampling prior to hysterectomy. Obstet Gynecol 1989; 73: 405–409

58 Pantaleoni D. On endoscopic examination of the cavity of the womb. Med Press Circ 1869; 8: 26–27

59 Taddei G L, Moncini D, Scarselli G, Tantini C, Bargelli G. Can hysteroscopic evaluation of endometrial carcinoma influence treatment? Ann NY Acad Sci 1994; 734: 482–487

60 Finikiotis G. Hysteroscopy: an analysis of 523 patients. Aust N Z J Obstet Gynaecol 1989; 29: 253–255

61 Parasnis H B, Parulekar S V. Significance of negative hysteroscopic view in abnormal uterine bleeding. J Postgrad Med 1992; 38: 62–64

62 Gimpleson R J. Panoramic hysteroscopy with directed biopsy versus dilatation and curettage for accurate diagnosis. J Reprod Med 1984; 29: 575–578

63 Lewis B V. Hysteroscopy in gynaecological practice: a review. J R Soc Med 1984; 77: 235–237

64 Loverro G, Bettocchi S, Vicino M, Selvaggi L. Diagnosis of endometrial hyperplasia in women with abnormal uterine bleeding. Acta Eur Fertil 1994; 25: 23–25

65 Karlsson B, Granberg S, Hellberg P, Wikland M. Comparative study of transvaginal sonography and hysteroscopy for the detection of pathologic endometrial lesions in women with postmenopausal bleeding. J Ultrasound Med 1994; 13: 757–762

66 Altaras M M, Aviram R, Cohen I, Markov S, Goldberg GL, Beyth Y. Microhysteroscopy and endometrial biopsy results following failed diagnostic dilation and curettage in women with postmenopausal bleeding. Int J Gynaecol Obstet 1993; 42: 255–260

67 Spiewankiewicz B, Stelmachow J, Sawicki W, Kietlinska Z. Hysteroscopy with selective endometrial sampling after unsuccessful dilation and curettage in diagnosis of symptomatic endometrial cancer and endometrial hyperplasia. Eur J Gynaecol Oncol 1995; 16: 26–29.

68 de Jong P, Doel F, Falconer A. Outpatient diagnostic hysteroscopy. Br J Obstet Gynaecol 1990; 97: 299–303

69 Cooper M J, Broadbent J A, Molnar B G, Richardson R, Magos A L. A series of 1000 consecutive out-patient diagnostic hysteroscopies. J Obstet Gynaecol 1995; 21: 503–507

70 Downes E, al-Azzawi F. How well do perimenopausal patients accept outpatient hysteroscopy? Visual analogue scoring of acceptability and pain in 100 women. Eur J Obstet Gynecol Reprod Biol 1993; 48: 37–41

71 Tanizawa O, Miyake A, Sugimoto K. Re-evaluation of hysteroscopy in the diagnosis of uterine endometrial cancer [English abstract]. Acta Obstet Gynaecol Jpn 1991; 43: 622–626

72 Gillespie A, Nichols A. The value of hysteroscopy. Aust N Z J Obstet Gynaecol 1994; 34: 85-87.

73 Peterson H B, Hulka J F, Phillips J M. American Association of Gynecologic Laparoscopists' 1988 membership survey on operative hysteroscopy. J Reprod Med 1990; 35: 590–591

74 van der Weiden R M, Arentz P W, Veselic M. Endometrial cells in the peritoneal cavity after laparoscopy and chromotubation. J R Soc Med 1992; 85: 397–398

75 Schmitz M J, Nahhas W A. Hysteroscopy may transport malignant cells into the peritoneal cavity. Eur J Gynaecol Oncol 1994; 15: 121–124

76 Sagawa T, Yamada H, Sakuragi N, Fujimoto S. A comparison between the preoperative and operative findings of peritoneal cytology in patients with endometrial cancer. Asia-Oceanic J Obstet Gynaecol 1994; 20: 39–47

77 Neis K J, Brandner P, Keppeler U. Tumour cell seedling caused by hysteroscopy? Geburtshilfe Frauenheilkunde 1994; 54: 651–655

78 Bourne T H, Campbell S, Steer C V, Royston P, Whitehead M I, Collins W P. Detection of endometrial cancer by transvaginal ultrasonography with color flow imaging and blood flow analysis: a preliminary report. Gynecol Oncol 1991; 40: 253–259

79 Varner R E, Sparks J M, Cameron C D, Roberts L L, Soong S J. Transvaginal sonography of the endometrium in postmenopausal women. Obstet Gynecol 1991; 78: 195–199

80 Dörum A, Kristensen B, Langebrekke A, Sörnes T, Skaar O. Evaluation of endometrial thickness measured by endovaginal ultrasound in women with postmenopausal bleeding. Acta Obstet Gynaecol Scand 1993; 72: 116–119

81 Tsuda H, Kawabata M, Kawabata K et al. Differences between occidental and oriental postmenopausal women in cut-off level of endometrial thickness for endometrial cancer screening by vaginal scan. Am J Obstet Gynecol 1995; 172: 1494–1495

82 Bockman J V. Two pathogenic types of endometrial carcinoma. Gynecol Oncol 1983; 15: 10–17

83 Cicinelli E, Romano F, Anastasio P S, Blasi N, Parisi C. Sonohysteroscopy versus hystero-scopy in the diagnosis of endouterine polyps. Gynecol Obstet Invest 1994; 38: 266–271

84 Gaucherand P, Piacenza J M, Salle B, Rudigoz R C. Sonohysterography of the uterine cavity: preliminary investigations. J Clin Ultrasound 1995; 23: 339–348

85 Cullinan J A, Fleischer A C, Kepple D M, Arnold A L. Sonohysterography: a technique for endometrial evaluation. Radiographics 1995; 15: 501—514

86 Parsons A K, Lense J J. Sonohysterography for endometrial abnormalities: preliminary results. J Clin Ultrasound 1993; 21: 87–95

87 Sheth S, Hamper U M, McCollum M E, Caskey C I, Rosenshein N B, Kurman R J. Endometrial blood flow analysis in postmenopausal women: can it help differentiate benign from malignant causes of endometrial thickening? Radiology 1995; 195: 661–665

88 Andolf E, Svalenius E, Astedt B. Ultrasonography for early detection of ovarian carcinoma. Br J Obstet Gynaecol 1986; 93: 1286–1289

89 MacFarlane C, Sturgis M C, Fetterman F S. Results of experiment in control of cancer of female pelvic organs and report of 15 years of research. Am J Obstet Gynecol 1955; 69: 294–298

90 Prys-Davies A, Oram D. Screening for ovarian cancer. Prog Obstet Gynaecol 1991; 9: 349–374

91 Bao R, Wu A, Ou Y. Magnetic resonance imaging in the diagnosis and staging of endometrial carcinoma. Chin J Obstet Gynecol 1995; 30: 215–217

92 Yamashita Y, Mizutani H, Torashima M et al. Assessment of myometrial invasion by endometrial carcinoma: transvaginal sonography vs contrast-enhanced MR imaging. Am J Roent 1993; 161: 595–599

93 Sironi S, Taccagni G, Garancini P, Belloni C, DelMaschio A. Myometrial invasion by endometrial carcinoma: assessment by MR imaging. Am J Roent 1992; 158: 565–569

94 Lien H H, Blomlie V, Trope C, Kaern J, Abeler V M. Cancer of the endometrium: value of MR imaging in determining depth of invasion into the myometrium. Am J Roent 1991; 157: 1221–1223

95 Minderhoud-Bassie W, Treurniet F E, Koops W, Chadha-Ajwani S, Hage J C, Huikeshoven F J. Magnetic resonance imaging (MRI) in endometrial carcinoma; preoperative estimation of depth of myometrial invasion. Acta Obstet Gynecol Scand 1995; 74: 827–831

96 Ind T E J, Iles R K, Carter P G et al. Serum placental-type alkaline phosphatase activity in women with squamous and glandular malignancies of the reproductive tract. J Clin Pathol 1994; 46: 1035–1037

97 El-Ahmady O, Gad M, el-Sheimy R et al. Comparative study between sonography, pathology and UGP in women with perimenopausal bleeding. Anticancer Res 1996, 16: 2309–2313

98 Indraccolo S R, Cecchi A, Thodos A, Brandi S, Carta G. Possibility of the combined use of tumour markers in endometrial carcinoma. Minerva Gynecol 1991; 43: 461–463

99 Grainger D A, DeCherney A H. Hysteroscopic management of uterine bleeding. In: Drife J O. (ed) Clinical obstetrics and gynaecology. Dysfunctional uterine bleeding and menorrhagia, Vol. 32. London: Baillière Tindall, 1989; 403–414

100 Margolis M T, Thoen L D, Boike G M, Mercer L J, Keith L G. Asymptomatic endometrial carcinoma after endometrial ablation. Int J Gynaecol Obstet 1995; 51: 255–258

Nicholas Panay   John Studd

Non-contraceptive uses of the hormone releasing intra-uterine systems

Until recently, approximately 100 000 hysterectomies were performed per annum for benign causes. Preliminary data are already showing that this figure can at least be halved by use of the levonorgestrel intra-uterine system and the progesterone releasing intra-uterine system. Add to this, the beneficial effects on dysmenorrhoea, fibroids, pelvic inflammatory disease, ectopic pregnancy and avoidance of progestogenic side effects in HRT users and you have one of the most significant developments in gynaecological management of the 20th century. Of course there is no such thing as the universal panacea and the systems are not without their own problems which will be discussed. However, this chapter hopes to show that these pale into virtual insignificance when you consider the benefit/risk ratio.

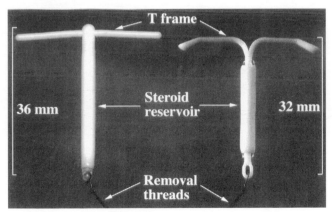

Fig. 25.1 Progesterone and levonorgestrel releasing intra-uterine systems.

Mr Nicholas Panay, Research Fellow in Obstetrics and Gynaecology, Academic Department of Obstetrics and Gynaecology, Chelsea and Westminster Hospital, 369 Fulham Road, London SW10 9NH, UK

Mr John Studd, Consultant Gynaecologist, Academic Department of Obstetrics and Gynaecology, Chelsea and Westminster Hospital, 369 Fulham Road, London SW10 9NH, UK

STRUCTURE AND MECHANISM OF ACTION OF INTRA-UTERINE SYSTEMS

Structure

There are two intra-uterine systems currently in usage (Fig. 25.1). The system currently licensed in the UK for contraception is the levonorgestrel intra-uterine system, Mirena® (LNG IUS). It consists of a plastic T-shaped frame with a steroid reservoir around the vertical stem of polydimethylsiloxane. The stem contains 52 mg of levonorgestrel, the levo-isomer of norgestrel, derived from the 19 nor-testosterone progestogens (Fig. 25.2), released at a rate of 20 µg per day. The Progestasert® intra-uterine progesterone system (PIPS) is not yet licensed in this country but is being used in phase III trials. It consists of a

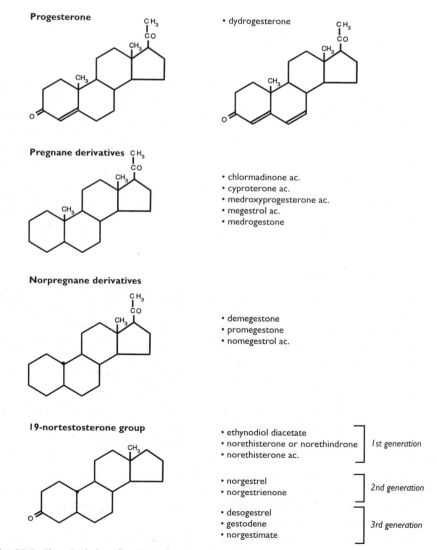

Fig. 25.2 Chemical classification of progestogens.

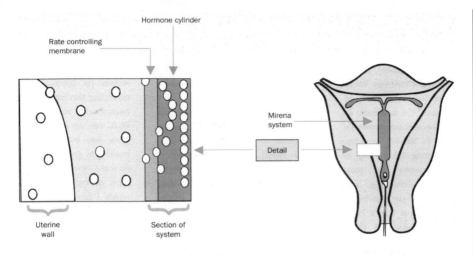

Fig. 25.3 The delivery of levonorgestrel from an intra-uterine system to the uterine wall (from Davie,[1] with permission).

polymeric T-shaped platform with a reservoir containing 38 mg of progesterone released at a rate of 65 μg per day. The total quantity of progesterone contained in one Progestasert system is less than the amount produced in one day by the corpus luteum during the latter part of the menstrual cycle. The drug is distributed in silicone (polydimethyl siloxane) fluid in both systems with a rate limiting membrane allowing slow diffusion of the drug into the endometrium (Fig. 25.3).[1] Both frames are rendered radio-opaque by impregnated barium sulphate. The LNG IUS is currently licensed for contraception for 3 years but there are data for 7 year bioavailability; the PIPS is licensed in the USA for 1 year's usage with up to 2 year bioavailability.

Endometrial effects

The effect of all progestogens on the endometrium is mediated via a decrease in oestrogen receptors and an increase in the 17α-oxoreductase activity that converts oestradiol to oestrone. Progestogens inhibit mitotic activity as evidenced by the decrease in number of mitoses in both the glandular epithelium and stroma. They also induce the secretory transformation. In women using oestrogen therapy, the incidence of hyperplasia is reduced to 4% with 7 days of oral progestogen and 0% with 12 days of oral progestogen if it is prescribed at an adequate daily dosage.[2,3] Although the effect of progestogen is protective to the endometrium in a dose and duration dependent manner, the exact relationship remains largely unknown because of considerable interindividual variability,[4] complex oestrogen/progestogen interactions[5] and the absence of an appropriate animal model. This would explain why some patients experience problems with heavy, prolonged periods and endometrial hyperplasia where the same duration, dose and type of progestogen would produce atrophy in another patient.

The LNG IUS has been shown to be effective at controlling endometrial hypertrophy by suppressing endometrial growth. After a few weeks the endometrial glands atrophy, the stroma becomes swollen and decidual, the mucosa thins and the epithelium becomes inactive. There is also suppression of spiral arterioles, capillary thrombosis and a local inflammatory response.[6] As a result of the suppression caused by the local release of hormone, also mediated by the regulatory action of high local levels of progestogen on endometrial oestrogen receptors,[7] the endometrium becomes unresponsive to oestrogen with no menstrual shedding. It has also been shown that there is no effect on endometrial endothelial factor VIII activity which is reduced by ordinary coils leading to a bleeding tendency.[8] The endometrial changes are uniform within three cycles after insertion of the system[7] with no further histological development over the long term.[9] After removal of the system, the morphological changes in the endometrium return to normal and menstruation returns within 30 days.[10] Endometrial suppression with decidual transformation is also the main mechanism of action with the PIPS, with equally rapid return to normal of the morphological changes.[11] The PIPS has been shown to be effective at controlling endometrial hypertrophy by suppressing endometrial growth[12–14] and can even be used to treat endometrial hyperplasia.[15] Endometrial biopsy studies indicate that continuous application of progesterone to the uterus results in changes indicative of an inactive endometrium. The changes appear to reverse rapidly after discontinuation. No cellular abnormalities were attributed to use of the system.[16]

Ovulation

During the first year of LNG IUS use, some women may experience changes in ovarian function but, after this, women usually have completely normal ovulatory cycles.[17] Menstrual bleeding does not reflect ovarian function, average oestradiol and progesterone levels being the same in amenorrhoeic and menstruating users (Table 25.1).[18,19] Studies of plasma hormone levels, menstrual patterns and blood chemistry in various patient groups using the PIPS demonstrated no systemic effects of the system, even on the progesterone-sensitive hypothalamic-pituitary-ovarian axis.[20,21]

Table 25.1 Mean plasma and E2 and LNG concentrations (pg/ml) in menstruating and amenorrhoeic women using the LNG IUS (Luukkainen et al)[18]

	E2	LNG
Menstruating	103.9 (n = 66)	175.2 (n = 62)
Amenorrhoea	132.7 (n = 20)	179.9 (n = 20)

Pharmacokinetics

The plasma concentrations achieved by the LNG IUS are lower than those seen with the LNG implant, the combined oral contraceptive and the mini-pill (Fig. 25.4).[22–25] Although there is marked interindividual variation in serum levonorgestrel levels (1–200 pg/ml), the serum and endometrial levels remain

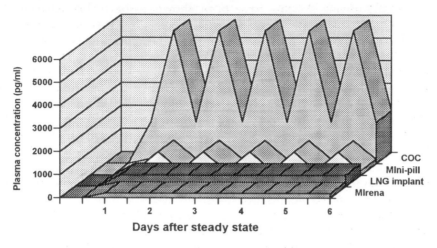

Fig. 25.4 Schematic comparison of levonorgestrel plasma concentrations for four different methods of contraception (adapted from Diaz et al,[22] Kuhnz et al,[23] Weiner et al[24] and Nilsson et al[25]).

stable for 6–7 years. Also, unlike the oral contraceptives, the levels with the LNG IUS do not display peaks and troughs. Endometrial concentrations after 6 years are still in excess of the capacity of the local progesterone receptors.

Results of studies with baboons show that intra-uterine systems delivering 65 µg/day of labelled progesterone do not produce detectable changes in concentrations of circulating progesterone. Progesterone released by the system is quickly metabolised to steroid intermediates. Unlike the metabolites of synthetic analogues, progesterone catabolites have little or no endocrine function and do not accumulate in the tissues.

NON-CONTRACEPTIVE BENEFITS OF HORMONE RELEASING INTRA-UTERINE SYSTEMS

Premenopausal bleeding problems and hysterectomy

Until recently, there was only a small range of medical treatments for menorrhagia, of limited or no benefit, usually failing, and leaving no option between putting up with the symptoms and hysterectomy. Most hysterectomies are performed for benign reasons, usually for intractable menorrhagia and pain where medical therapy has failed. For a while, there was optimism that the hysterectomy rate could be dramatically reduced by resection or ablation of the endometrium, but enthusiasm waned when it was realised that the procedure was not without its own complications. Bleeding problems returned in over a third of cases, often necessitating hysterectomy to solve the problem, and women wishing to use oestrogen therapy still needed progestogenic opposition. There is a new enthusiasm that the hysterectomy rate can be reduced with hormone releasing intra-uterine systems. Originally developed for use as contraceptives, it was realised that these systems could dramatically reduce the amount of blood loss and lead to amenorrhoea in a substantial number of cases.

The intra-uterine systems have been shown to be highly effective in reducing menstrual loss in premenopausal women. In a study by Andersson and Rybo,[26] menstrual loss was significantly reduced in women with dysfunctional menorrhagia (80 ml loss per period). After 3 month's usage, there was an 85% reduction in menstrual loss and 97% after 12 month's LNG IUS usage as measured by extraction of blood. There was a significant increase in serum ferritin in the first year of use. 35% of women were amenorrhoeic at one year. In a more recently reported study by Andersson et al,[27] it was shown that haemoglobin concentrations increased as a result of the reduction in menstrual loss produced by the LNG IUS demonstrating another positive health benefit for the system. The progesterone releasing system has also been shown to reduce menstrual blood loss[28] but not to the same extent as the LNG IUS (65% reduction 12 months post-insertion).

A reduction in menstrual loss by the LNG IUS was also demonstrated by Barrington and Bowen-Simpkins[29] in a group of 50 women who had failed medical therapy and were awaiting hysterectomy or trans-cervical resection of the endometrium. The treatment was so effective that it was possible to take 41 of these women off the waiting list, i.e. 82% were able to avoid major surgery. In another prospective study of 54 women on the waiting list for hysterectomy for menorrhagia, 67% came off the waiting list because they were satisfied with their treatment compared to only 15% of those on medical therapy.[30]

The reduction in menstrual blood loss with the hormone-releasing intra-uterine systems is far superior to anything achieved by medical treatments such as the prostaglandin inhibitors and the anti-fibrinolytics which at very best reduce blood loss by 50% (Effective Health Care).[31] Although amenorrhoea can be achieved with the gonadotrophin-releasing analogues and danazol, their side effects and risks associated with a long term hypo-oestrogenic state make them unacceptable for long term usage.

Although the hormone releasing systems are not strictly speaking licensed for treatment of menorrhagia, there is no reason why a pre-menopausal non-sterilised woman could not be given the LNG IUS for contraception which coincidentally might have a beneficial effect on her heavy periods. Also, there is a large and ever growing number of gynaecologists and GPs who are using the LNG IUS on a 'named patient basis' for non-contraceptive indications such as menorrhagia and as progestogenic opposition to oestrogen therapy. It is important to note that it is legal for a practitioner to prescribe an unlicensed product to a fully informed and consenting patient if he/she is adopting a practice that would be endorsed by a responsible body of professional opinion.[32] However, we look forward to the day when the hormone systems can be officially registered for indications we already know them to benefit.

Dysmenorrhoea

There is evidence that other gynaecological conditions which could necessitate hysterectomy are resolved by the intra-uterine systems. Both Sivin and Stern[33] and Barrington and Bowen-Simpkins[29] reported that, in their group of patients, dysmenorrhoea was alleviated by the LNG IUS. 80% of patients had improvement in the latter study group.

Endometrial hyperplasia

Workers first used the PIPS to reverse endometrial hyperplasia.[15] In a subsequent study, the PIPS was found to be successful in 81% of cases but there was quite a high recurrence rate after removal.[34] There are also good data for regression of endometrial hyperplasia[35,36] by the LNG IUS which can be achieved quicker than with the PIPS probably due to the greater efficacy of androgenic progestogens over progesterone in achieving secretory transformation. The LNG IUS would, therefore, be the IUS of choice for this indication unless the woman is severely progestogen intolerant, in which case the PIPS would be a better choice.

The hormone releasing intra-uterine systems may also have a preventative and therapeutic role in women using tamoxifen for breast cancer. It is a well recognised complication of tamoxifen therapy that the partial oestrogenic agonistic effect of the drug often induces endometrial hyperplasia and can cause uterine cancer.[37] Studies are currently being conducted to determine the effectiveness of the LNG IUS in both preventing and treating hyperplasia in this situation.

Prevention and treatment of uterine fibroids

Prevention of fibroid growth with long term usage was suggested by the Population Council Study which detected a significantly lower incidence of fibroids in LNG IUS users in comparison with copper IUCD users.[33] A prospective pilot study of five women, reported in the same year,[38] suggested not only a preventative but also a therapeutic effect for the LNG IUS in that fibroids were actually reduced in size after 6–18 month's usage. It has been postulated that these findings may be due to the effect of levonorgestrel on insulin-like endometrial growth factors and their binding proteins.[39,40]

Menopausal bleeding problems and progestogenic side effects on HRT

Oral progestogens can also have significant negative mood effects.[41–45] They can also have adverse androgenic effects both on the skin and cardiovascular risk markers. About 20% of women will have significant progestogen intolerance with about half this number having serious effects which will prevent them from continuing with treatment. This intolerance of progestogenic effects is one of the main reasons for poor compliance with HRT[46,47] leading to high discontinuation rates of prescribed hormone replacement therapy.[48] Not infrequently, women request hysterectomy so that unopposed oestrogens may be used.[49]

In principle, the lowest effective dose of progestogen should be used for opposition to oestrogen therapy.[50,51] The hormone releasing intra-uterine systems, rather than an oral progestogen, to prevent menorrhagia and endometrial hyperplasia in women receiving oestrogen therapy, should be an ideal way of avoiding progestogenic side-effects. In the last few years, workers have also shown that the LNG IUS can be used to provide progestogenic opposition for oral,[52] transdermal[53] and implanted oestrogens.[54] Transvaginal ultrasound and endometrial biopsy were used in the studies to confirm atrophy – there were no cases of endometrial hyperplasia in any of the LNG IUS users. The proportion of amenorrhoeic IUS users after 1 year was high, Raudaskoski's[53] patients achieving an 80% and Suhonen's[54] a 75% rate of amenorrhoea. In spite of the favourable bleeding and progestogenic side effect data in HRT usage, the LNG IUS is currently licensed only as a contraceptive in the UK. Finland allows its use for up to 5 years as progestogenic opposition for oestrogen therapy. There appears to be no lipid metabolic advantage of the LNG IUS compared to cyclical oral administration of progestogen in hormone replacement therapy though data are scarce.[55,56]

Results of two recent studies[57,58] indicate that the PIPS also suppresses endometrial proliferation in postmenopausal women taking 0.625 mg oral conjugated oestrogen daily. Shoupe et al[57] reported a progestational effect of the system on the endometrium (late secretory changes, decidualised stroma, atrophic glands) after 12 months; prior to the study, biopsy had shown a proliferative endometrium. Archer et al[58] reported similar progestational effects after 18 months use of the system with oestrogen therapy. In these studies, there was no systemic absorption of progesterone; both Shoupe et al[57] and Archer et al[58] reported unchanged levels of serum progesterone compared with baseline during use of the system with oestrogen therapy. This differs from the LNG IUS where some systemic absorption of levonorgestrel does occur producing levels of around 200 pg/ml.[53] Shoupe et al[57] reported a beneficial effect on lipids with a 22% increase in HDL levels and a 21% decrease in LDL from baseline with the combined regimen.

Work recently completed in our unit showed that both adverse progestogenic effects and severity of bleeding were reduced to a minimum when patients using mainly oestradiol implants who were progestogen intolerant were switched from oral progestogens to the LNG IUS (Fig. 25.5A). Endometrial suppression was uniform with no cases of endometrial proliferation or hyperplasia at 1 year (Fig. 25.5B) and a greater than 50% rate of amenorrhoea. At time of data analysis, all but one of the 20 women who said they wanted hysterectomy, either because of bleeding problems or progestogenic side effects, were able to avoid this by LNG IUS usage.[59]

Premenstrual syndrome

Although the underlying cause of PMS remains unknown, cyclical ovarian activity appears to be an important factor. A logical treatment for severe PMS, therefore, is to suppress ovulation and thus suppress the cyclical endocrine/ biochemical changes which cause the cyclical symptoms. A treatment of proven efficacy in a placebo controlled trial which appears suitable for long term usage is continuous 17β-oestradiol combined with cyclical progestogen. 100–200 mcg transdermal oestradiol is currently used.[60,61] Unfortunately, oestradiol treatment in non-hysterectomised women necessitates the taking of cyclical oral progestogens, usually norethisterone, medroxyprogesterone acetate or dydrogesterone to prevent endometrial hyperplasia. Workers have shown that PMS-like side effects from the progestogens are the most frequently encountered problem with this treatment, leading to reduced treatment efficacy and high discontinuation rates. In a study by Smith et al,[61] 44% of patients receiving either dydrogesterone 10 mg for 10 days each month or medroxyprogesterone acetate

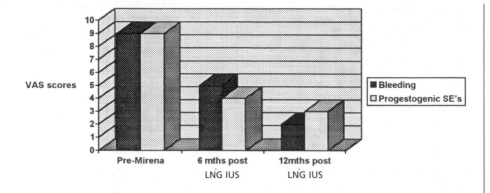

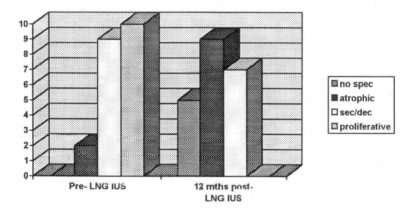

Fig. 25.5 (**A**) Visual analogue scales (VAS) of global progestogenic side effects and bleeding severity in women using oestrogens with the levonorgestrel intra-uterine system for progestogenic opposition. (**B**) Effect of LNG IUS on endometrium after 1 year.

dydrogesterone 10 mg for 10 days each month or medroxyprogesterone acetate (MPA) 5 mg for 10 days each month experienced side effects attributable to the progestogen. An even higher incidence of side effects (58%) been observed in women using cyclical norethisterone.[62] Work is currently being undertaken to show that use of hormone releasing intra-uterine systems rather than oral progestogens should maximise the treatment efficacy of transdermal oestrogens for PMS by minimising the incidence of progestogenic PMS-like physical and psychological side effects. The PIPS should be particularly effective as the systemic levels of hormone are undetectable and natural progesterone has few side effects anyway. There is also work to suggest that the LNG IUS on its own may benefit premenstrual symptoms.[29] This effect may possibly be due to improvement in menorrhagia and dysmenorrhoea which reduces the depression associated with the premenstrual expectancy of these symptoms.

Prevention of ectopic pregnancy

The absolute ectopic rate is extremely low with the LNG IUS being the lowest of any intra-uterine method of contraception. In one study by Andersson et al,[27] the rate of 0.02 per 100 woman years compared very favourably with Nova T users (0.25 per 100 woman years) and sexually active women not using contraception (1.2–1.6 per 100 woman years). However, because the LNG IUS is so effective at preventing intra-uterine pregnancy, if a pregnancy does occur with the IUS in situ then there is a high risk of this being ectopic (1 out 5 pregnancies in the Andersson et al[27] study of 1821 coil insertions). The risk of an ectopic pregnancy with the PIPS appears to be higher than other non-hormone releasing IUDs; about the same level as non-contracepting women. However, if used as progestogenic opposition for oestrogen therapy in perimenopausal women, particularly with patches and implants which can inhibit ovulation, the ectopic rate should be negligible.

Prevention of pelvic inflammatory disease

The system appears to be protective because of the thickening effect on cervical mucus preventing ascending infection, endometrial suppression and reduced bleeding. The incidence of PID with the LNG IUS is very low: at 5 years the rate is less than 1 per 100 women years. The difference in PID incidence between the LNG IUS and copper IUCD was greatest in women less than 25 years of age, the age group most associated with an increased risk of PID.[27,63] However, not all studies have confirmed these findings but at worse they have found the incidence of PID to be comparable to traditional IUCDs.[7,33] The PIPS does not appear to have this protective effect, the relative risk of PID being the same as other IUDs at approximately 1.6. In view of the favourable PID data for the LNG IUS, one might have a slightly lower threshold for using this system where there is a past history of PID.

PROBLEMS OF THE HORMONE RELEASING INTRA-UTERINE SYSTEMS

Fitting of systems

The initial drawback of both systems is their slightly wider diameter vertical stem which is a consequence of the steroid reservoir. This necessitates a wider insertion tube in the case of the LNG IUS. The insertion diameter is even greater in the case of the PIPS because the arms are initially folded down against the stem. These features can lead to difficulty in fitting of the systems, particularly in nulliparous women and may require some cervical dilatation prior to insertion. The requirement for dilatation can usually be determined at time of uterine sounding by judgement of the ease with which the sound passes. Should it be deemed necessary to dilate the cervix it is vital that adequate analgesia is administered first if the patient's confidence is to be retained and insertion is not to fail. This can usually be achieved either by the administration of a non steroidal analgesic, e.g. mefenamic acid 500 mg, 1 h before insertion, or by use of a para-cervical block via a dental syringe of either 1% lignocaine or xylocaine without adrenaline 5 min before insertion. The same care should be taken when inserting the intra-uterine systems as with other IUDs and complications such as perforation, embedment, expulsion and fragmentation are all possible. Interestingly, the expulsion and perforation rates of the LNG IUS are not significantly different to the Nova T IUCD.

Bleeding problems

A problem with both the currently available intra-uterine systems is that it takes approximately 3 months for the endometrium to atrophy under the influence of the released hormone. During this time, bleeding can be very erratic and heavy at times but almost always settles after 3–6 month's usage.[64] Pre- and perimenopausal women experience more episodes of spotting and bleeding. Good counselling is vital if treatment discontinuation is to be avoided. In the PIPS studies by Wan et al,[21] Shoupe et al[57] and Archer et al,[58] bleeding and spotting were common in patients during the first 3 months following insertion but diminished substantially thereafter. No patients withdrew from the studies because of adverse events. It may be of benefit to use tranexamic acid for the first 3 months to reduce bleeding until atrophy of the endometrium has occurred under the influence of the IUS hormone.

Adverse progestogenic effects – physical and metabolic

In spite of the very low constant serum levels of progestogen produced by the LNG IUS, some women still seem to experience adverse progestogenic effects. These can be both physical, such as oedema, headache, breast tenderness, acne and hirsuitism[18,27] and metabolic such as decreased LDL levels.[56] This is probably because the progestogen within the LNG IUS is derived from the 19-nortestosterone group of progestogens which have more physical and metabolic side effects than the C21 progesterone group of progestogens (Fig. 25.2). There appears to be no significant effect on carbohydrate metabolism, coagulation parameters or liver enzymes.[65] The physical effects have been shown to subside after the first few months of usage. It is important that patients are sympathetically counselled and reassured that most side effects are transient and reminded that the serum hormone levels are much lower than those produced by other hormonal contraceptives such as the progestogen-only pill. Side effects related to fluid retention, such as oedema and bloating, may respond to a mild diuretic such as 25 mg of either spironolactone or hydrochloro-thiazide.[66] Addition of an androgen (e.g. a 100 mg testosterone implant every 6 months) may occasionally ameliorate breast tenderness. Headaches are unlikely to occur if oestrogens are used continuously but if they do occur they may be improved by the addition of a mild diuretic or of androgen.

From studies of plasma hormone levels, menstrual patterns and blood chemistry in various patient groups[20,21] it was found that the PIPS produced no significant systemic effects. Shoupe et al[57] reported serum HDL increased 22% and LDL decreased by 21% from baseline with the combined oestrogen/PIPS regimen. Archer et al[58] and Spellacy et al[67] reported no change in total cholesterol, although triglycerides did increase between 6 and 12 months in

Archer's study. Spellacy et al[67] surprisingly detected an increase in insulin secretion suggesting a systemic effect from the progesterone released by PIPS. However, there do not appear to be adverse physical or psychological progestogenic side effects with the PIPS and as such it is ideal for women who are exquisitely progestogen sensitive.

Functional ovarian cysts

Functional ovarian cysts have been shown to be commoner in LNG IUS users than copper IUCD users (1.2 versus 0.4 per 100 woman years).[33] This finding is not surprising considering the higher incidence of cysts in progestogen only pill users. What must be remembered is that these cysts can almost always be managed conservatively.

Amenorrhoea

If inadequately counselled prior to insertion, a woman may regard the reduction in bleeding or cessation of periods as being pathological. This has lead to unnecessary system removal in some cases.[27,33] It is vital that patients and practitioners are aware that the amenorrhoea is purely due to a local effect of hormone on the endometrium producing atrophy. Patients should be made aware of the health benefits of reduced bleeding. If a woman feels strongly about maintaining regular bleeds then the hormone releasing intra-uterine systems are an inappropriate therapeutic option. As discussed earlier, ovulation is only rarely affected and oestrogen levels are identical in menstruating and non-menstruating users.[18,19]

COST EFFECTIVENESS

The cost of the LNG IUS to the NHS is £99.25, an initially high price. However, to make its use cost effective as treatment for menorrhagia, which might otherwise have lead to hysterectomy (costing the NHS approximately £4000) only 1 in 40 hysterectomies would have to be saved. Also, the longer the duration of use of hormone replacement therapy, the greater the cost effectiveness.[68] Since bleeding problems and progestogenic side effects are the biggest reasons for women dropping out from therapy, the hormone releasing coils easily justify their initial expense by increasing continuation rates, preventing hysterectomy to allow the use of unopposed oestrogens and ultimately maximising the cost effectiveness of HRT. It is unfortunate, therefore, that many trusts, gynaecologists and GPs still object to the initial cost of the systems when they have the potential to be cost effective by reducing patient morbidity, and specifically, the need for hysterectomy.

CONCLUSIONS

The progesterone and progestogen releasing intra-uterine systems substantially reduce menorrhagia in premenopausal women. The recent Government funded

Table 25.2 Summary of possible non-contraceptive uses of the hormone releasing intra-uterine systems

Potential application	Most appropriate IUS
Menorrhagia	LNG IUS
Dysmenorrhoea	LNG IUS / PIPS
Endometrial hyperplasia	LNG IUS / PIPS
Prevention / treatment fibroids	LNG IUS
HRT bleeding problems	LNG IUS
HRT progestogenic side effects	PIPS / LNG IUS
Progestogenic opposition for E2 in PMS	PIPS / LNG IUS
Prevention of ectopic pregnancy	LNG IUS
Prevention of PID	LNG IUS

PIPS == Progestasert intra-uterine progesterone system; LNG IUS = Levonorgestrel intra-uterine system.

Effective Health Care Bulletin – The Management of Menorrhagia stated that data from Scandinavia pointed to the effectiveness of the hormone releasing intra-uterine device as a first line treatment for menorrhagia. The systems can also be used in HRT regimens to minimise adverse progestogenic effects, improve the benefit/risk ratio and maximise compliance. In addition, there is evidence that dysmenorrhoea may be improved, PID and ectopic rates reduced and fibroid growth inhibited (Table 25.2). They are not without their own problems; insertion can be difficult, bleeding can be heavy and erratic in the

Table 25.3 Summary of potential problems with hormone releasing intra-uterine systems and possible solutions

Potential problem	Relevant IUS	Possible solution(s)
Difficulty fitting	PIPS / LNG IUS	1) Premedicate with non- steroidals 2) Paracervical block 3) Cx dilation 4) Consider GA
Bleeding problems	PIPS / LNG IUS	1) Pre and post insertion counselling 2) Tranexamic acid
Progestogenic side effects	LNG IUS	1) Pre and post insertion counselling 2) Reassure that usually transient 3) Symptomatic relief, e.g. (i) Evening primrose oil/low dose androgen for breast tenderness (ii) Mild diuretics for fluid retention
Functional cysts	LNG IUS	Manage conservatively if possible Ultrasound follow-up
Amenorrhoea	LNG IUS / PIPS	Pre and post insertion counselling
Perforation/ embedment/expulsion	LNG IUS /PIPS	Manage as with other IUCDs
Pregnancy with IUS in situ	PIPS / LNG IUS	Manage as with other IUCDs (no evidence of fetal abnormality)

PIPS = Progestasert intra-uterine progesterone system; LNG IUS = Levonorgestrel intra-uterine system.

first three months and progestogenic side effects can still occur (Table 25.3). In spite of this, the hormone releasing systems provide the first true alternative to hysterectomy for intractable menstrual and HRT-associated bleeding problems and progestogen intolerance. Future work should focus on confirming the efficacy, safety and cost-effectiveness of these systems, thus building confidence amongst medical practitioners as to their non-contraceptive uses. Registration of the systems as treatments for menorrhagia and as progestogenic opposition for oestrogen therapy, will increase their usage, bring down their costs and, inevitably, reduce the hysterectomy rate. Until we can convince practitioners as to the benefits of the hormone releasing intra-uterine systems we will not be able to dispel the prejudice which many patients have against coils which tars these systems with the same brush.

REFERENCES

1 Davie J. New hormone delivery systems. Diplomate 1996; 3: 184–190
2 Sturdee D W, Wade-Evans T, Paterson M E L, Thom M, Studd J W W. Relations between bleeding pattern, endometrial histology and oestrogen treatment in menopausal women. BMJ 1978; i: 1575–1577
3 Paterson M E L, Wade-Evans T, Sturdee D W, Thomas M H, Studd J W W. Endometrial disease after treatment with oestrogens and progestogens in the climacteric. BMJ 1980; i: 822–824
4 Lane G, Siddle N C, Ryder T A, Pryse-Davies J, King R J B, Whitehead M I. Dose dependent effects of oral progesterone on the oestrogenised postmenopausal endometrium. Acta Obstet Gynaecol Scand 1983; 106: 17–22
5 Henderson B E, Ross R K, Lobo R A, Pike M C, Mack T M. Re-evaluating the role of progestogen therapy after the menopause. Fertil Steril 1988; 49: 9S–15S
6 Zhu P, Hongzhi L, Ruhua X et al. The effect of intra-uterine devices, the stainless steel ring, the copper T220 and releasing levonorgestrel, on the bleeding profile and the morphological structure of the human endometrium – a comparative study of three IUDs. Contraception 1989; 40: 425–438
7 Luukkainen T, Allonen H, Haukkamaa M et al Five year's experience with levonorgestrel releasing IUDs. Contraception 1986; 33: 139–148
8 Zhu P, Hongzhi L, Wenliang S et al. Observation of the activity of factor VIII in the endometrium of women pre- and post-insertion of three types of IUDs. Contraception 1991; 44: 367–387
9 Silverberg S G, Haukkamaa M, Arko H et al. Endometrial morphology during long-term use of levonorgestrel-releasing intra-uterine devices. Int J Gynaecol Pathol 1986; 5: 235–241
10 Nilsson C G, Lahteenmaki P. Recovery of ovarian function after the use of a d-norgestrel releasing IUD. Contraception 1977; 15: 389–400
11 Hagenfeldt K, Landgren B M, Edstrom K, Johanisson E. Biochemical and morphological changes in the human endometrium induced by the progestasert device. Contraception 1977; 16: 183–197
12 Martinez-Manautou J, Aznar R, Maqueo M, Pharriss B B. Uterine therapeutic system for long term contraception: II. Clinical correlates. Fertil Steril 1974; 25: 922–926
13 Martinez-Manautou J, Maqueo M, Aznar R, Pharriss B B, Zaffaroni A. Endometrial morphology in women exposed to uterine systems releasing progesterone. Am J Obstet Gynecol 1975; 121: 175–179
14 Sievers S. Dallenbach-Hellweg clinical and morphological studies in patients following insertion of progesterone containing IUD (Progestasert system). Geburtshilfe Frauenheilkd 1976; 36: 334–340
15 Volpe A, Botticelli A, Abrate M et al An intra-uterine progesterone contraceptive system (52 mg) used in pre- and peri-menopausal patients with endometrial hyperplasia. Maturitas 1982; 4: 73–79

16 Erickson R E, Mitchell C, Pharriss B B, Place V A. The intra-uterine progesterone contraceptive system. In: Advances in planned parenthood. Princeton: Exerpta Medica, 1976; 167–174.

17 Luukkainen T. Levonorgestrel-releasing intra-uterine device. Ann NY Acad Sci 1991; 626: 43–49

18 Luukkainen T, Lahteenmaki P, Toivonen J. Levonorgestrel-releasing intra-uterine device. Ann Med 1990; 22: 85–90

19 Nilsson C G, Lahteenmaki P L A, Luukainen T. Ovarian function in amenorrhoeic and menstruating users of a levonorgestrel-releasing intra-uterine device. Fertil Steril 1984; 41: 52–55

20 Tillson S A, Marian M, Hudson R et al. The effect of intra-uterine progesterone on the hypothalamic-hypophyseal-ovarian axis in humans. Contraception 1975; 11: 179–192

21 Wan L S, Ying-Chih H, Manik G, Bigelow B. Effects of the Progestasert® on the menstrual pattern, ovarian steroids and endometrium. Contraception 1977; 16: 417–434

22 Diaz S, Pavez M, Miranda P et al. Long term follow-up of women treated with Norplant® implants. Contraception 1987; 35: 551–567

23 Kuhnz W, Al-Yacoub G, Fuhrmister A. Pharmacokinetics of levonorgestrel and ethinylestradiol in 9 women who received a low-dose oral contraceptive over a treatment period of 3 months, and, after a washout phase, a single oral administration of the same contraceptive formulation. Contraception 1992; 46: 455–469

24 Weiner E, Victor A, Johansson E D B. Plasma levels of d-norgestrel after oral administration. Contraception 1976; 14: 563–570

25 Nilsson C G, Lahteenmaki P L A, Luukkainen T et al. Sustained intra-uterine release of levonorgestrel over five years. Fertil Steril 1986; 45: 805–807

26 Andersson J K, Rybo G. Levonorgestrel releasing intra-uterine device in the treatment of menorrhagia. Br J Obstet Gynaecol 1990; 97: 690–694

27 Andersson K, Odlind V, Rybo G et al. Levonorgestrel-releasing and copper-releasing IUDs during 5 year's of use: a randomised comparative trial. Contraception 1994; 49: 56–72

28 Bergkvist A, Rybo G. Treatment of menorrhagia with intra-uterine release of progesterone. Br J Obstet Gynaecol 1983; 90: 255–258

29 Barrington J W, Bowen-Simpkins P. The levonorgestrel intra-uterine system in the management of menorrhagia. Br J Obstet Gynaecol 1997; 104: 614–616

30 Puolakka J, Nilsson C, Haukkamaa M et al. Conservative treatment of excessive uterine bleeding and dysmenorrhoea with levonorgestrel intra-uterine system as an alternative to hysterectomy. Acta Obstet Gynaecol Scand 1996; 75 (Suppl): 82

31 The Management of Menorrhagia Effective Health Care: Bulletin No.9. Leeds: University of Leeds, 1995

32 Mann R. Unlicensed medicines and the use of drugs in unlicensed indications. In: Goldberg A, Dodd-Smith I. (eds) Pharmaceutical Medicine and Law, Vol 8. London: Royal College of Physicians, 1991; 103–110

33 Sivin I, Stern J. Health during prolonged use of levonorgestrel 20 µg/d and the Copper T Cu 380 Ag intra-uterine contraceptive devices: a multicentre study. Fertil Steril 1994; 61: 70–77

34 Gasparri L, Scarselli G, Colofranceschi M, Taddei G, Tantini C, Savino L. Management of precancerous lesions of the endometrium. In: Ludwig H, Thomsen K. (eds) Gynaecology and obstetrics. Berlin: Springer, 1986

35 Perino A, Quartararo P, Catinella E et al. Treatment of endometrial hyperplasia with levonorgestrel releasing intra-uterine devices. Acta Eur Fertil 1987; 18: 137–140

36 Scarselli G, Tantini C, Colafranceschi M et al Levonorgestrel-Nova T and precancerous lesions of the endometrium. Eur J Gynaecol Oncol 1988; 9: 284–286

37 Neven P, De Muylder X, Van Belle Y, Campo R, Vanderick G. Tamoxifen and the uterus. BMJ 1994; 309: 1313–1314

38 Singer A, Ikomi A. Successful treatment of fibroids using an intra-uterine progesterone device [abstract]. 14th World Congress of Gynaecology and Obstetrics (FIGO); Montreal, Canada; 24–30 September 1994

39 Pekonen F, Nyman T, Lahteenmaki P et al Intra-uterine progestin induces continuous insulin-like growth factor binding protein-1 production in the human endometrium. J Clin Endocrinol Metab 1992; 75: 660–664

40 Sturridge F, Guillebaud J. Gynaecological aspects of the levonorgestrel-releasing intra-uterine system. Br J Obstet Gynaecol 1997; 104: 285–289

41 Hammarback S, Backstrom T, Holst J, von Schoultz B, Lyrenas S. Cyclical mood changes as in the premenstrual tension syndrome during sequential estrogen-progestagen post-menopausal replacement therapy. Acta Obstet Gynaecol Scand 1985; 64: 393–397

42 Holst J, Backstrom T, Hammarback S et al. Progestogen addition during oestrogen replacement therapy – effects on vasomotor symptoms and mood. Maturitas 1989; 11: 13–20

43 Backstrom T, Bixo M, Seippel L, Sundstrom I, Wang M. Progestins and behaviour. In: Gennazzani A R, Petraglia F, Purdy R H. (eds) The Brain: Source and Target for Sex Steroid Hormones. New York: Parthenon, 1996; 277–291

44 Smith R N J, Holland E F N, Studd J W W. The symptomatology of progestogen intolerance. Maturitas 1994; 18: 87–91

45 Magos A L, Brewster E, Singh R, O'Dowd T, Brincat M, Studd J W W. The effects of norethisterone in postmenopausal women on oestrogen replacement therapy: a model for premenstrual syndrome. Br J Obstet Gynaecol 1986; 93: 1290–1296

46 Ferguson K J, Hoegh C, Johnson S. Estrogen replacement therapy: a survey of women's knowledge and attitudes. Arch Intern Med 1989; 149: 133

47 Studd J W W. Complications of hormone replacement therapy in post-menopausal women. J R Soc Med 1992; 85: 376–378

48 Barlow D H, Grosset K A, Hart H, Hart D M. A study of the experience of Glasgow women in the climacteric years. Br J Obstet Gynaecol 1989; 96: 1192–1197

49 Studd J W W. Shifting indications for hysterectomy. Lancet 1995; 345: 388

50 Rozenbaum H. How to choose the correct progestogen. In: Birkhauser M H, Rozenbaum H. (eds) Menopause. European Consensus Development Conference, Montreux, Switzerland. Paris: Editions ESKA, 1996; 243–256

51 Panay N, Studd J W W. Progestogen intolerance and compliance with HRT in menopausal women. Hum Reprod Update 1997; 3: 159–171

52 Andersson K, Mattsson L-A, Rybo G et al Intra-uterine release of levonorgestrel – a new way of adding progestogen in hormone replacement therapy. Obstet Gynecol 1992; 79: 963–967

53 Raudaskoski T H, Lahti E I, Kauppila A J et al. Transdermal estrogen with a levonorgestrel-releasing intra-uterine device for climacteric complaints: clinical and endometrial responses. Am J Obstet Gynecol 1995; 172: 114–119

54 Suhonen S P, Holmstrom T, Allonen H O et al. Intra-uterine and sub-dermal progestin administration in postmenopausal hormone replacement therapy. Fertil Steril 1995; 63: 336–342

55 Andersson K, Stadberg E, Matsson L A et al. Intra-uterine or oral administration of levonorgestrel in combination with estradiol for climacteric complaints. Effects on lipid metabolism during 12 months of treatment. MD Thesis 1992; 1–12

56 Raudaskoski T H, Tomas E I, Paakkari I A, Kauppila A J, Laatikainen T J. Serum lipids and lipoproteins in postmenopausal women receiving transdermal oestrogen in combination with a levonorgestrel intra-uterine device. Maturitas 1995; 22: 47–53

57 Shoupe D, Meme D, Mezro G, Lobo R A. Prevention of intra-uterine hyperplasia in postmenopausal women with intra-uterine progesterone. N Engl J Med 1991; 325: 1811–1812

58 Archer D F, Viniegra-Sibai A, Hsiu J G et al. Endometrial histology, uterine bleeding and metabolic changes in postmenopausal women using a progesterone-releasing intra-uterine device and oral conjugated estrogens for hormone replacement therapy. Menopause 1994; 1: 109–116

59 Panay N, Studd J W W, Thomas A, et al. The levonorgestrel intra-uterine system as progestogenic opposition for oestrogen replacement therapy. Presentation at Annual Meeting of the British Menopause Society Exeter, July 1996

60 Watson N R, Studd J W W, Savvas M et al Treatment of severe premenstrual syndrome with oestradiol patches and cyclical oral norethisterone. Lancet 1989; ii: 730–734

61 Smith R N J, Studd J W W, Zamblera D et al. A randomised comparison over 8 months of 100 µg and 200 µg twice weekly doses of transdermal oestradiol in the treatment of severe premenstrual syndrome. Br J Obstet Gynaecol 1995; 102: 475–484

62 Watson N R, Studd J W W, Savvas M et al. The long term effects of oestradiol implant therapy for the treatment of premenstrual syndrome. Gynaecol Endocrinol 1990; 4: 99–107

63 Haukkamaa M, Stranden P, Jousimies-Somer P et al. Bacterial flora of the cervix in women using different forms of contraception. Am J Obstet Gynecol 1986; 154: 520–524

64 Nilsson C G, Lahteenmaki P, Luukainen T. Levonorgestrel plasma concentrations and hormone profiles after insertion and after one year of treatment with a levonorgestrel – IUCD. Contraception 1980; 21: 225–233

65 Luukkainen T. Levonorgestrel-releasing IUCD. Br J Family Plan 1991; 19: 221–224

66 Gambrell R D. Progestogens in estrogen replacement therapy. Clin Obstet Gynecol 1995; 38: 890-901

67 Spellacy W, Buhi W C, Birk S A. Carbohydrate and lipid studies in women using the progesterone intra-uterine device for 1 year. Fertil Steril 1979; 31: 381–384

68 Cheung A P, Wren B G. A cost-effectiveness analysis of hormone replacement therapy. Med J Aust 1992; 156: 312–316

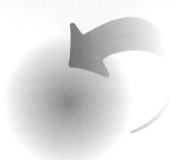

Index

Progress in Obstetrics and Gynaecology
Edited by John Studd

All backlist volumes are available. You can place your order by contacting your local medical bookseller or the Sales Promotion Department, Harcourt Brace and Company Ltd, 24–28 Oval Road, London NW1 7DX, UK

Contents of Volume 1

ISBN 0443 02178 3

Progress in Obstetrics and Gynaecology
Edited by John Studd

Contents of Volume 2

ISBN 0443 02396 4

Progress in Obstetrics and Gynaecology
Edited by John Studd

Contents of Volume 3

ISBN 0443 02665 3

Progress in Obstetrics and Gynaecology
Edited by John Studd

Contents of Volume 4

ISBN 0443 03054 5

Progress in Obstetrics and Gynaecology
Edited by John Studd

Contents of Volume 5

ISBN 0443 03268 8

Progress in Obstetrics and Gynaecology
Edited by John Studd

Contents of Volume 6

ISBN 0443 03572 5

Progress in Obstetrics and Gynaecology
Edited by John Studd

Contents of Volume 7

ISBN 0443 03885 6

Progress in Obstetrics and Gynaecology
Edited by John Studd

Contents of Volume 8

ISBN 0443 04170 9

Progress in Obstetrics and Gynaecology
Edited by John Studd

Contents of Volume 9

ISBN 0443 04412 0

Progress in Obstetrics and Gynaecology
Edited by John Studd

Contents of Volume 10

ISBN 0443 04754 5

Progress in Obstetrics and Gynaecology
Edited by John Studd

Contents of Volume 11

ISBN 0443 05059 7

Progress in Obstetrics and Gynaecology
Edited by John Studd

Contents of Volume 12

ISBN 0 443 05307 3

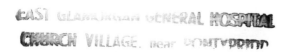